English language contact-induced features in the language of medicine

European University Studies

Europäische Hochschulschriften

Publications Universitaires Européennes

Series XXI **Linguistics**

Reihe XXI Linguistik

Série XXI Linguistique

Volume/Band **381**

Csilla Keresztes

English language contact-induced features in the language of medicine

An investigation of Hungarian Cardiology discharge reports and language attitudes of physicians and patients

PL ACADEMIC RESEARCH

Bibliographic Information published by the Deutsche Nationalbibliothek
The Deutsche Nationalbibliothek lists this publication in the Deutsche Nationalbibliografie; detailed bibliographic data is available in the internet at http://dnb.d-nb.de.

This book was originally handed in and defended as a PhD dissertation under the following title: "Investigation of English language contact-induced features in Hungarian cardiology discharge reports and language attitudes of physicians and patients" in the English Applied Linguistics PhD Program, University of Szeged, Hungary, supervised by Anna Fenyvesi PhD.

The publication of this book was sponsored by RAPIKER Ltd.

ISSN 0721-3352
ISBN 978-3-631-62564-4

www.peterlang.de

Acknowledgements

During the years I was working on this study, I have learnt that academic work is not a lonely endeavor. There have been many people who I wish to thank for contributing ideas and offering support.

First of all, I would like to thank my supervisor, Anna Fenyvesi, Interim Director of Institute at the Department of English Studies, University of Szeged for the expertise, help and encouragement offered throughout the designing and implementation of the study.

I am also grateful to Erzsébet Barát, Director of Gender Studies Track and Deputy Head of Department at the Department of English Studies, University of Szeged for her ideas in developing the semi-structured interviews, to Professor Miklós Kontra, Head of the PhD Program in English Applied Linguistics and of the English Language Teacher Education and Applied Linguistics Department, University of Szeged for continuously recommending me the relevant literature, and to Eszter Szabó-Gilinger, assistant professor at the English Language Teacher Education and Applied Linguistics Department, University of Szeged for both academic and spiritual support.

I am indebted to Professor Tamás Forster, M. D. Head of the Second Department of Internal Medicine and Cardiological Center, University of Szeged for providing me the discharge reports, and letting me interview his colleagues and patients at the department, as well as to head physicians Györgyi Piros, M. D. and Piroska Túri, M. D. for letting me interview their colleagues.

I wish to thank assistant professor Kálmán Havasi, M. D. and Gábor Marton, M. D. resident at the Department of Cardiology, University of Szeged, and Balázs Sinkovics, assistant professor at the Department of Hungarian Linguistics, University of Szeged for valuable communication on terminology.

I am also grateful to Zoltán Domokos, program developer for developing a word-search and -analyzing program for my study, and to Edit Paulik, M. D. associate professor and Imre Gera, informatics manager at the Department of Public Health, University of Szeged for help in statistics.

Thanks are also due to Judit Kozma, head nurse at the Department of Cardiology for her help in organizing the patient interviews.

I owe special debt to my colleagues at the Department of Medical Communication and Translation Studies, University of Szeged, especially to Éva Demeter, Head of the Department, and Vanda Varga, who supported me throughout the years of investigation and while I was writing the book.

Finally, I am most grateful to my parents and my family, especially my husband Istvan Rapolti and our children Nora and Gergely for their patience, support and encouragement.

Table of Contents

1. Introduction

Since the 1950s English has become not just an important language in the field of medicine but the predominant language of health sciences. Even in countries that strictly stick to the use of their native tongue (for example Germany), English has been put into the foreground in health sciences since the 1970s, overtaking the role of the native language. The dominance of the English language as a second language can be observed in Austria, Switzerland and France (Fehér 1997; Ammon 2001), as well as in Hungary,[1] especially in the language of sciences, including health sciences.

Contact linguistics is an interdisciplinary branch of multilingualism research, the study of language contact and interferences in the language use of bilingual/multilingual speakers. Half of the world's population is bilingual, and bilingualism is present in practically every country in the world (Grosjean 1982). Bilinguals are people employing two languages, who recognize themselves and are recognized by others as using two languages (Pauwels 1986).

The aim of this book is to describe a subregister of the Hungarian language of medicine, to reveal and analyze the English contact-induced features in this specific purpose language, and to investigate the attitude of various discourse communities affected by it towards the English language.

The impact of some major European languages, among them the English language on Hungarian and its lexicon has already been investigated (e.g. Országh 1968, 1977; Csapó 1971; Magay 1977; Kontra 1992, 2001; Grétsy 1996; Farkas and Kniezsa 2002; Zimányi 2004; Fenyvesi 2005), however, studies, surveys and lists of English contact-induced features in the language of medicine are rare compared to those of other European languages (Kontra 1981, 1982; Keresztes 2003, Grétsy 2004).

After World War II much of the world's scientific potential became concentrated in the United States. One of the consequences was the leading position acquired by that country in scientific publishing and in the storage and dissemination of scientific and technical information (Truchot 2002). Since the middle of the 1980s English has become the universal language of research publications playing an influential role in researchers' careers (Ammon 2001), imposing serious restrictions on the free flow of scientific information without a high level of English knowledge (Medgyes and László 2001). Therefore, there might be widespread asymmetrical bilingualism/multilingualism among the non-native English speakers of the medical community worldwide.

1 English is the first choice to learn as a foreign language for the majority of Hungarian schoolchildren (Medgyes and László 2001).

English language competence has risen substantially also among Hungarian scientists, including physicians, and especially those under age 65 since the 1980s (Medgyes and László 2001). Chandler-Burns (1997: 2) points out the importance of English among medical doctors by claiming that "it is a fact of life that one does not need to know English to be a successful physician; however, to be a successful physician–researcher it will be incumbent upon the person to read and write English fluently".

For scientists, publications are vital means of communicating research results and of investigating and/or contributing to knowledge capital. They traditionally have also been indicators of productivity and prestige. The dominance of English is present in certain written registers: 89% of all science and technology articles, 80% of databases and 62% of CD-ROMs are in English (Bilan 1996: 173), thus, being able to write and publish in English plays an influential role in researchers' careers. The Dutch physician, Vandenbroucke (1989) claims that "not to have been born with English as your mother tongue is a major hereditary occupational handicap for a medical scientist". However, the elimination of a language (i.e. one's native language) from certain domains can threaten social cohesion and the vitality of a language (Phillipson 2008: 3).

English language medical research articles have been studied from various linguistic aspects (Bazerman 1988; Myers 1990; Swales 1990; Atkinson 1992, 1996; Rébék-Nagy 1997; Gunnarson 2006; Taaivitsainen 2006), but the impact of the requirement on physicians that they should be able to communicate their findings in English and express themselves in that language properly if they want to be fully accepted members of the international academic community has been investigated only by few researchers (Ong et al. 1995; Ammon 2001; Taaivitsainen and Pahta 2003).

The present book reports on a study designed to investigate how Hungarian physicians[2] are influenced by the English language in their professional lives, and what types of interference[3] can be found in the Hungarian documents written by them. Such interferences have been looked at mainly from a puristic aspect so far (Keszler 2004; Grétsy 2004; Balázs 2005), and little sociolinguistic or contact linguistic research has been done on them to date.

Nevertheless, this book aims at going beyond general conclusions about the phenomenon of interference in the language of medicine by investigating not only written documents to identify features due to contact with English, but also by exploring the attitude of the members of certain speech communities towards

---

2 The term physician is used in this book to refer to doctors who have specialized/subspecialized in a medical subject, e.g. cardiology or family health care.

3 The linguistic term interference is used in this book synonymously with contact induced features. A detailed description of the phenomenon is provided in section 2.1 below.

the English language and interference phenomena, which may or may not have become inherent elements of this specific purpose language.

To achieve this aim, a triangulation of two methods is adopted in the present study (Figure 1): the investigation of medical documents is complemented by carrying out structured interviews with members of the medical community and patients. The combination of data collected by the two methods, hopefully, compensates for the weaknesses and blind spots of each single method and provides better insight into present day Hungarian for medical purposes.

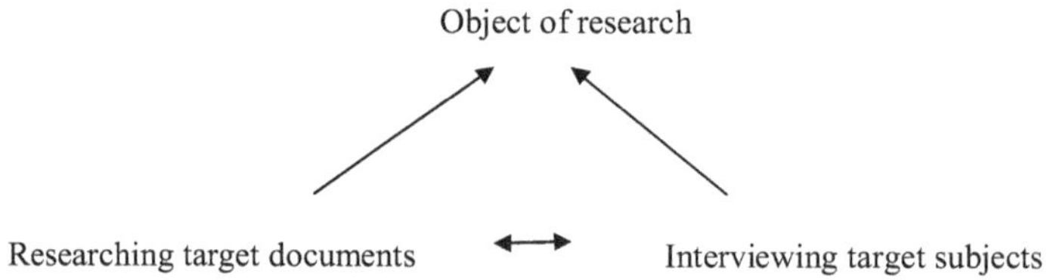

Figure 1. Triangulation of methods used in the research.

Since the field of medicine is diverse and subdivided into various specialties, from a methodological aspect it would be difficult to draw far-reaching conclusions about the language of health sciences as a whole or to interpret linguistic data in each medical subdiscipline. Thus, the research reported on here is focused on only one field of medicine, cardiology, attempting to give an overview of the linguistic interferences in this subdiscipline in a complex, detailed manner, and examining the attitudes of both health professionals and patients towards the impact that English has on this special purpose language of Hungarian.

Cardiology is a subdiscipline of Internal Medicine (Figure 2). Cardiologists study the heart and the vascular system of the human body and deal with the diagnosis and management[4] of cardiovascular diseases. When narrowing down the targeted area of research, cardiology was selected for a closer investigation, on the one hand, as it is a technologically sophisticated, professionalized, institutionalized, and highly invasive medical discipline. There have been great innovations and scientific progress in this medical field since the last decade of the 20th century. On the other hand, cardiovascular diseases are the leading

---

4 Management is the term used in health care to refer to the treatment of the patient in general.

causes of death in several countries of the world,[5] including Hungary, since more people die annually from cardiovascular diseases (29% of all global deaths) than from any other single cause (WHO 2009), thus, the language used by cardiologists and its manifestation in the discharge reports written by them is, by definition, of general interest.

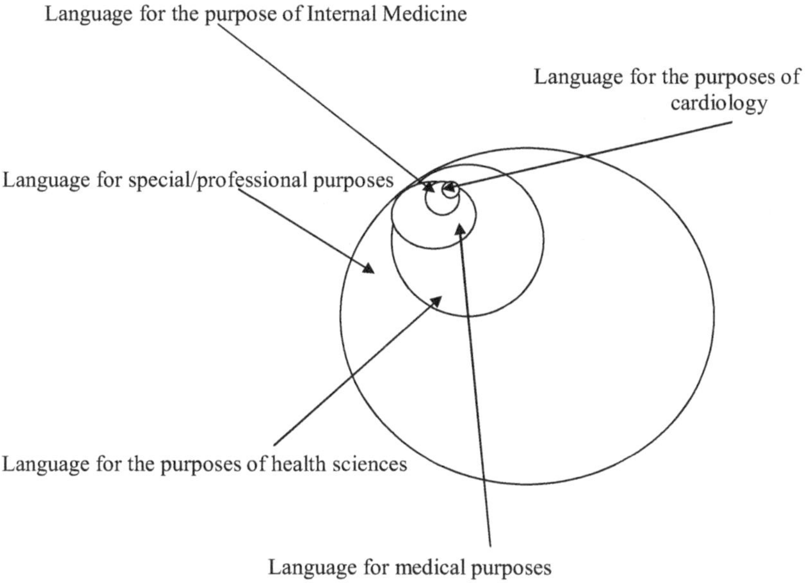

Figure 2. The integration of the language of cardiology into special/professional languages (Keresztes 2003).

Numerous studies have been published on medical English[6] but studies on medical Hungarian are limited in number, and very little has been published on the language of cardiology. To date, however, no research on the effect of the English language on the Hungarian medical language in the field of cardiology has been carried out.

Hospital discharge reports[7] are written documents prepared when the patient is discharged from a health institution after receiving management. It is a well-

---

5 70 million Americans suffer from cardiovascular diseases and cardiovascular-related deaths account for 40 percent of annual deaths in the USA (Zhang 2008: 168)

6 A review of papers and books on medical English is provided in section 2.3.1.

7 These reports are also referred to as discharge summaries.

defined genre of medical writing, a narrative recounting of a single case of a disease or injury. In its typical form, the discharge report records the course of a patient's disease(s) from the onset of symptoms to the outcome, usually either recovery or death. It comprises the patient's personal data, diagnoses, applied procedures, past medical history, history of present illness, relevant family and social history, course of hospitalization and instructions for the future.[8] From a linguistic point of view discharge summaries are distanced and objective. The physician may be present only in metacomments, the narrative is in the third person and focuses on clinical facts (Taaivitsainen and Pahta 2003), and conventions help to record details in an economical form.

Writing these documents is part of the daily routine of Hungarian practising physicians, as each discharged patient in Hungary receives such a document before leaving the health institute (WHO Regional Office for Europe, Declaration on the Promotion of Patients' Rights in Europe 1995; MEES[9] 2007). This is the very document in which the physician sums up the history of the patient's disease(s) and gives guidance about further management to the primary care physician. [10]

There is a constant debate going on among health care providers and patients' rights activists in Hungary nowadays whether these documents should be "translated" into a language comprehensible for patients or not, whether these documents are addressed to the patient as well or only to the attending family practitioner, and whether the patient is only entitled to deliver the document to the primary care provider or has the right to understand it fully. These issues however essential from a sociological aspect will be discussed only briefly in this book. Nevertheless, attitudes of patients undergoing cardiological management at a university clinic towards this specific purpose language are investigated in the present study, together with the attitude of primary, secondary[11] and tertiary care[12] physicians involved in the clinical and community care[13] provided for the patient.

---

8 A detailed description of the components of Hungarian and English hospital discharge reports is given in Appendix 1.

9 MEES stands for Magyar egészségügyi ellátási standardok [Hungarian health care standards] cf. website http://www.eum.hu. Access: 19 August, 2008.

10 The term primary care physician refers to the family/general practitioner.

11 Secondary care comprises healthcare services provided by specialists, such as cardiologists, dermatologists, and others working at an outpatient department, to whom patients are referred by their primary care providers.

12 Tertiary care provides healthcare services for hospitalized patients who require treatment from highly specialized providers, which often involves highly sophisticated technology.

13 The term community care is used in medical literature for care provided for the patient at a primary level.

Hospital discharge summaries are rarely studied from a linguistic aspect, since these documents are not readily available for the public. It is recorded in the Hungarian *Rights and Obligations of Patients*[14] that "each patient shall have the right to become acquainted with the data contained in the medical record prepared about him/her, and shall have the right to request information on his/her health care data". A patient "shall also have the right to have persons involved in his/her health care disclose his/her health care and personal data [...] and to have them handle such data confidentially".

The discharge report is the (tertiary) physician's major tool of written communication towards colleagues in primary and secondary care involved in the further management of the patient and towards the patients themselves[15]. It is essential that the target groups (cardiologists and family physicians) share a great deal of special knowledge, use the same specialized vocabulary, and can decode the message in a precise way. By investigating a yet rarely studied text type in medicine, the hospital discharge summary, this study may contribute to a better understanding and a more complex analysis of the medical language used by Hungarian physicians.

---

14 Rights and Obligations of Patients (According to Act CLIV of 1997 on Health) www.szoszolo.hu/50english, date of access: Febr 16 2007 (English text is given on the website).

15 It is not compulsory, however, to hand this document to discharged patients in all countries, e.g. in the UK it is sent to the family physician of the patient by mail.

2. Literature review

This multidisciplinary study describes the Hungarian language of cardiology through investigating English language contact-induced features in Hungarian hospital discharge reports, and physicians' and patients' attitudes towards the English language globalization in the field of sciences, the presence of the English language in the Hungarian language of medicine, and the English language contact-induced features present in the Hungarian hospital discharge reports. The literature review gives an insight into the various disciplines that are dealt with in the book: language contact (Section 2.1), globalization, especially language globalization (Section 2.2), the language of medicine (Section 2.3), genres in medicine (Section 2.4), patient's rights (Section 2.5), cardiology (Section 2.6), and methodology (Section 2.7).

2.1. Language contact

On of the main sources of language change general in language contact, and the changes that can be investigated are the ones that have spread in a speech community (or subcommunity), and the process of spread is a function of contact between these speakers (Thomason 2003). Milroy states (1992: 84–85) the following:

"When linguists speak of a close contact situation, they are usually thinking of contact between *systems*, but what actually occurs is contact between *speakers* of different languages: the changes that result and which are then observed in the system have been brought about by the speakers, who form weak and uniplex ties when two populations first come into contact. So, strictly speaking, it isn't really *language*-contact at all, but *speaker*-contact."

Weinreich also places emphasis on the speakers of a language when giving his definition of language contact: "two or more languages will be said to be IN CONTACT if they are used alternately by the same persons. The language-using individuals are thus the locus of contact" (1953: 1; emphasis in the original). It is important to note here that not only spoken contact, but also written contact is a factor contributing to language change. In fact, it is the written contact between English and Hungarian found in a corpus of Hungarian cardiology discharge reports (USZCCDR)[16] that is investigated and analyzed in this book.

16 The initialism of USZCCDR (University of Szeged Corpus of Cardiological Discharge Reports) is used in the present book to refer to the analyzed corpus.

Contact linguistics is an interdisciplinary branch of multilingualism research involving the study of language contact, and as a result of this contact, the interferences in the language use of bilingual speakers. Physicians worldwide are typically bilingual or multilingual speakers of their native tongue and English, and, usually, Latin. Language contact is "the alternate use of two or more languages by the same persons" (Haugen 1958: 771), and such persons are referred to as bilinguals. In the mind of these bilingual speakers two or more distinct linguistic systems exist, and the point where a speaker switches from one system to the other can be identified (Haugen 1958). These systems are overlapping and result in interference, "instances of deviations from the norms of either language, which occur in the speech of bilinguals as a result of their familiarity with more than one language" (Haugen 1958: 772).

Contact linguistics receives various stimuli from the sociology of language (Fishman 1971), sociolinguistics (Labov 1972), ethnography (Gumperz 1962; Hymes 1964), social psychology (Lambert 1967; Giles 1977), and language ecology (Haugen 1972) as well as from numerous other neighboring disciplines.

Three major areas of investigation in contact linguistics are language use, the language user, and the language sphere. According to Nelde (2002: 326), "the significant parameters of contact linguistics are linguistic levels (phonology, syntax, and lexicon) and also discourse analysis, stylistics and pragmatics". But there are several external linguistic factors that also have a role in language change, such as nation, language community, language boundaries and migration (Nelde 2002).

In the past two decades the following research topics have been elaborated in the fields of code-switching: code-switching and universal constraints (e.g. Poplack and Meechan 1998; Sankoff 2004), the development of theoretical frameworks and processing models (de Groot and Kroll 1997; Nicol 2001), the Matrix language frame model (Myers-Scotton 1993, 1997; Myers-Scotton and Jake 2000), grammatical aspects of 'code-switching' (Jacobson 1989), code-switching in conversations (Auer 1998), the reversing of language shift (Fishman 2000), and the refinement of Poplack and Sankoff's model based on borrowing.

Current research on language contact comprises the psychological and neurological aspects of bilingualism, the sociological characters of bilingual communities (stable and endangered), the acquisition of two or more languages, the linguistic consequences of contact: the relationship between language contact and language change, linguae francae, language alternation, language maintenance and loss, pidgins and creoles, borrowing and code-switching.

Cultures and languages are not isolated, but they are constantly changing due to internal forces or contacts with other cultures and languages (Foley 1997). Language contact occurs when speakers of distinct speech varieties interact and their languages influence each other. Language contact can occur at language borders between adstratum languages, or as the result of migration with an intrusive language acting as either a superstratum or a substratum. This change is often one-sided, or it may affect only a particular segment of a discourse community, with the change, thus, appearing only in a particular dialect, jargon or in a specific register (Maclean and Maher 2001).

Language contact can have various linguistic consequences: it may result in the borrowing of words, or it may even lead to the creation of a new language. Moravcsik highlights that "the characterization and explanation of what can be borrowed from one language into another is [...] a complex task" (1978: 120). Winford (2003: 2) argues that "between these two extremes lies a wide range of possible outcomes involving varying degrees of influence by one language on the other". He claims that it is the speakers of those languages who are in contact with each other and who use a certain mixture of elements from the languages involved.

Traditionally, the phenomenon of language contact is "the use of more than one language in the same place at the same time" (Thomason 2001: 1). Bussman gives a much narrower definition for language contact by claiming that it is "a situation in which two or more languages coexist within one state and where the speakers use these different languages alternately in specific situations" (1996: 260).

However, language contact nowadays does not have to imply the coexistence of two languages within one state. In fact, English–Hungarian contact, for example, may mostly take place via the Internet, television, cinema, the press and the process of learning and teaching English (Dörnyei 2006). As Hungarian–English bilingualism, in general, is unbalanced, we do not witness mutual influence between the languages in contact. It is restricted to one direction only (the English language has its influence on the Hungarian language of the bilinguals), and is manifested in the appearance of loan words mostly, with the more prestigious language being the donor. As Jespersen (1964: 208–209) pointed out, "loan-words always show a superiority of the nation from whose language they are borrowed, though this superiority may be of many different kinds".

Cultures and languages are constantly in flux (Foley 1997), and the end-results are manifold. Nevertheless, it is actually not the languages that come into contact with each other, as it was pointed at above, it is always the speakers of the languages who are in contact. Their attitudes towards each other will affect the way they speak; however, it is frequently more convenient to simply talk about the languages as though they had a life of their own.

Thomason (2001) expresses that language contact between the speakers can be described as a result of internal (linguistic) and external (social and psychological) factors. Linguistic factors involve e.g. the degree of typological similarity between the languages in contact. Other linguistic constraints are specific to particular areas of linguistic structure (e.g. phonology, morphology) and some of them are of more general, perhaps universal in nature.

Social factors include the length and intensity of contact between the groups, their respective sizes, the power and prestige relationships, and patterns of interaction between them, and the functions that are served by intergroup communication (Winford 2003).

Generally, language contacts have taken place under conditions of social inequality (war, conquest, colonialism, slavery, or migration, etc.) or urbanization or trade (Sankoff 2004). Thus, language contact should be considered as the historical product of social forces (Heine et al. 2005). Contact situations can be varied, among the factors that contribute to greater intensity of contact are a high level of bilingualism, socioeconomic and/or political pressure on one speaker group in a two-language contact situation to shift to the other language, length of contact, and relative sizes of speaker populations. Great intensity of contact is a necessary but not a sufficient condition for interference (Thomason 2003).

In some cases externally induced changes do not require speakers of the different languages to have actual social contact, the influence of a language can also be accomplished e.g. by learning, reading books, or certain texts; thus, sociopolitical factors can also play a role in the attitudes towards the languages and in the motivations to use one language or another (as we can see, for instance, in case of physicians).[17]

According to historical linguists, language changes have four major causes. The first one is drift (Sapir 1921) – that is the structural tendencies inherent in a given language resulting from pattern pressures or structural imbalances. The second cause is dialect borrowing (Ross 1988), a phenomenon that refers to the process of one dialect copying an element or structure from another dialect the long-term result of which can be the convergence of the recipient dialect with the source dialect, and the third cause is foreign interference. The last two, however, are not separable as they are points on the same continuum (Thomason 2009): it is difficult to draw a line between situations in which only dialects influence each other and other situations in which separate languages have an impact on each other. A fourth cause of change can be deliberate change by groups of speakers, usually in languages of small speech communities, or through formal language-planning activities.

17 Literature on language attitudes is discussed below in 2.7.1.

In most cases, language contact results in contact-induced language change(s), i.e. the linguistic results of contact between two or more languages (Thomason and Kaufmann 1988), in either (any) or both (all) languages in contact. A contact-induced language change can be any linguistic change that would have been less likely to occur outside a particular contact situation (Thomason 2001). These changes are mostly, however not exclusively, externally motivated (Thomason 2001). All languages constantly undergo alterations, and that can formulate constraints on the transition from one state of a language to an immediately succeeding state (Weinreich et al. 1968). On the other hand, contact-induced language changes are processes confined to certain areas resulting from specific historical events (Kuteva and Heine 2003).

Myers-Scotton (2002) examines the nature of major contact phenomena, especially lexical borrowing, grammatical convergence, code-switching, first language attrition, mixed languages, and the development of creoles. She argues forcefully that types of contact phenomena often seen as separate, in fact, result from the same processes and can be explained by the same principles.

Johanson (2002) highlights that language contact phenomena are results of intraclausal code copying, i.e. he assumes that a speaker does not use different codes in one utterance alternately. His model focuses on the concept that an element of one language serves as a model that is copied into a second language. Copies can be global or selective, the former being elements copied as a whole with all their structural properties, while the latter is the result of copying only certain structural properties of the model into genuine units.

Thomason (2001: 11) postulates that "all aspects of language structure are subject to transfer from one language to another, given the right mix of social and linguistic circumstances". The most frequent phenomenon is borrowing, which should be distinguished from code-switching and from interference through shift. It is the transfer of mainly lexical elements from other languages or other varieties (dialect or register) of the same language. Mainly words, primarily nouns are borrowed or new meanings of old words, or sometimes derivational morphemes. Calques or loan translations are also referred to as borrowings, when a language uses its own elements to 'translate' a foreign word or phrase (or even an instance of grammar).

Mechanisms of interference can be categorized: the implementers of change are bilinguals, second language acquirers. Third category is negotiation and the last category is conscious and deliberate decisions by speakers to implement language change (Thomason 2003).

Haugen (1950) divides borrowed elements into classes with various phonological and semantic characteristics: loanwords, loanblends, loanshifts (including loan translations and semantic loans). Loanwords can be subdivided into additions and substitutions (Field 2002).

Sankoff (2004) discusses the linguistic outcomes of language contact in terms of five major domains: the phonetic/phonological level, the lexical level, syntax and discourse/pragmatics and morphology/grammatical and semantic categories. She claims that the first two are the major 'gateways' to all of the other aspects of contact influenced change.

Weinreich (1953) describes phonic, grammatical and lexical interferences. Referring to Haugen (1950), Kontra (1981) distinguishes between direct, indirect borrowing/transfer and hybrid borrowing. Lanstyák (2000) also differentiates between indirect and direct borrowings when describing majority language elements in minority languages. Zsilinszky (2003) follows this categorization when studying English elements in Hungarian etymological dictionaries.

The influence of medical English on other European medical languages affects all linguistic subsystems: from lexis through semantics and syntax to rhetorico-pragmatics, but the most common is still borrowing of vocabulary items (Alcaraz and Navarro 2006). When investigating English language contact-induced features in the Hungarian language of medicine, the lexico-semantic level, semantic level, syntactic level, phonemic level, typographical level, and rhetorico-pragmatic levels should be considered separately.

Motivations for borrowing can be various, involving prestige (individual or collective), and need (objective need to express new ideas or name scientific and technological innovations). Both reasons for borrowing can be identified in the Hungarian language of medicine and cardiology (see 2.3.2 below).

Apart from the very general distinction between 'necessity borrowing' and 'luxury borrowing' and the two frequently named motives 'the need to designate new (imported) things' (Weinreich 1953; Bellmann 1971; Campbell 1998) and 'prestige' (Weinreich 1953, Scheler 1977), the following aspects, among others, have been mentioned as causes for lexical borrowing: the need to differentiate between special nuances of expression, including stylistic variation, the need to play with words, homonymic clashes, loss of effectiveness of words or, seen from a juxtaposed viewpoint, emotionality of a specific concept, feeling of insufficiently differentiated conceptual fields or rise of a specific conceptual field, attraction of a borrowing due to an already borrowed word, the general attraction of borrowing an etymological doublet, political or cultural dominion of one people by another, the bilingual character of a society, the need for a euphemistic expression, and 'laziness' of the translator or lack of lexicographical means, or temporary lack of remembering the indigenous name (Grzega 2002).

Language contacts have, historically, taken place in large part under conditions of social inequality resulting from wars, conquests, colonialism, slavery, and migrations – forced and otherwise. Relatively benign contacts involving urbanization or trade as a contact motivation are also documented, as are some situations of relative equality (Sorensen 1967; Sankoff 1980).

Language contacts have in some periods and places been short-lived, with language loss and assimilation a relatively short-term result, whereas "other historical situations have produced relative long-term stability and acceptance by the bi- or multilingual population" (Sankoff 2004: 641).

Hungarian physicians and, especially, cardiologists who work at university clinics[18] are influenced by their knowledge of English in their daily professional activities when they speak and write in Hungarian. One of the main aims of this book is to investigate the affects of the English language contact that can be detected in the hospital discharge reports written by them.

2.1.1. History of contact linguistics

The study of effects of language contact has been the focus of investigations of linguists since the 19th century; a great deal of interest was devoted to it by Paul (1880), Schmidt (1872), and Schuchardt (1884). Schuchardt pointed out the close connection between code-mixing and multilingualism in 1884, and emphasized the importance of research on code-mixing. In the 20th century these effects were discussed by Sapir (1921), Bloomfield (1933) and other early pioneers of structuralism.

Contact linguistics in its narrow sense goes back to the early 1950s. During the decades before then, cultural-linguistic contacts such as lexical borrowing had been in the centre of research (Goebl et al. 1996). The two-volume handbook of contact linguistics (Goebl et al. 1996) is an international, European oriented state-of-the-art coverage of the field of language contact at the time (Clyne 1991). In the 1950s, research developed into two major trends: the investigation of the results of language contact on the languages involved and on its speakers or society. Language contact continues to enjoy a rather separate life within historical linguistics (Thomason and Kaufman 1988) as well as in creole studies.

The analysis of linguistic contact of classical languages and its, mostly lexical, effects had been in the forefront of the investigations for a long time. Sociological and psychological aspects were also introduced as a focus of investigation by Haugen (1950), Weinreich (1953), and Fishman (1964), who attributed special attention to external linguistic factors. In this way, the originally interlingual character of research shifted towards interethnic contacts, interference and transference analyses, the social and situational elements of the language, and areas of language use and attitudes.

---

18 These physicians are regularly involved in research, they read and publish in English, and they take part in international conferences where the language of work is mainly English (see details in Section 2.3.1).

Clyne (2003) suggests that Weinreich's and Haugen's works can be considered as the beginning of American sociolinguistics. They also established the position of language contact among topics of central importance and made it a subdiscipline of linguistics. They established a comprehensive framework for the study of language contact in its social setting. The goals of this subdiscipline, according to Weinreich (1953: 86), are the following: "to predict typical forms of interference from the sociolinguistic description of a bilingual community and a structural description of its languages is the ultimate goal of interference studies" and "instances of deviation from the norms of either language which occur in the speech of bilinguals as a result of their familiarity with more than one language, i.e. as a result of language contact, will be referred to as interference phenomena" (1953:1).

Though Weinreich focuses on the phenomenon of bilingualism, his statement can apply equally well to the study of all contact situations. Moreover, the field of contact linguistics is not limited just to the study of 'interferences' but "covers all the linguistic consequences of contact, including phenomena such as simplification and various other kinds of restructuring that characterize the outcomes of contact" (Winford 2003: 209).

Some scholars devote their attention to the problems of ethnic minorities who are under the influence of a majority language. A systematic study of language maintenance began with Kloss (1929), while other scholars became interested in the immigrant languages in North America and elsewhere (cf. Herzog 1941; Reed 1948; Pap 1949; Haugen 1953). Studies like these created the foundation for the discipline known as the sociology of language, focusing, among other matters, on language maintenance and shift (Fishman 1964; Fishman 1966).

Several historical linguists stressed the importance of social factors in language contact including Whitney (1881) and Schuchardt (1884). Much of Schuchardt's discussion of the linguistic aspects of language contact is accompanied by details of the social context, the groups in contact, and other relevant sociocultural data. As Winford (2003: 10) claims:

"We need to distinguish among the various social contexts of language contact if we are to understand the nature and direction of contact-induced change [...]. It is necessary to examine, where possible, the actual speech behavior of persons in each contact situation in order to uncover the factors that motivate them to change their language in one way or another."

In Europe in the 1960s, the emphasis in language contact research was mainly put on psycholinguistic and sociolinguistic problems, analyzed, for example, by Weiss (1959) and Vildomec (1963).

The term contact linguistics (Figure 3) was introduced at the First World Congress on Language Contact and Conflict in 1979, according to Nelde (1997).

Contact linguistics is now recognized as a branch of sociolinguistics (Nelde et al. 1996). The consequences of language contact can be language generation, i.e., pidginization and creolization (Mühlhäusler 1986; Bickerton 1981); language degeneration, i.e., language displacement (Dorian 1989); and/or novel patterns of language use, i.e., code-switching (Myers-Scotton 1993).

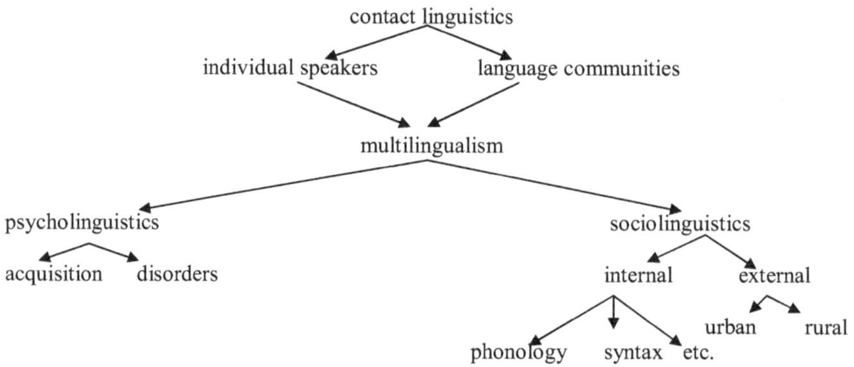

Figure 3. The relation of contact linguistics to multilingualism (Nelde 2002: 326).

Another term, conflict, was also discussed at the First World Congress on Language Contact and Conflict in 1979 in close relation to language contact. This latter term, however, remains ambiguous, especially when it refers generally to social conflicts which can arise in multilingual situations (Hartig 1980). The notion that neither contact nor conflict can occur between languages appears essential here: they are conceivable only between speakers of languages.

Hartig (1980) distinguishes between interlingual and interethnic language conflicts. Conflicts should not be condemned as only negative, since new structures that are more advantageous than the foregoing ones can be the result of these conflicts (Nelde 2002).

Thomason and Kaufman (1988) study a wide variety of contact phenomena, and attempt to lay the foundations for both a typology of contact outcomes and an empirical and theoretical framework for analyzing such outcomes. They also emphasize the need for an interdisciplinary approach and refine the terminology and descriptive framework used in previous works.

Currently, work on language contact includes psychological and neurological aspects of bilingualism, sociological characterization of bilingual communities (both stable and endangered), acquisition of two or more languages, the linguistic consequences of contact, the relationship between language contact and language change, linguae francae, language alternation, language maintenance and loss, pidgin, creole, borrowing and code-switching (King 2000).

Seeking the best explanation for a given linguistic change we must consider potential internal motivations as well as potential external motivations. Thus, we should add another case of linguistic change to the causes, the deliberate change by groups of speakers (Thomason 1997b), as we can find it in certain speech communities e.g. among scientists and physicians.

The relation between internal and external motivations of change has also been discussed extensively in historical linguistics (cf. Harris and Campbell 1995), whereas Silva-

Corvalan (1994) and others have shown the duality of internal and external influences.

Hawkins (1986) provides a framework for contrastive typology in establishing underlying generalizations about a language following Sapir's notion of drift – the way a language keeps changing in the same direction.

Fishman in 1966 developed a new area of research, language maintenance and shift, and described the qualitative and quantitative paradigms and models linking language with the nation and nationalism (Fishman 1985, 1989, 1991). Studies on language maintenance and shift are described in many immigrant countries (Clyne 1982, 1991; Gardner 1985; Kontra 1990; Fishman 1991, 1997; Hoffman 1991; Bartha 1998, 1999; De Vries 1999; Fenyvesi 2005).

The field of language contact has changed considerably in recent years, and more discussion has gone into the formulation of constraints and the development of theoretical frameworks and processing models (Clyne 2003). Works in the 1990s were devoted to developing the Matrix language frame model (Myers-Scotton 1993, 1997; Myers-Scotton and Jake 2000) and the refinement of Poplack and Sankoff's model based on a borrowing vs. code-switching dichotomy and universal constraints (Poplack and Meechan 1998; Sankoff 1998).

A relatively new and partly overlapping field of contact linguistics is intercultural communication. Most of the progress has been achieved in contrastive and intercultural pragmatics (Blum-Kulka et al. 1989; Wierzbicka 1991; Kasper and Blum-Kulka 1993), but the literature in crosscultural discourse is also increasing (Connor and Kaplan 1987; Duszak 1997; Coupland 2007).

Linguistic research into borrowing has a long tradition in Hungarian historical linguistics: lexical borrowing has been in the focus of the studies in the field. Sajnovics (1770) and Gyarmathi (1799), who discovered the genetic relationship of Finno-Ugric languages, are the forerunners of Hungarian contact linguists. Keresztes (1975) describes English–Hungarian word order interference, and Csapó (1971) investigates English–Hungarian loanwords in the language of sports. In the 1970s most Hungarian studies published in the field described interference (especially lexical borrowing, i.e. 'foreign words') as a frightening phenomenon which should be eliminated, and the purity of the Hungarian language should be defended against Anglicisms. Országh (1977) provides a historical overview of this phenomenon, Magay (1977) reveals the English elements in the Hungarian lexicon, and Kontra (1981) describes interferences in a specific register, in the Hungarian language of medicine. Since the 1990s language contact has been discussed on two major aspects in Hungary: sociolinguistic analysis of the language of bilingual ethnic minorities living outside Hungary (cf. Bartha 1993; Fenyvesi 1995a, 2006; Kontra 1990, 1997c, 2009; Péntek 1997; Csernicskó 1998; Göncz 1999; Benő 2000; Lanstyák 2000, 2006; Sándor 2000), and the language, especially some specific purpose languages of bilingual Hungarians discussed from a puristic aspect (cf. Fábián 1993; Grétsy 2002a; Balázs 1998; Tóthfalusi 1998; Grétsy 2004; Zimányi 2006; Bősze 2009).

In minority situations where language contact with majority language is less intense, "extensive lexical borrowing is coupled with less structural borrowing and results in only minor typologically relevant change" (Fenyvesi 2005: 5). In specific purpose languages, and among them in the language of medicine, purists urge language reform and language planning to stop the corruption of the Hungarian language caused mainly by the English language (Zimányi 2006). As the Hungarian language is extremely flexible and able to accept and integrate new terms, a balance should be found between puristic approach to use only Hungarian terms and the adoption of foreign items (Grétsy 2002a).

2.1.2. Terminology of contact-induced language change

Studying the concepts of the above linguists on contact linguistics, we may come to the conclusion that the terminology they use is still incoherent. Traditionally contact-induced language changes are considered and termed 'borrowings', whereas Winford (2003) calls them 'interferences' in a wider sense. Ross (2003) introduces a new term for the same phenomenon, 'metatypy', which means restructuring of certain language elements under intense language contact, a type of morpho-syntactic and semantic language change brought about by language contact involving some multilingual speakers. Some linguists strictly use the term interference for 'substratum interference', whereas others speak about 'transfer'.

Interference was introduced by Weinreich (1953: 1) as a neutral term: "those instances of deviation from the norms of either language which occur in the speech of bilinguals as a result of their familiarity with more than one language, i.e. as a result of language contact".

Sankoff (2004) uses both borrowing and substratum interference when describing the results of contact-induced language change. Van Coetsem (1988) distinguishes between two types of transfer: borrowing under recipient language agentivity vs. imposition under source language agentivity (in second language acquisition transfer). Van Coetsem affirms that in all cases of cross-linguistic influence, there is a source or donor language and a recipient language. The direction of transfer of material is always from the source language to the recipient language, and the agent of the transfer is either the recipient language speaker (recipient language agentivity) or the source language speaker (source language agentivity). In the former case, he speaks about borrowing, in the latter, imposition. However, he adds that borrowing and imposition are not the only types of contact-induced change, but they are the main ways in which languages in contact can directly influence each other. The processes of simplification, internal innovation and others can result from language contact as well, particularly in cases where a speaker is acquiring a language, or is not fully proficient in a secondary language. Van Coetsem (1988: 3; emphasis in the original) defines borrowing as follows:

"If the recipient language speaker is the agent, as in the case of an English speaker using French words while speaking English, the transfer of material (and this naturally includes structure) from the source language to the recipient language is *borrowing (recipient language agentivity)*."

It is important that linguistic dominance and social dominance should be differentiated clearly. The former refers to the fact that a speaker is more proficient in one of the languages involved in contact, which is typically the speaker's first or primary language, whereas social dominance refers to the social and political status of a language (van Coetsem 1988).

Van Coetsem (1988) argues that there are two main 'mechanisms', imitation and adaptation, which are associated with the two main transfer types. Both mechanisms are at work in both of the transfer types, but in borrowing, imitation comes into play before adaptation, while the reverse is obtained in true imposition.

Some other linguists, especially in the context of creole formation, use the term 'substratum influence' referring to interference via shift, and 'transfer', in the context of second language acquisition. Yet others use the term interference to refer to any type of cross-linguistic influence, including borrowing, while others use transfer in the same broad sense.

Haugen (1950: 213) points out that "borrowing as here defined is strictly a process and not a state, yet most of the terms used in discussing it are ordinarily descriptive of its results rather than of the process itself". The classifications of borrowings into loanwords, loan translations and the like "are merely tags that various writers have applied to the observed results of borrowing". In his definition of loan word vs. foreign word, he noted that German linguists differentiate between two types of borrowing for simple loans. He states that "the Germans here make a distinction between the *Lehnwort*, a historical fact, and the *Fremdwort*, a contemporary fact" (1972: 104). Directly translated, a *Lehnwort* is a 'loan word' and *Fremdwort* means 'foreign word'. There is disagreement among linguists regarding what exactly qualifies a word as a loan word or a foreign word.[19] The general consensus is that the difference between the two terms lies in the given word's degree of integration into the receiving language. Loan words are usually more integrated than foreign words: they have been in the receiving language for a longer period of time. The origin of these words is not readily apparent. On the other hand, foreign words and many internationalisms can be more easily identified because they are integrated to a lesser degree; there is no assimilation or only partial assimilation.

Yang (1990) gives a more complex definition for both terms, describing how they differ from each other with regard to their differing degrees of integration. He accentuates that foreign words are "lexemes or connecting lexemes which are borrowed from a foreign language and are used in German without any orthographical, morphological or semantic change and whose foreign origin is clearly and easily recognizable, like for example Callgirl, Cowboy, Jeans" (1990: 11). On the other hand, his definition for loan words is that "a loan word is similar to a foreign word as it is also a word borrowed from a foreign language, but it has been adapted phonologically and/or morphologically and/or orthographically to the borrowing language" (1990: 11).

Therefore, the integration of a borrowing, whether on a phonological, morphological or orthographical level, plays a key role in differentiating between a loan word and a foreign word. Betz's (1939, 1974) system for borrowing was divided into two main categories, loan words and loan substitutions. His loan substitution category was further divided into loan shifts and loan meanings. Loan shifts are further subdivided into loan formations and loan creations.

It is clear that loan creations do exist, but whether they are a phenomenon of borrowing or not is debatable. The main argument put forward is that loan creations are in fact just new recipient language words and not borrowings at all. The important counterargument for the case against this, and, in favor of loan creations as an aspect of borrowing, is that loan creations are filling a gap in the recipient language's vocabulary. This gap corresponds to terms which exist in

19 The term *foreign word* is not used in Anglo-American literature.

the source language that have no equivalent in the recipient language. Therefore, loan creations are a valid category because even if they do not borrow the terminology they still borrow the concept.

Haugen (1950) takes a slightly different approach. Unlike Betz, his system consists of three categories – complete importation, partial importation and no importation. Fink (1968) and later Viereck (1986) use similar terminology to that of Haugen. Fink divides his categories into no substitution, partial substitution and full substitution.

A further category of borrowing which has been introduced is that of pseudo-loans (Yang 1990). Pseudo-loans occur where a lexeme of the source language is used to produce a word in the recipient language. The resulting word looks like a word from the source language, but it does not actually occur in the source language. There is some disagreement, however, about whether or not pseudo-loans should be included as a category of borrowing. A few linguists including Kirkness (1984) dismiss them as not being a valid category due to the fact that pseudo-loans do not actually occur in the source language. Here, the counterargument is that pseudo-loans would not occur at all in the recipient language, but for the existence of the word in the source language from which they are derived, therefore, pseudo-loans are in fact a valid category of borrowing.

Thomason and Kaufman (1988: 37) define borrowing as "the incorporation of foreign features into a group's native language by speakers of that language: the native language is maintained but is changed by the addition of the incorporated features". When the influence goes the other way, and native language structures influence the second language, the phenomenon is termed substratum interference.

As Haugen (1953: 383) points out the difficulty in defining the phenomenon with a single term is associated with the following:

"Unfortunately, we are unable to watch the mental processes directly, and can only guess at them by observing their results and comparing those results with what the speakers themselves report about their own mental experience."

It has long been debated whether, and under what conditions, languages can borrow structural features. Thomason and Kaufman (1988) highlight that there is a scale of borrowing with slight lexical borrowing at one extreme and extensive grammatical replacement at the other, with varying degrees of structural borrowing in between. Certain structural innovations in a recipient language appear to be "mediated by lexical borrowing, and are therefore not clear cases of direct structural borrowing" (King 2000: 136). In other cases, where direct borrowing of structural elements occurs, it typically involves free morphemes such as prepositions and conjunctions (Thomason and Kaufman 1988). Bound morphemes appear to be borrowed only in cases where they substitute for the recipient language morphemes that are semantically and structurally congruent with them.

Thomason and Kaufman argue that direct borrowing of structural elements can occur only when the languages involved are typologically very similar, allowing for the substitution of a recipient language morpheme by a close counterpart in the source language. Structural borrowing is subject to much stricter constraints than structural imposition, and has much less impact on the grammar of the recipient language.

A non-established borrowing (mostly of words/terms) is also sometimes called a 'foreignism' (see discussion above). Foreignisms are said to be used for a particular purpose, for instance, to make a connection with a specific culture by means of its language. However, any word can be used for a particular purpose, so the boundary between foreignism and lexical borrowing is almost indistinct. Since the two concepts cannot be kept strictly apart, it seems best to avoid the technical term foreignism.

Whether a word is perceived as new (or foreign) or not is also related to its degree of adaptation or nativization. Both terms refer to the adjustment of spelling, pronunciation and morphology of loan words to the native structure of the recipient language. Though institutionalization does not necessarily go together with adaptation, it often does. The degree of adaptation also reflects the attitudes of the affected speech community (Fischer 2008).

'Adaptation' is sometimes distinguished from 'adoption', which is defined as mainly unmodified borrowing (Hock 1991). However, in practice, many scholars use adaptation and adoption synonymously, since few completely non-adjusted borrowings exist, at least regarding pronunciation.

The term 'interlanguage' was first used in studies of second language acquisition (SLA), in the works of Selinker (1972) and Schumann (1975). It was introduced in an effort to conceptualize the linguistic system of the second language learner as rule-governed and orderly, rather than an error-ridden version of the target language. In this respect the concept of interlanguage in SLA parallels to some extent the notion of the 'vernacular' in sociolinguistics.

Interlanguage is the result of the interaction among the many language acquisition device factors in any two (or three in multilingual situations) languages developing more or less simultaneously. According the Hamers and Blanc (1990), between the choice of one language and the other, there exists for the bilingual speaker a whole range of intermediary strategies which include the modification of either code and the relative use of both.

Interlanguage may be viewed as an adaptive strategy in which the speaker tries to speak the interlocutor's first language, although he has little proficiency in it. This strategy uses simplification, reduction, overgeneralization, transfer, formulaic language, omissions, substitutions, and restructurings (Selinker 1972).

Ellis (1985) describes interlanguage as the theoretical construct which underlies the attempts of SLA researchers to identify the stages of development through which second language (L2) learners pass on their way to L2 or near L2 proficiency.

Interlanguage is described by many as permeable, dynamic, changing, and yet systematic (Selinker 1972; Corder 1975). It may undergo relative fossilization and relative change, but it reveals an underlying cognitive process even though its surface structure seems the opposite because it does not match conventional forms of what is linguistically correct.

However, while interlanguage is the language constructed before arriving at more ideal forms of the target language, code-switching may occur during and after the interlanguage phase. For Corder (1981) it is a working model, a grammar, a system which can be used quite effectively for communicative purposes. It presupposes that the language learner at all points of his learning career has a language. Corder created a visual symbol to portray the interlanguage notion with three overlapping circles (Figure 4). This model was further developed by Duran (1981) claiming that “whatever theory (Universal Grammar types or General Learning types) explains language best is not the issue here but the point is that whatever theory is operating, this theory will explain the growth of all three: Language A, Interlanguage, and Language B” (1981: 87). She highlights that there might be a new phonology, morphology, syntax, and semantics created which differ to different degrees from Language A and Language B (Figure 5). The relationship of Languages A and B creates new forms of language which are not normative or conventional forms of either language, “the interlanguage form will be perceived as non-normative and ‘strange’ [and] negative labels such as fossilization, interference, semilingualism, debased, confused, unbalanced, anomalous, pseudolingual, incorrect” (Duran 1981: 88) will be attached to the new forms.

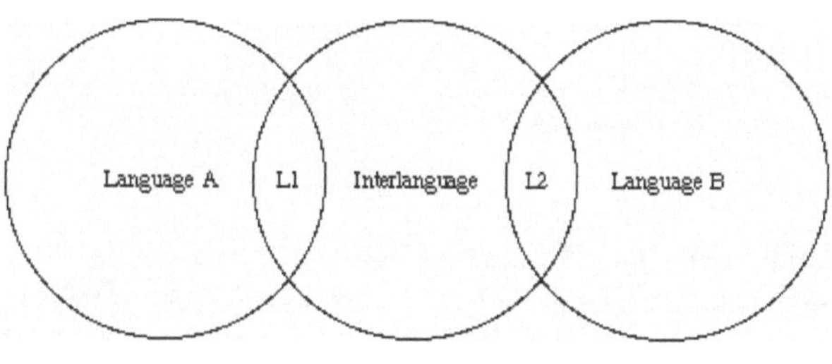

Figure 4. Corder's visual model of interlanguage notion (Corder 1981).

Code-switching (see Section 2.1.2) is the mixture of the elements of two languages in conversations among bilinguals. There has been some disagreement about the distinction between code-switching and borrowing, but "no hard and fast criteria have been found that would distinguish the two" (Winford 2003: 107–108). The distinction has more to do with the greater frequency and perhaps transitory nature of single word switches than with the process of transfer itself. In each case, the transfer type is the same. While code-switching is a syntactic process retaining the structural markings of the source language, borrowing is said to be a lexical process, structurally integrating lexical units. Moreover, code-switching mostly consists of multi-word sentential units, in contrast to borrowings, which are usually considered mono-lexical. However, these distinctions fail to account for the possibility of single-word code-switches and multi-word borrowed units. It is probably best to consider code-switching and borrowing as a cline of usage (Onysko 2005).

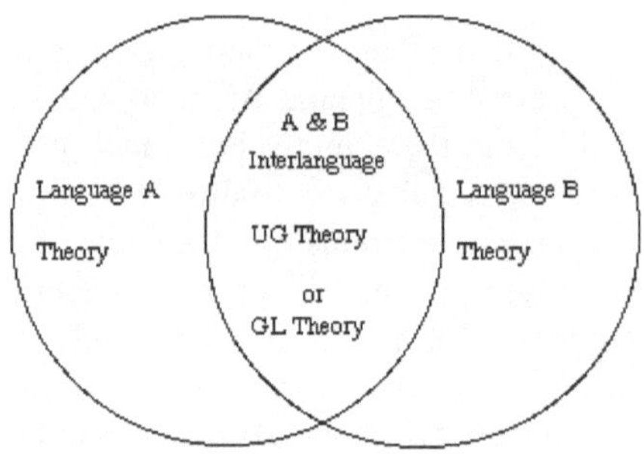

Figure 5. Duran's adaptation of Corder's (1981: 87) interlanguage notion (UG: universal grammar, GL: general learning types)

Some scholars deny any connection between borrowing and code-switching (they accentuate that code-switched elements will never turn into borrowings), whereas others consider code-switching to be the only mechanism through which foreign morphemes are incorporated into a language. Heath (1989) concludes that there is a transition between code-switching and permanent interference, as nouns and discourse markers are the most frequent code-switched elements and these are also among the most common types of borrowings. Therefore, we should accept the argument that, if the code-switched element is very common and if monolingual speakers of a language have adopted it from bilinguals, it must be assumed to have become a loanword (Heath 1989).

2.1.3. Code-switching

Code-switching refers to the mixing, by bilinguals (or multilinguals), of two or more languages in discourse often with no change of interlocutor or topic. Such mixing may take place at any level of linguistic structure (Poplack 1980).

Thomason (2001: 132) defines code-switching as "the use of material from two or more languages by a single speaker with the same people in the same conversation". It includes both switches from one language to another at sentence boundaries (intersentential switching) and switches within a single sentence (intrasentential switching). The latter is called code-mixing by some scholars.

Poplack (1980, 2000) argues that code-switching includes extra-sentential switching as well as tag- or tag-like switching that involves an utterance and an interjection (a tag).

MacSwan (2005) describes code-switching in a narrower sense by claiming that code-switching is the alternate use of two (or more) languages within the same utterance. Therefore, code-switching is a mechanism of interference (the most studied of all mechanisms) that is especially noticeable in many bilinguals' conversations.

As vital components of a bilingual's verbal repertoire, code-mixing and code-switching have received considerable attention in sociolinguistics. Consequently, several sociolinguists have attempted to grapple with these linguistic phenomena through various definitions and characterizations. For example, Di Pietro (1977: 3) defines code-switching as "the use of more than one language by communicants in the execution of a speech act".

Valdes-Fallis (1976: 877) refers to code-switching simply as "the alternation of two languages," and Scotton and Ury (1977: 5) propose that "code-switching [is] the use of two or more linguistic varieties in the same conversation or interaction." Hymes (1974: 103) states that it has "become a common term for alternate use of two or more languages, varieties of a language, or even speech styles."

Grosjean defines code-switching as "the alternate use of two or more languages in the same utterance or conversation" (1982: 145). Although there is no embracing definition for this phenomenon, there is one streak running through these various definitions: at least two languages or two varieties of a language must be involved.

Code-switching carries particular socio-interactional purposes, which has been an interesting research issue in sociolinguistics. Most researches examine its motivations, settings, rules and uses from many aspects. The main strength of code-switching is that it is primarily for sociolinguistic purposes, which implies that the code-switching functions should be within the grasp of average members in the speech community. In this regard, it is less of a simple phenomenon of linguistic inadequacy, but more of a combination of linguistic insights and socio-cognitive and cultural interpretation.

The functional and interactional view of code-switching was initiated by Gumperz (1964). In his definition (1982: 98), code-switching is seen as the "juxtaposition with the same speech exchange of passages of speech belonging to two different grammatical systems or subsystems" and as a type of "contextualization cue" which facilitates listeners to interpret speakers' intentions:

"Code switching signals contextual information equivalent to what in monolingual settings is conveyed through prosody or other syntactic or lexical processes. It generates the presuppositions in terms of which the content of what is said is decoded."

From the perspective of communicative function, Myers-Scotton (1993) suggests the objective of the markedness model is to explain the social motivation of code-switching. In her markedness model, code choices vary along a markedness continuum, ranging from marked to unmarked, and are indexical of the rights-and-obligations sets between interlocutors in a given interaction type, which is also known as the 'negotiation principle'. In addition, she affirms that speakers are creative and rational actors.

Code-switching was also researched in the field of medicine and health care. Crane (1997) evaluates the effectiveness of doctor–patient communication at a hospital in Bakersfield, California. The doctor–patient communication, as measured by patient understanding of diagnosis and treatment, appears to be compromised by language barriers. However, the bilingual doctors use language switching to improve communication with patients. Another relevant study conducted by Roberts (1994) is an ethnographic investigation of nurse–patient interaction at a hospital ward in West Wales where English and Welsh are spoken interchangeably. The study measures the effects of code-switching on patient satisfaction and nurse–patient relationships and demonstrates how bilingual skills can be effectively used to increase rapport in the clinic inpatient encounters:

"Code-switching in itself is perhaps not a linguistic phenomenon, but rather a psychological one, and its causes are obviously extralinguistic. But bilingualism is of great interest to the linguist because it is the condition of what has been called interference between languages." (Vogt 1954: 368)

Vogt stresses that all languages and almost all language users experience language contact, and that contact phenomena are important elements of language change.

Heller's ethnographic observations and sociolinguistic study in Quebec and Ontario have led her to consider the economics of bilingualism, and to view code-switching as a political strategy (Heller 1988, 1999). Since languages tend to become associated with idealized situations and groups of speakers, the use of multiple languages "permits people to say and do, indeed to *be* two or more things where normally a choice is expected" (Heller 1988: 93).

Auer and Myers-Scotton seem to describe how or why code-switching occurs differently. Auer (1984: 1) refers to "the alternating use of more than one language," while Myers-Scotton (1993: vii) mentions "the use of two or more languages in the same conversation." Romaine (1989) cites Gumperz as the source of this definition. However, these definitions introduce an element not strictly present in Gumperz's (1982: 59) definition:

"Conversational code switching can be defined as the juxtaposition within the same speech exchange of passages of speech belonging to two different grammatical systems or subsystems."

A significant breakthrough was achieved in resolving the question of single-word tokens as 'code-switches' versus 'borrowings' in 1998 by the introduction of quantitative sociolinguistic methodology to several corpora of spontaneous bilingual discourse. Poplack and Meechan (1998) outlined a quantitative methodology that rendered operational the clear conceptual distinction between code-switching and borrowing. According to their method, bilingual discourse was analyzed according to five main accountable components: (1) unmixed Language 1; (2) unmixed Language 2; (3) multiword alternations (code-switches); (4) attested loanwords; and (5) ambiguous lone items. Their methodological innovation was to statistically compare the patterning of these items with analogous, identified items in the same corpus.

Studies of identity and code-switching show that a close observation of discourse can yield both empirically and theoretically rich understanding of the functions of language variation in social interaction. By tying observations to particular speakers and social actors, rather than moving too readily to discussions of cultural or linguistic norms, scholars can come to reliable understandings of the place of language in the construction and transmission of social traditions (Lee et al. 2006).

Even though early studies in linguistics argued that there are no syntactic restrictions in code-switching, Labov (1971) claimed that code-switching was the irregular mixture of two language systems and Lance (1975) explained that there are no syntactic restrictions in code-switching. In the past 20 years, most studies on the grammatical constraints on code-switching (Pfaff 1979; Poplack 1980) were devoted to the problem of how to distinguish a single word code-switch from a borrowing:

"In virtually all bilingual corpora empirically studied, mixed discourse is overwhelmingly constituted of lone elements, usually major-class content words, of one language embedded in the syntax of another." (Poplack and Meechan 1998: 127)

Sankoff (2004) highlights that there has been much debate about the formal linguistic constraints that condition or regulate switching, and also which grammatical sites accept or constitute barriers to switching, and whether in the formal model of code-switching it is useful to construct a matrix language (di Sciullo et al. 1986; Myers-Scotton 1993; Mahootian 1993).

Several constraints were established by linguists on code-switching: the two best-known are the free morpheme constraint, which highlights that a switch may not occur between a bound morpheme and a lexical form unless the latter has been phonologically integrated into the language of the bound morpheme (Sankoff and Poplack 1981), and the equivalence constraint, which emphasizes that switches tend to occur at points in discourse where juxtaposition of Language 1 and Language 2 elements does not violate a syntactic rule of either language, i.e. at points around which the surface structure of the two languages map onto each other (Poplack 1980).

Some further constraints discussed by contact linguists in the past 30 years have been the Clitic Pronoun Constraint (Pfaff 1979), the Dual Structure Principle (Sridhar and Sridhar 1980), Woolford's Model (Woolford 1983), the Closed Class Constraint (Joshi 1985), the Government Constraint (di Scuillo et al. 1986) and among others the Functional Head Constraint (Belazi et al. 1994), etc.

Auer (1995: 120) offers a list of "conversational loci in which switching is particularly frequent". He sets up a list of the conversational situations in which code-switches are commonly used: reported speech, change of participant constellation, parentheses or side-comments, reiterations, change of activity type, topic shift, puns, language play, shift of 'key', topicalisation, and topic/comment structure.

Sociolinguistic research in this area has concentrated on trying to establish what factors in the social and linguistic context influence switching: one language might typically be associated with one set of domains (Trudgill 1992). Research has also focused on what the grammatical rules are for where switching can and can not take place, and the extent to which it is possible to distinguish between code-switching and borrowing (Thomason 2001).

Mahootian (1993) assumes that code-switching is a socially stigmatized behavior, so switchers may be influenced by this stigma in rendering judgments on sentences. Indeed in many settings code-switching is regarded as a prestigious display of linguistic talent.

Code-switching may serve three main purposes (Crystal 1987), the first of which is filling a linguistic or conceptual gap when a lexical item is not available in one language, thus, the speaker is not able to express him/herself in one language, and thus, switches to another language to compensate for this deficiency. The second purpose may be of social origin; the speaker wants to express solidarity with or affiliation to a particular social group, or intends to exclude others from a conversation who do not speak his/her second language. And thirdly, other conversational purposes can also be identified, such as conveying the speaker's attitude to the listener, emphasizing a point made in the other language, indicating a change in the conversation or quoting another conversation. In most cases code-switching conveys an attitude and other emotives; therefore, it should be viewed as providing a linguistic advantage rather than an obstruction to communication (Cook 1991).

2.1.4. Borrowing

Linguistic borrowing is a very common and intensively studied phenomenon. The term 'borrowing' is usually applied to words and their meanings, though there can be phonological, morphological and syntactic borrowing as well. In spite of our familiarity with 'words', it is not always easy to say what a word is. Certain scholars have suggested that a word can occur in isolation. Others have suggested that a word contains one unit of meaning. A better approach to defining words is to acknowledge that there is no one totally satisfactory definition, but that we can isolate four of the most frequently implied meanings of 'word': the *orthographic* word, the *morphological* word, the *lexical* word and the *semantic* word (Todd, 1987: 49). An *orthographic* word is one which has a space on either side of it. A *morphological* word is a unique form. It considers form only and not meaning. A *lexical* word comprehends the various forms of items which are closely related by meaning. A *semantic* word involves distinguishing between items which may be morphologically identical but differ in meaning (Todd 1987). Lexemes are the units listed in a dictionary; more technically a lexeme is a set of related meanings (semanteme) associated with a set of related word forms (lemmata).

When a word has been borrowed, it becomes integrated into the receiver language with varying extent. Görlach distinguishes three main degrees of acceptance: in the first case the word is fully accepted – "either the word is not (or no longer) recognized as English, or is found in many styles and registers but it is still marked as English in its spelling, pronunciation or morphology" (2002b: xxi). In the second case the word is in restricted use and in the third case "the word is not part of the language – it is either a calque or a loan creation, or mainly known to bilinguals, or used only with reference to British or American contexts" (Görlach 2002b: xxiv).

Borrowing denotes the process as well as the object: as a process it usually refers to the importation of a word or a term (multiword expression) from one language into another[20] (Fischer 2008).

The process of borrowing can be very selective, adopting a foreign form but assigning it a new meaning, or adopting a foreign meaning or concept and assigning it to a native form. As an object, it denotes the form of the item that originally was not part of the vocabulary of the recipient language but was adopted from another language and made part of the borrowing language's vocabulary. Many of the outcomes of lexical borrowing involve innovations or creations that have no counterpart in the donor language. Some of these innovations may be created of donor materials, others may be created of native materials, and still other creations may be blends of native and foreign items (Winford 2003).

Haugen's influential 1950 article on linguistic borrowing can still be considered as central for current studies of loanwords and loanword integration. Haugen distinguishes loanwords, loanblends and loanshifts. Loanwords proper are words and phrases that were transferred from the source language with no or minimal morphemic substitution.

Haugen introduced the concepts of importation and substitution; if the loan is similar enough to the model so that a native speaker would accept it as a native word, the borrowing speaker has imported the model into this language, provided it is an innovation in that language. If the speaker has reproduced the model inadequately, he has substituted a similar pattern from his/her own language. This distinction between importation and substitution can apply not only to a given loan as a whole but to its constituent patterns as well, since "different parts of the pattern may be treated differently" (1950: 212).

---

20 Borrowing can also refer to the importation of a word's meaning from one language into another or the meaning of the item that originally was not part of the vocabulary of the recipient language but was adopted from some other language. This aspect of borrowing will be discussed in section 5.1.3.

Haugen mentions a third option as well, which is characterized by partial correspondences between the languages, so that it becomes impossible to decide whether it is a case of importation or substitution: “if the loan contains patterns that are not innovations in the borrowing language, it becomes impossible to distinguish the two kinds of reproduction” (1950: 213).

Lexical borrowing is a common form of cross-linguistic influence, which can occur under a variety of conditions ranging from superficial familiarity of the source language, even without real contact with the source language’s speakers, to “close interaction between recipient and source language speakers in bilingual communities” (Winford 2003: 29).

The continuum of borrowing can spread from relatively slight lexical borrowing to extreme structural borrowing; the borrowing scale of Thomason and Kaufman (1988) is presented in Table 1. This scale consists of five stages representing the increasing intensity of contact and the increasing typological distance. Features at the top (i.e. lexical features) are borrowed first, and they are borrowed during each further stage.

Table 1. Borrowing scale (based on Thomason and Kaufman 1988, and modified by Winford 2003)

Stage	Features
1. casual contact	only lexical borrowing
2. slightly more intense contact	slight structural borrowing; conjunctions and adverbial particles
3. more intense contact	slightly more structural borrowing; adpositions, derivational affixes
4. strong cultural pressure	moderate structural borrowing (major structural features that cause relatively little typological change)
5. very strong cultural pressure	heavy structural borrowing (major structural features that cause significant typological disruption)

In the linguistic literature loans are classified according to different aspects concerning the way they are borrowed, the way speakers use them, and their stage of conventionalization. Regarding the way of borrowing, loans are classified as direct borrowing – the results of direct contact between two language (cf. Haugen, Kontra, Lanstyák) and indirect – via other languages (Winford 2003). Table 2 gives one possible overview of the various types of borrowing. Not only may the terminology vary (cf. the alternative terms given above), but also other categorizations are possible, and differ from scholar to scholar. While, for instance, Yang (1990) incorporates lexical borrowing, hybrid formation, and pseudo-borrowing into one category, Onysko (2007) argues that pseudo-borrowing is actually no borrowing at all.

Direct loans can be subclassified according to the speaker who uses these features: a native or a non-native speaker. So loans can be categorized as "proper loans (features taken over from the source language into the target language where the target language is the native tongue or first language of a speaker) and retents, retention of first language features in the second language due to inadequate language knowledge" (Semenets 1985: 94–95).

Since the process of borrowing is not reduced to the simple transferring of features of one language into the other language, the borrowed feature can go through stages of assimilation: occasional use in the speech of bilinguals, appearing in the written language (probably together with different types of explanations), and phonological assimilation and morphological integration into the borrowing language.

Table 2. Types of borrowing (based on Fischer 2008: 7).

1. Lexical borrowing	
2. Semantic borrowing	Loan meaning Loan formation: Loan translation / Loan rendition / Loan creation
3. Hybrid formation	
4. Pseudo-borrowing	Lexical pseudo-borrowing Semantic pseudo-borrowing

According to the stage of assimilation of loans in the receiving language two large classes of loans are distinguished: conventionalized (integrated, assimilated) words and non-conventionalized (heterogeneous, foreign, nonce) words. The assimilated words, as a rule, are "registered in lexicographical sources while the heterogeneous ones appear in rare occasional uses in texts without being fixed in the language" (Proshina 2001: 185).

As a result of the review of Haugen's distinction, two criteria were obtained in the Hungarian language concerning borrowing, which can each take two values: (1) conformity versus non-conformity to the source language form (importation versus substitution), and (2) conformity versus non-conformity to the target language system. If the loanword is kept in its foreign phonetic form, it can be classified as a foreign word, if it is phonetically adapted to its new environment, a loanword in the proper sense. The term *foreign word* is used in Hungarian literature, especially by language purists (e.g. Balázs, L. Grétsy, Zs. Grétsy, and Zimányi); however, it has not been so widely used in the Anglo-American literature, at least not in recent sociolinguistic studies.

Assimilated borrowings can be referred to as loanwords, and non-assimilated borrowings as borrowed words. It is very difficult to draw the line between foreign words and borrowed words. Various possible criteria have been discussed: sociolinguistic and stylistic criteria (which are adopted by von Polenz 1967, but rejected by Duckworth 1977), the question whether the words are borrowed for the first time or already lexicalized in the target language, and structural factors. In the latter case, foreign words are defined as words containing non-native sounds, sound combinations, stress patterns, graphemes, while no such elements appear in assimilated loanwords. Duckworth (1977: 46) claims that "a word borrowed from another language is a *foreign word* if the pronunciation and the spelling do not correspond to the pronunciation rules of the receiving language, while it is a *loanword* if they correspond to these rules".

Kabakchi (1998) categorized borrowings according to their appearance in dictionaries: basic (lexical units registered in abridged dictionaries and known to an average language speaker); special (lexical units registered in unabridged dictionaries and known to the domain specialists); and occasional (lexical units not registered in dictionaries but appearing in the texts devoted to the external culture).

Table 3. Common types of lexical change (Fischer 2008: 5).

Onomasiological	**Semasiological**	
	denotational meaning	connotational meaning
word-formation	narrowing	pejoration
borrowing	widening	amelioration
	metonymy	
	metaphor	

Another type of distinction was set up in cognitive linguistics by distinguishing onomasiological change and semasiological change (Table 3). Word-formation and borrowing are onomasiological changes, whereas changes in meaning belong to semasiology. The semasiological changes can be further divided into denotational meaning changes, such as narrowing, widening, metonymy and metaphor, and connotational meaning changes, such as pejoration and amelioration (Geeraerts 1997).

Regarding the integral phase of borrowing, the borrowing process implies an onomasiological change. In addition, however, a semasiological change also takes place, since not all meanings of the word in the source language are generally taken over into the target language. In the post-integral phase, further semasiological changes and also onomasiological changes (e.g. new compounds or derivatives) are likely to happen. Thus in borrowing onomasiological and semasiological changes are closely intertwined.

In immigrant or minority languages nonce borrowings are the route for the later adoption or integration of lexical items as loan words (Poplack and Sankoff 1984). Along with numerous lexical borrowings, they "usually ensue phonological changes in the recipient language" (Sankoff 2004: 643). Such alterations may include processes that apply only to the foreign-origin vocabulary, but may also spread to native vocabulary. The introduction of foreign lexical material is accompanied by not only phonological changes, but often by morphological and/or syntactic changes as well.

Adhering to both van Coetsem's 1988 and Thomason and Kaufman's 1988 concept of borrowing as, by definition, involving speakers' importing features from other languages into their native language, various studies describe the influence of native phonological patterns on foreign lexical items borrowed into the language.

The main process that is involved in the lexical aspects of languages in contact is borrowing. In the majority of contact situations, borrowing occurs most extensively on the part of minority language speakers from the language of wider communication into the minority language. On the other hand, we can also identify words that have become accepted within majority language communities that derive from language shift by various immigrant groups and would thus clearly fall under the definition of 'substratum influence' (Sankoff 2004).

Though most language contact situations lead to unidirectional rather than bidirectional linguistic results conditioned by the social circumstances, it is also the case that linguistic structure overwhelmingly conditions the linguistic outcomes. Morphology and syntax are clearly the domains of linguistic structure least susceptible to the influence of contact, and this statistical generalization is not vitiated by a few exceptional cases. On the other hand, lexical items are clearly the most readily borrowable elements, and borrowing lexicon can lead to structural changes at every level of linguistic structure (cf. Muysken 1985, 1999).

Grammatical replication (Figure 6) is part of a network of types of linguistic transfer. Grammatical replication, widely referred to as 'structural borrowing' or 'grammatical calquing', is "a process whereby speakers of a language, called the replica language, create a new grammatical structure on the model of some structure of another language, called the model language" (Heine and Kuteva 2008: 59). It concerns meanings and the structures associated with them, but not forms, that is, phonetic substance is not involved. Like other cases of replication, grammatical replication contrasts with borrowing, which involves phonetic substance, that is, either sounds or form-meaning units such as morphemes, words, or larger entities. Both replication and borrowing are manifestations of contact-induced transfer or code-copying (Johanson 1992, 2002).

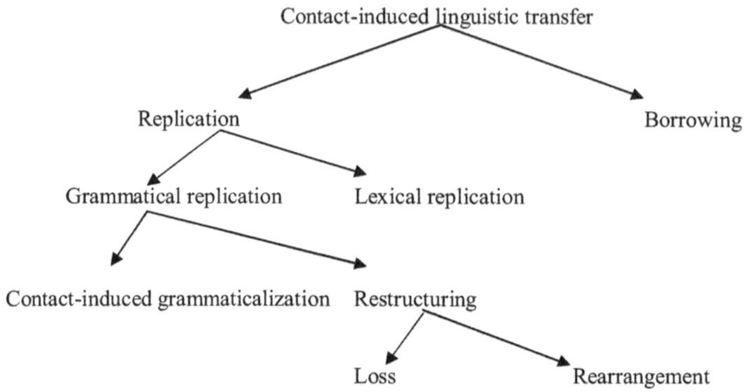

Figure 6. The main types of contact-induced linguistic transfer (Heine and Kuteva 2008)

2.1.5. English contact-induced language change (Englishization)

The term *Anglicism* was first used in the 17th century and refers to a linguistic feature of English used in another language. The term has commonly been associated with the increasing influx of English borrowings since the middle of the 20th century, with loanwords related to the international role of mainly the United States, and to English as a lingua franca. The term *Anglicism* is often used derogatively by language purists.

Although Anglicism is connected to the word *England* etymologically, it is generally not only used for contact-induced features of British English but also for English loans from all varieties of the English language.

The study of lexical borrowings has a long tradition going back at least to the historical comparative language studies of the 19th century and extending over all philologies. While the comparison of languages and their history was the focus of language studies in the 19th century and descriptive–structural approaches prevailed until the middle of the 20th century, the cognitive–semantic view has achieved wide acceptance recently, with prototype semantics having paved the way. Research on Anglicisms concentrates on several main areas. A number of empirical–descriptive studies describing Anglicisms are mostly based on print media as general text corpora (cf. Görlach 2002a). Lexicographical description of Anglicisms was presented in various dictionaries of Carstensen, Görlach and Busse. Some historical studies deal with the increasing influence of the English language, accompanied by research on attitudes towards Anglicisms and on language policies. Opinions range from an open disparagement of Anglicisms to a differentiated assessment of facts and problems, pointing to solutions and future perspectives (cf. Spitzmüller 2005; Görlach 2002b). Anglicisms have been explored with respect to certain language registers and technical languages as well. While Anglicisms in news language and in the language of advertisements have been extensively studied for several decades (Rando 1973; Fairclough 1989, 2006; Gottlieb 1997; Onysko 2007), other specialized discourses have gained an importance in European research since the 1990s, for instance the language of computer technology, business or medicine (Dürmüller 1992; Ammon 2001; Truchot 2001; Taavitsainen and Pahta 2003). The preoccupation with Anglicisms always involves the consideration of English in a global context, which, at least indirectly, influences the borrowing of English words or word elements into other languages (Fischer 2008).

Stanforth (1984) makes a distinction between British English and American English in his summary of contact between German and various other languages. This topic is quite controversial at the moment, as academics disagree on whether Anglicisms should be classified into separate subcategories according to their origins from either British English or American English. However, two complications arise if one attempts this further division: the first is defining what actually qualifies as British English, and the second is differentiating between this and American English. Hansen and Uwe (1996: 28) attempt to clarify this, but only succeed in demonstrating the inherent confusion:

"British English is used explicitly or implicitly to refer to the type of English spoken and written in England [...], British English occurs as a cover term for the variety of English used in Great Britain [...]. Even more broadly, British English is used as a cover term for the varieties of English in the British Isles [...]. British English occurs as a label to refer to the British (or, more precisely, English) branch of varieties of English (as opposed to the American branch)".

In this study the term *Englishism* will be used as an umbrella term. It should be noted, however, that most English language contact-induced features in the language of sciences are due to contact with American English rather than British English (the reasons are discussed in Section 2.2).

An Englishism (used in the broad sense) may undergo certain phases of integration into a language. First, it is not known to and not used by many speakers of the recipient language. Eventually, it may spread and take part in a process of institutionalization. This process is "brought to a close when the word has become part of the common core of the language" (Fischer 2008: 16). Nevertheless, it is usually difficult to decide whether an Anglicism has become a fully accepted linguistic phenomenon of the recipient language. The only objective method for solving this dilemma may be to check whether the lexeme under investigation is listed in the dictionary of foreign words or the monolingual dictionary of the language concerned. Dictionaries, however, contain only lexemes and do not assist the researcher in deciding about other contact-induced features (e.g. grammatical features), thus corpus studies can be more helpful in this case. The problem of selecting Englishisms is not easily solved and is also dependent on the focus and the data of a study.

The majority of Englishisms often seem to have a distribution restricted to particular sciences or subject areas (cf. English technical terms can often be found in the written discourse of medicine), whereas English colloquialisms tend to occur in advertising, in journalism and in youth language.

In some contact linguistic studies the distinction is made between Englishisms and internationalisms, for instance Görlach (2001) emphasizes that internationalisms are words of Latin or Old-Greek, and therefore they should be excluded from the category of Anglicisms/Englishisms. However, whether the form of a word looks or sounds English often depends on the differences or similarities of the linguistic structures of the source and the target language. Görlach claims that many of these words look very similar to their English counterparts, but this similarity might be due to the fact that the English language had also borrowed substantially from Latin.

When analyzing data found in USZCCDR, I did not exclude words that may have a Latin origin in general as medical terminology rests on a fundamentally Latin nomenclature with roots, prefixes and suffixes drawn from Greek and Latin. Most twentieth century additions to the language of medicine are English words built of Latin word roots and affixes (Dirckx 1983, 2006), thus, it is almost impossible to say whether a Hungarian medical word containing Latin or Greek elements was directly borrowed from Latin, or it was indirectly borrowed from Latin via English. Another process within contact-induced changes in the language of medicine is that recently, former Latin loanwords are used more extensively than earlier due to English language contact since the English language of medicine use the Latin loanwords more frequently and the speakers of the medical discourse community make use of Latin morphemes in coining new terms (see Section 2.4).

2.2. Globalization

Globalization was described in the Statement of UN Committee on Economic, Social, and Cultural Rights on May 11, 1998, as a "phenomenon which has brought fundamental changes within every society". The world seems to be getting smaller because of communication technologies, increasing contact with distant parts of the world, an increase in mobility, and the rise of transnational corporations and organizations.

Beck, a German social scientist, has remarked that the word globalization is "the most used – and misused – and least often defined, probably most misunderstood, most nebulous and politically charged catchword, which has caused much debate in recent years and will continue to do so in years to come" (1997: 42, translation by Erling 2004: 2). Steffen suggests that "we currently lack the means of analyzing the globalization process appropriately and this, of course, only adds to the misuse of the term" (2002: 92) and there is a need for further investigation into the significance of globalization – especially within the realm of applied linguistics.

The most recent stage of globalization can be attributed to the situation formed after World War II. The term 'global village' was first used by McLuhan (1969), and he used it to refer to the "compression of the world and the intensification of consciousness of the world as a whole" (Robertson 1992: 8).

The concept of globalization has often been connected with standardization (Levitt 1983: 92–93), and globalization is sometimes seen as a process that leads to the homogenization of cultures and languages in a system where all institutions come to be dominated by the same principle.

2.2.1. Language globalization

Crystal points out that translation and interpreting have limits in international communication, and "the more a community is linguistically mixed, the less it can rely on individuals to ensure communication between different groups" (1997: 11). To solve this problem, a common language, a lingua franca should be used. In some communities a simplified language, a pidgin is developed combining the elements of two languages, and in other cases the more powerful language becomes the lingua franca.

The language and culture which serve as the main homogenizing forces of globalization come from the United States. Since 1945, the US has become the most important economic and cultural power, and used its power to internationalize its own economy. Moreover, the dominance of the US in the media and cultural industries has resulted in the fact that American products can be consumed in English around the world.

At the end of the 20th century "a rough but reasoned estimate yields about 1.3 billion more or less fluent speakers of English" (Crystal 1997: 53–63) in the world, the great majority of whom are non-native speakers of the language. The new developments require at least basic but, in most cases, advanced knowledge of English for getting a good job, studying at university, and staying informed of science, literature, or various fields of culture.

Globalization and language spread go hand in hand and language is not regarded as a neutral player in the globalization formula. Two conflicting conceptions of the role of global English are described in literature: the diffusion of language paradigm, which attributes the spread of English to its hybridity and regards this spread as natural and beneficial, and the ecology of language paradigm, which primarily highlights the maintenance of indigenous languages and cultures (Tsuda 1994). The diffusion of language paradigm is associated with linguistic genocide, subtractive learning, imperialism, hierarchisation, polarization, and gaps, whereas the ecology of language paradigm is associated with equality, maintenance, diversity, and growth (Skutnabb-Kangas 2001). These two paradigms have opposing views on several concerns, among which is whether the ascendancy of the English language as the international language of communication occurred naturally or was a calculated effort (Kachru 1986; Graddol 1997; Phillipson 2001; Skutnabb-Kangas 2001). This is important because it signals whether this spread is related to the imposition of power or not. The concept of 'linguistic imperialism' was first used by Phillipson (1992), and the debate about the global use of English has become politicized (Erling 2004).

It is in the economic and political interest of the United States to ensure that if the world is moving toward a common language, it be English; that if the world is moving toward common telecommunications, safety, and quality standards, they be American; and that if common values are being developed, they be values with which Americans are comfortable. English in several aspects links the world (Rothkopf 1997).

There can be no real economic growth and development where:

"a whole people are denied access to the latest developments in science, technology, health, medicine, business, finance, and other skills of survival because all these are stored *in foreign languages*. [...] there can be no democracy where a whole people have been denied the use of *their languages*, where they have been turned strangers in their own country." (Ngũgĩ 1998: 90–91, original emphasis)

The prevailing use of English in high-prestige domains such as scholarship has main implications for democracy, a well-informed public sphere and population, and social cohesion, if local, more accessible languages are not also used. "It is important not to think of democracy in purely western terms" (Phillipson 2009: 11).

2.2.2. English as an international lingua franca

The term *lingua franca* has been used in widely different senses. Crystal points out that "a language achieves a genuinely global status when it develops a special role that is recognized in every country. […] To achieve such a status, a language has to be taken up by other countries around the world" (Crystal 1997: 3–4) either by making it the official language, or by giving it a priority in the country's foreign language teaching.

A language can be considered global on the basis of the number of its speakers, or the power of its speakers (economic, technological or cultural, political or military), in most cases a language cannot be considered independently, only in accordance with its speakers' power and their dominant role (Crystal 1997).

English as a lingua franca stands for a special type of communication (Lesznyák 2004). The increased contact between certain speech communities that evolved because of globalization affects "more people communicating over more language boundaries therewith increases the need for a common code" (Erling 2004: 19). It is the English language that often fulfills this need for a global lingua franca. Therefore, English is nowadays considered to be "both a consequence of and a contributor to globalization" (Fishman 1998: 27). Bamgbose outlines that recently there has been an "over-whelming acceptance of the global dominance of English" (2001: 357), as speakers of English use this language both to take part in and profit from globalization.

Joseph (2001) gives a detailed overview of English becoming an international language, and traces the origin of this process back to 1873. The linguistic literature recognizes English as the most prominent international language from the 1930s (Richards 1943). Nevertheless, postcolonial varieties of English were recognized only after World War II, and sociolinguistic studies started to assess the impact of the English language on other languages in the 1940s (Wright 2003).

English has become the lingua franca of the 20th century, "a language used for convenience", and relied on as "a medium of communication for people who speak different first languages" (Crystal 1995: 454). It is a "language, no longer the domain of a specific country, culture, race, or religious group, [it] is not geographically restricted" (Modiano 1999: 12).

English has also become a lingua franca to the point that literate, educated people are in a very real sense linguistically deprived if they do not know English. Poverty, famine, and diseases are instantly recognized as the cruelest and least excusable forms of deprivation. "Linguistic deprivation is a less easily noticed condition, but one of nevertheless great significance" (Burchfield 1985: 160).

English is considered as a symbol of modernization, the key to expanded functional roles (Kachru 1986). Knowing English opens the linguistic gates to international business, technology and science, and travel, and lacking this knowledge closes these gates. Thus, we can conclude that English provides linguistic power. Because of its status as a powerful global language relied on for many purposes and under many circumstances, the use of English as a language of wider communication has been seen as a main source of communicative inequality, as nonnative speakers of English can be at a disadvantage if they have to struggle to express themselves when communicating in it.

Pennycook (1995) uses a critical and multifaceted approach to show how imperialism is far more complex on the linguistic and cultural level. She claims that "we should be acutely aware of the implications of this spread for the reproduction and production of global inequalities" (1995: 54). The spread of English in all main areas of life is considered as a significant side effect of globalization. Thus, the English language empowers those who speak it and discriminates against those who do not. Indeed, Pennycook (1995: 186) summarizes it succinctly when he states that:

"English functions as a gatekeeper to positions of prestige in society. With English taking up such an important position in many educational systems around the world, it has become one of the most powerful means of inclusion into or exclusion from further education, employment, and social positions."

Hence, linguistic discrimination becomes a reality and English remains mandatory for the global workplace.

On the other hand, in international communication there are modifications in 'world Englishes' of a minor type in lexis, syntax, and discourse patterns, and more major ones in pronunciation. There is substantial variation in the use of English within and across countries, but, especially in writing, there is a standardized product that ensures intelligibility (Rajadurai 2007).

Phillipson claims that *lingua franca* is "a pernicious, invidious term" if the language in question is a first language for some people but for others a foreign language, such communication typically being asymmetrical (2008: 14).

In fact, the discourse on world English(es) changed gear dramatically in 1992 with the publication of Phillipson's book *Linguistic Imperialism*. Whereas the 1980s saw relatively restrained arguments from Kachru and other enthusiasts in the world English(es) 'movement' on the need for a paradigm shift in the study of English as an international language, this discourse was formulated according to the game-rules of an essentially western liberal perspective (Bolton 2004).

The nature of this relationship, Phillipson argues, is one of structural and systemic inequalities[21], in which the political and economic hegemony of western anglophone powers is established or maintained over scores of developing nations, particularly former colonies of European powers. The political and economic power of such nations in the Third World is, moreover, accompanied by 'English linguistic imperialism', defined by Phillipson in the following terms:

"A working definition of *English linguistic imperialism* is that *the dominance of English is asserted and maintained by the establishment and continuous reconstitution of structural and cultural inequalities between English and other languages* [...] English linguistic imperialism is seen as a sub-type of linguicism." (1992: 47, original emphasis)

Partly in response to Philippson's *Linguistic Imperialism* (1992), Fishman also discusses English in the context of economic globalization:

"Economically unifying and homogenizing corporate and multinational forces are increasingly creating a single market into which all societies – former colonial and non-colonial states alike – can be and, indeed, for their own self-interests' sake, usually seek to be integrated. The language of these forces is now most frequently English . . . On the other hand, a similarly powerful trend is occurring in the opposite direction, in the direction of asserting, recognizing, and protecting more local languages, traditions, and identities – even at the state level – than ever before in world history." (Fishman 1996: 639)

Raley (1998) recognizes that globalization is not only a social, political, economic and cultural phenomenon, but now also an academic one. A lingua franca is most appreciated in certain communities, e.g. international academic and business communities (Crystal 1997). The globalization of the international academic communities promotes an intensified interaction between scholars and disciplines.

2.2.3. The English language in Europe

The motto 'unity in diversity' of the European Union also accounts for the language needs and desires described earlier in Section 2.2.1. The native tongues of Europe are perceived as a source of wealth and as a bridge to greater solidarity and even mutual understanding. The Union's objectives are to respect and promote the rich cultural and linguistic diversity of Europe, and to safeguard

---

21 Thus, it is surely not language itself that exerts hegemonic control but its users, who might see language as an instrument of domination.

and enhance Europe's cultural heritage, as expressed in Article I-3 in the Treaty Establishing a Constitution for Europe, as well as in other documents (cf. website http://eur-lex.europa.eu). Since the 1990s many actions have been undertaken to improve communication and increase individual multilingualism among European citizens.

In 2005, a new framework strategy for multilingualism was developed, promoting the learning of at least two foreign languages, i.e. not only English but another language in addition to one's mother tongue (Peckham et al. 2008). All these activities, which are apparently deemed necessary, signal a challenge for Europe: the challenge that economic, political and juridical convergence does not facilitate cultural streamlining.

Not only Anglicisms and English as an international means of communication but also the increasing interconnectedness and confluence with all parts of the world should be regarded as a necessary incentive to concerning oneself with one's own cultural identity and heritage, leading to its appreciation, promotion and protection (Fischer 2008).

Europe, where the ideal of one national language per nation-state became a central feature of modernity, is reinventing itself. The Council of Europe's language policies have provided a new focus for foreign language learning across Europe. The new European model provides more than a means of standardizing approaches to language education through mechanisms such as the Common European Framework. It represents a wider ideological project to improve citizens' awareness of the multilingual nature of Europe, to encourage a positive attitude towards linguistic diversity, and to promote the learning of several languages.

The European project is to foster large-scale multilingualism in Europe (or 'plurilingualism' as the Council of Europe prefers to call it). European citizens should ideally learn two languages in addition to their mother tongue. The expected benefits of such a program include a better understanding between neighboring nations, improved mobility of people in work and study, and an enhanced sense of a shared European identity (Graddol 2006).

One of the weaknesses of the European project is that all languages are positioned as having a 'home' in one or more member countries. In theory, English has no greater status, in European terms, than, say, French or Swedish. In practice, however, within many large companies, and even in parts of the European governmental institutions, English has become a common working language. In some quarters the de facto special status of English in Europe is causing resentment (cf. Phillipson 2003).

Not surprisingly, English has acquired a special place in school timetables in most countries (Dörnyei 2006). Steadily, across Europe, English has become the 'first foreign' language in education systems, often replacing another language from that position. For example, in Switzerland, some German-speaking cantons have controversially decided that English will be introduced at an earlier age than French, the second national language of Switzerland (Dürmüller 1992).

In the Baltic States and post-Soviet countries, English has, in many cases, now replaced Russian as the main foreign language. In Estonia, for example, the 2000 census asked citizens which foreign languages they could speak. It found that the decline of Russian speaking was exactly matched by rise in English amongst young people. English is also being introduced in primary schools (Rannut 2004). The regular Eurobarometer surveys, which ask EU citizens in which foreign languages they can hold a conversation, indicate, not surprisingly, that the numbers of people claiming to be able to speak English have been rising in the last couple of years in most countries surveyed (Graddol 2006).

Since the end of the Cold War in the late 1980s and the development of the EU, there has been a need for a new European lingua franca.[22] Increased contact between communities has required that more people communicate across more boundaries, and, as a result, people rely more and more on English. Phillipson (2001) claims that "in reality English is no longer a foreign language in several member states [...] it is a fact of working and social life for many EU citizens". English is now being used alongside native languages in almost every European country and several studies have shown that its domains of use have expanded (cf. Coulmas 1991; Hartmann 1996).

English has become the most widely spoken second and foreign language throughout Europe as more than 30% of EU citizens state that they have sufficient skills in English to have a conversation (Table 4). Generally, there was an increase in foreign language learning in the EU in the last forty years, and there were also observable increases in learning French and German, but English is the language whose status has progressed most. "When English is used so extensively, confirming its dominance in many domains, this serves to make the learning of English more attractive than learning other languages" (Phillipson 2008: 11). English is not only the most important language of world communication, but it is the main language of intra-European communication.

22 The Latin language was the lingua franca of educated people in Europe in the Middle Ages for centuries until French took over this role in the 18th century.

Table 4. Proportion of EU population who speak the three most commonly spoken languages (Eurobarometer 2001: 53, cf. Europeans and their languages 2006)

Language	Proportion of **L1** speakers in EU	Proportion of **L2** speakers in EU	**Total** Proportion of L1 and L2 speakers in EU together in EU
English	16%	31%	47%
German	24%	8%	32%
French	16%	12%	28%

In 19 out of 29 countries polled, English is the most widely known language apart from the mother tongue, this being particularly the case in Sweden (89%), Malta (88%) and the Netherlands (87%) (*Europeans and their Languages* 2006: 4).

English has progressively, over a thirty-year period, taken over the role that French played earlier as the key language of the internal affairs of the Union. This can be seen in the figures for the language of initial drafting of EU texts. They reveal a dramatic decline in the use of German and French, and an increase in the use of English as the default in-house language. This clearly strengthens the interests of proficient users of English, whether as a first or second language.

70–80% of all TV fiction shown on European TV is American. “American movies, American TV and the American lifestyle for the populations of the world and Europe at large have become the lingua franca of globalization, the closest we get to a visual world culture” (Bondebjerg 2003: 79–80).

Other languages that aspire to ‘global’ importance, including French, function in similarly hegemonic ways. Cohabitation or partnership between ‘big’ languages and demographically or politically smaller languages is typically asymmetrical. Partnership between former colonial languages and local languages is invariably unequal. There are, however, viable strategies for attempting to achieve equitable linguistic power-sharing (Phillipson 2009).

Hartmann (1996) examines the use of English in various domains such as academia, education and EU administration, and he also discusses European bilingualism, diglossia and the adoption of English lexis into European languages. He claims that “the future looks as though it belongs to the English language, even though it [the English language] could itself be transformed in the process” (1996: 2).

Several linguistic studies have described and analyzed the growing use of English in Europe (cf. Filipović 1990), and in 1997, a special edition of the journal *World Englishes* (Volume 16) was dedicated to this subject, publishing the papers of ten European scholars presenting different aspects of the functions of English in Europe.

Although many Europeans accept the practical necessity of English, there is also widespread fear about the damage it might do to other European languages. Görlach has undertaken an extensive survey of English in Europe that has resulted in the publication of *English in Europe* (Görlach 2002a), the *Dictionary of European Anglicisms* (Görlach 2001) and the *Annotated bibliography of European Anglicisms* (Görlach 2002b). In these volumes he records the lexical impact of English on selected European languages including the Hungarian language. These works analyze the presence of English in sixteen European languages in the last five decades, and consider the reaction across Europe to the influx of Anglicisms. Görlach claims that "Anglicisms will continue to increase, [and] not only in the countries that have been retarded by political and ideological restrictions, mainly in Eastern Europe" (2001: 11–12).

English language globalization has led to the development of stabilized bilingualism in Europe at least in certain speech communities (sciences, information technology, and business). There are two different types of bilingual speech communities: the first are multilingual settings where English is used as a lingua franca, so the primary input is not from native speakers. The language becomes a unifying source, and users not only acquire the language but also make it their own (Lesznyák 2004). In such settings New Englishes have emerged. The second type is settings where there already exists a national language, so when English is introduced, the community becomes bilingual. Code-switching and code-mixing are common in these settings.

Various studies have been published on globalization to give insight into it; however, they do not describe all of its implications. Research is still needed which "geopoliticiz[es] the national and locat[es] it in large (and unequal) histories and geographies of global power and structure" (Shome and Hegde 2002: 253). No one listens to what you say "if you do not speak English because English is the language of power and, by speaking another language, you show you have no power. [...] It is therefore reasonable to suppose that the tendency to use English as a *lingua franca* is not motivated by practical considerations alone" (Truchot 2002: 18).

Phillipson and Skutnabb-Kangas highlight that "evidence in western and Eastern Europe shows that diglossia, with English as the intrusive dominant language, may be imminent" (1996: 446). The term diglossia refers here to two distinct languages (Fishman 1972) rather than two dialects.

In the European context, the parameters determining hierarchies of language are multiple and mobile: there is "an unresolved tension between the maintenance of the autonomy of national languages and the hegemonic consolidation of English both in the supranational institutions and within each state" (Phillipson 2008: 13).

How far domain loss is a reality in Scandinavia has yet to be researched adequately and preliminary surveys are of limited theoretical and empirical validity. Existing diagnostic efforts are hampered by loose terminology, in that 'domain' may refer to a vast range of activities or to a narrow spectrum, and 'loss' is inappropriate in that it obscures the agency of both the losers and the gainers. In reality, domains are not 'lost', specific spoken or written activities are subjected to linguistic capital accumulation by dispossession due to forces behind an increased use of English, the result being the marginalization of other languages (Phillipson 2006, 2008).

Although the Hungarian language literature targeting the effects of globalization is growing, language globalization is only discussed by few (e.g. Kontra 1997a, 2001, 2009; Sándor 2001; Kozma and Fóris 2002; Péntek and Benő 2003).

2.2.4. The English language in Hungary

Hungarian is a Finno-Ugric and agglutinative language that has been in contact with Indo-European inflectional languages during its history in the Carpathian Basin. The social circumstances of contacts between Hungarian and other languages vary widely. Some of the contacts are within the borders of Hungary and others are in either neighboring countries or in countries with a large number of Hungarian immigrants (Fenyvesi 2005).

In the twentieth century a much closer contact developed between English and other languages of Europe due to new means of communication (Odlin 1989). The result was a very free and versatile linguistic borrowing of English words by European languages, including the Hungarian language (Kontra 1982).

Every language (with very few exceptions) borrows and assimilates words and other linguistic features from other languages. The Indo-European English language has assimilated vocabulary among others from European languages such as Latin, Greek, French, Dutch, Spanish and a few items even from Hungarian, not to mention the languages of the other four continents (including America with all its indigenous languages). The list of Hungarian contact-induced features in English is relatively short, involving mainly (or I may say only) lexical items such as *coach* (<*kocsi*), *czardas* (<*csárdás*), *hussar* (<huszár) or *vizla* (<*vizsla*).

On the other hand, Finno-Ugric Hungarian has also assimilated words from various languages, from e.g. German, Greek, French, Italian, Latin, Lovari, different Slavic languages and Turkish, and quite a few English words were also borrowed during the last three centuries (e.g. E *club* > H *klub,* E *sandwich* > H *szendvics,* E *sport* > H *sport,* E *whisky* > H *viszki*[23]).

The geographical situation of Britain and Hungary excluded a close contact between speakers of the two languages until recently (Farkas and Kniezsa 2002), and English contact-induced language features remained sporadic until about the past 30 years. However, Országh (1968) describes that a kind of 'Anglomania' developed in Hungary in the second quarter of the 19th century in 'educated classes'. Borrowing was focused mainly on words for machinery and tools, communication and transportation, some political expressions, commercial and financial terms. At the end of the 19th and beginning of the 20th centuries a number of sports and games were introduced from Britain with their terminology and certain vocabulary of upper class social life and amusement. However, the majority of the borrowings from English were via French or German due to the given geographical and political factors. Hundreds of English words have been documented (Országh 1968) from the Hungarian press in the 19th century, however, only few of them have stayed and assimilated to be the 'active member' of the current Hungarian language. These 'active members' have undergone a process of phonological, orthographic, morphemic and semantic adaptation, thus, becoming assimilated loanwords.

The first purist publications pointing to the 'threat of the English language' appeared in the 1920s and 1930s. After the Second World War, the influx of English words increased dramatically, but there was a strong tendency to purge English elements for obvious political reasons (Farkas and Kniezsa 2002: 280). In the early 1930s, a campaign organized by the Hungarian sporting press succeeded in eliminating about 50 English sporting terms (Csapó 1970) being the only successful attempt yet, to eliminate the Anglicisms from Hungarian or at least reduce their number.

Then, with the growing influence of the Soviet Union at the end of the 1940s, a new, politically motivated purism developed in Hungary against English contact-induced features with the ban on Western European books and journals, and restrictions on mobility (Huszár 1985). Negative attitudes emerged toward everything of foreign origin, including foreign words. Few words were borrowed at the time. Among them were technical terms (*bulldozer, grader*), including land-lease cars and truck names (Ford, Dodge, Willis). Popular non-fiction used quite a number of Americanisms, mostly in a negative light. English studied at school and English texts published for readership abroad reflected Soviet reality and were full of politicized clichés. English was almost completely

23 See Országh (1968) for a detailed list of borrowings through the mid-1960s.

expelled from school curricula, and partially returned to secondary and higher education only in the 1960s.

The decline and subsequent end of the Cold War have changed both the geopolitical and linguistic landscape. The emergence of a unipolar world, in which the United States is the dominant political force, has arguably led to the ascendancy of English as the language of diplomacy. The United States' global economic strength has served as a vehicle for the export of American culture via the entertainment industry and various corporate brands. Without doubt, one of the most significant technological and cultural advancements of the past fifteen years was the development of the Internet. This phenomenon has two sides. On the one hand, no other technology has brought people around the world into closer contact. On the other hand, the undeniable lingua franca of the Internet continues to be English. For all of the above reasons, "globalization has allowed English to penetrate all societies, if not as a foreign language then as the source for significant linguistic borrowing" (Proshina 2005: 442).

However, since the development and global spread of the Internet, English has become the main source of contact-induced features in the Hungarian language. There is almost no domain in Hungarian without English lexemes and other linguistic features leading to Anglophilia (affiliation for everything that is English) in various fields of life. The fields that are mostly affected by this phenomenon are catering, tourism, information technology, economics, medicine, sports and youth culture (Petzold and Berns 2000; Farkas and Kniezsa 2002).

Since the late 1980s English has become the most popular foreign language in Hungary, and now it is the first (and in many schools the only) choice in the school curriculum (Medgyes 1993; Petzold and Berns 2000). English has taken the first position as the most popular language, and has been followed by the traditional regional lingua franca, German, in the second place, and French in the third place (Dörnyei 2006). What is perhaps even more important is the fact that English started to be considered not only a very useful, but also a fashionable language. The development of modern technology, especially the Internet, as well as the dominant position of the United States in the present-day world, is of great significance here as well. Moreover, the contacts between English and Hungarian have become closer than ever before due to the opening of the British (and Irish) labor market for Hungarians, following the entrance of Hungary to the European Union.

This spreading of the English language is, however, looked at as a "mixed blessing" (Kontra 2001), and harmful effects of globalization on life in Hungary are also, to some extent, associated with English. Language purists consider only the harmful effects of globalization and the spread of the English language, and they want to 'defend our language' against these 'harmful and threatening' effects. Grétsy and Kemény (1996) highlight that using English terms means only showing off one's knowledge and Minya (2003) refers to the present language situation as an era for a new neologist movement.

There is no sufficient information concerning the sociolinguistic aspects of English language contact in Hungary, as only few studies are available yet. Országh (1968) highlighted the presence of English words in the Hungarian language, and he set up categories to classify Anglicisms in Hungarian (1977). He was followed by Kontra (1981), who focuses on Anglicisms in one special language, the Hungarian language of medicine.

Sociolinguistic studies describe language contact of Hungarians living outside Hungary. Gal (1979) writes about language contact of Hungarian with (Austrian) German of Hungarians living in Felsőőr (Oberwart), while Fenyvesi (1998, 2005, 2006) reveals patterns of borrowing and language attrition of two generations of American Hungarian speakers. Kontra has edited a Special Issue of *Multilingua* on Language Contact in East-Central Europe in 2000. This comprehensive volume contains, among other things, reviews on Hungarian minority language use in Slovakia (Lanstyák, Kontra), Subcarpathia, Ukraine (Csernicskó and Fenyvesi), and the Hungarian speaking areas of Moldova, Romania (Sándor) with respect to intergroup contacts and conflicts. Language is the central symbol of national identity for both Hungarians and the speakers of the majority languages. The authors of the above mentioned Special Issue also highlight the differences in the Hungarian language use between bilinguals in these areas and monolingual speakers in Hungary.[24] Fenyvesi (2005) has edited a comprehensive collection of sociolinguistic works on Hungarian in contact with other languages containing a wealth of information on many bilingual communities involving Hungarian as a minority language. The communities covered in the book are located in countries neighboring Hungary (Austria, Serbia, Slovakia, Slovenia, Romania and Ukraine) as well as overseas (Australia and the United States). The language use of Hungarian Americans has been studied by Kontra (1990), Bartha (1993) and Fenyvesi (1995b, 2006). The above mentioned studies are mostly interview-based, whereas Fenyvesi (2006) has used a questionnaire to investigate American English language contact-induced features in Toledo, Ohio, which is a novel method in the field of contact linguistics, and is particularly applicable to Hungarian, which is rich in morphology.

24 See also Keresztes (2006a) on these differences between Hungarian physicians in Romania and in Hungary.

2.3. The language of medicine

Langslow (2000: 5) describes technical languages as "varieties of a language with their own history, with areas of overlap with non-technical varieties which may have influenced them and been influenced by them". A technical language is limited in use not only to certain discourse communities but also to certain registers. A technical language has considerable overlap with the standard language, although it typically has non-standard features at all linguistic levels (with the probable exception of phonology), too. The lexicon is by far the most prominent and most fully researched and documented aspect of technical languages. The terminology used to refer to certain phenomena or methods in the technical language may be unfamiliar to speakers who are not members of that discourse community.

Sager et al. (1980: 69) highlight the fact that:

"special languages are semi-autonomous, complex semiotic systems based on and derived from general language: their use presupposes specific education and is restricted to communication among specialists in the same or closely related fields."

There are certain technical terms the proper use of which (i.e. knowledge of the distinctions and oppositions) may require specialized knowledge in the given discipline. But, while the lexicon of the technical language may be different from that of everyday language because of the different things to which it makes reference, deviation from the standard (general) language in spelling, inflectional morphology, syntax or style is not prerequired. Nevertheless, such deviations from the standard language are common in several technical languages (Langslow 2000). Thus, it may be of interest to characterize a technical language by studying these linguistic aspects.

Medicine is the science and 'art' of maintaining and restoring human health through the study, diagnosis, and treatment of patients. It encompasses the fields of clinical medicine and surgery, medical research, biomedicine, and other health sciences as well. The language of medicine is one of the technical languages that are investigated for their instrumental role both in medical diagnosis and in treatment. Social and interactional research has been carried out on medical discourse since the 1970s (e.g. Engel 1977; Fisher and Todd 1983). Recent research topics include physician–patient interaction, medical socialization, medical ethics, and the representation of science and medicine in literature, whereas the social and cultural determinants of diseases are also explored through language use (Putnam 1975; West 1990).

Medical terminology, medical text patterns, and medical text and discourse content have been developed as a means of dealing with reality in a way that is appropriate for medical purposes (Gunnarson 2006). A specialized technical language, such as the language of medicine, can be defined as a "restricted repertoire of words and expressions selected from the whole language to cover every requirement within a well-defined context" (Maher 1986: 117). Medical terminology is a vocabulary for accurately describing the human body and associated components, conditions and processes in a science-based manner. Technical terminology consists largely of nouns. Many of the terms used in gross anatomy are taken from the vernacular in most languages: e.g. arm, back, breast, head or skull. Physicians rarely call these structures by any other names. For some parts of the body there are no 'polite words', so they use either a Latin term (e.g. *anus*) or an English one adapted from Latin (e.g. *testicle*) (Dirckx 2006).

Current medical English makes wide use of words borrowed from Latin: e.g. *defecation, eructation, micturition, regurgitation.* Although a few modern concepts are expressed by Anglo-Saxon words: e.g. (friction) *rub* or *frozen* (section).

Euphemisms and other forms of verbal sanitization have a long history and typically take two semantic forms: the metaphorical use of root terms (e.g. *pass water* instead of *piss* and *break wind* instead of *fart*), or the substitution of so-called 'Anglo-Saxon' words by polysyllabic abstract formulations using classical vocabulary. Examples range from *terminated pregnancy* instead of *abortion*, *erectile dysfunction* for *impotence*, through to *liquidate*, *neutralize*, or *terminate with extreme prejudice* instead of *kill*. While the first examples are natural and have a long history in the discourse community, the latter are more institutional in the sense of disguising violence by means of bland abstraction (Dirckx 1983).

Sooner or later, euphemisms come to be so closely linked to the things named that they themselves become offensive and must be replaced in their turn. *Alcoholism*, for example, has been renamed *ethanolism*, which is slightly equivocal since most recent terms on this pattern (*atropinism, iodism*) denote acute intoxication, no habituation.

Jespersen claims (1955: 230) that:

"this is the usual destiny of euphemisms; in order to avoid the real name of what is thought indecent or improper, people use some innocent word. But when that becomes habitual in this sense it becomes just as objectionable as the word it has ousted and now is rejected in its turn".

Physicians sometimes use metaphores or similes when describing an abnormal appearance, sound or odor: e.g. *air hunger, rusty sputum* and *napkin-ring obstruction*. Abnormal structures or movements are depicted by terms like *bamboo spine, cogwheel rigidity, flame hemorrhage* or *greenstick fracture*.

Some other medical terms refer to food or drink: e.g. *rice-water* stool in cholera, *strawberry* hemangioma, *bread-and-butter* heart in fibrinous pericarditis, or *coffee-ground* emesis. Another large class of metaphors includes words referring to animals: *staghorn* calculus, *spider* angioma, *hare*lip, *camel-*hump wave of the electrocardiogram or *butterfly* rash (cf. Dirckx 1983).

In English medical terminology the basic vocabulary is composed of word roots[25] derived mostly from Latin or Greek. A prefix can be added to modify the word root by giving additional information about the location of an organ, the number of parts, or time involved, and suffixes are used to add meaning such as condition, disease process or procedure. The word root usually cannot be used alone as most word roots in modern standard English. If the medical word root is borrowed from Latin or Greek, it will remain meaningless as a stand-alone term. A suffix or a prefix must be added, for example English *cardi-* from the Greek *kardía* cannot be used alone to mean *heart.* The addition of a suffix e.g. *-ac, -ology* is needed for the proper form to mean pertaining to the heart (*cardiac*) or a specialist who examines the heart (*cardiologist*).

The development of new terminology in a language that does not possess adequate technical description is a powerful force in the formation of the medical register (Maher 1986). Lewis (1975) describes the special characteristics of adjectives in descriptive anatomy in English, and de Bakey (1966) has revealed the tendency in medical discourse (defined by de Bakey as the 'restricted language of the medical community') to turn nouns into verbs (e.g. *to hospitalize* from the noun *hospital*). Further morphological particularities involve word coinage and syllabic contraction (e.g. *urinalysis* instead of *urinoanalysis*).

Dubois (1981) has pointed out the characteristic use of noun compounds in medical discourse. Compounding, which is also termed complex nominalization, refers to the relative proportion of attributive nouns and adjectives that modify the head of the nominal group (e.g. *human blood group B cell-immune*). Other common features of the medical register are the use of abbreviations in physician-to-physician conversation, e.g. *We had a DOA in the afternoon. DOA* in medical discourse means *dead on arrival*, elliptic features, e.g. *giving the patient oids*, which refers to *steroids/corticosterioids*, and the frequent use of slang and euphemisms (Crichton 1975; Christy 1979; Johnson and Murray 1985).

The most obvious feature of medical English is the extensive use of expert terms referred to as 'medical jargon', and the passive and impersonal style that focuses on measurable phenomena, i.e. the use of nominalizations, passive clauses and third person pronouns instead of first person ones (Zethsen and Askehave 2006).

---

25 I use 'word root' to designate a lexical element that carries a broad range of meanings and may appear in related words functioning as various parts of speech.

Medical discourse analysis is of interest to the applied linguist as it makes medical talk 'visible' as recognizable conversation with its full repertoire of analytic features. Cicourel (1981: 84) claims that:

"the medical interview is of value to the applied linguist because it highlights conditions that exist in the study of discourse but which are not always addressed, [...] the physician and the linguist face similar problems: how to make visible those aspects of discourse and textual materials that seem intended, implied and misleading."

Hedging is a common discoursive feature of medical writing (Skeleton 1997). It is the expression of tentativeness and possibility (Myers 1989; Salager-Meyer 1994). It is central to academic writing where statements are rarely made without subjective assessments of their reliability and the need to present unproven propositions with caution and precision (Hyland 2000). Hedges play an important role in gaining ratification for claims from a powerful peer group by allowing writers to present statements with appropriate accuracy, caution, and humility. They rather express possibility and prudence than certainty and overconfidence (Warta 2006).

Another discoursive feature of medical writing is the progressive moderation of the author's own voice; the focus is placed on facts. To some extent, the pronoun 'I' is replaced by 'we', neither because of involving the reader, nor because of co-authorship. It could rather be linked to the "progressive phasing out of authorial identity in scientific prose" (Gunnarson 2006: 714).

Medical language is traditionally regarded as the language used by medical experts when communicating in an expert-to-expert context. It is the language of the 'specialist', a special language as opposed to general language used by the general public. Medical terminology evolves due to the need for physicians in a field to communicate with precision and brevity, but this often has the (usually) undesired effect of excluding those who are unfamiliar with the particular specialized language of the group. This can cause difficulties when, for example, patients are unable to follow the discussions of physicians, and, thus, cannot understand information about their own condition and treatment.

2.3.1. English as a lingua franca of medicine

At present, English is the most widespread lingua franca of the western world used in sciences, and among them in medicine. Different sciences use English to various degrees, but English is considered to be the only language of wider communication within medicine and mathematics[26] (Medgyes and Kaplan 1992; Ammon 1994). As Ammon and Hellinger point out, "English has become so dominant as the international language of science, especially of scientific publications, that its use seems to be necessary if one wants to be read or discussed outside of one's own country" (1992: viii). This dominance, however, has developed only in the past 50 years.

Five periods can be distinguished in the history of the language of medicine in Europe (Fehér 1997). Medical historians write that in Ancient Times, around 500 B.C., it was the Old Greek language that dominated medical science. This role was partly overtaken by Latin in approximately 100 B.C., as the Roman Empire was gradually rising; however, the Hellenistic influence was still very decisive among physicians, and the Greek language also kept its leading role in medical sciences (Dirckx 1983).

In the Middle Ages there was no single lingua franca in medicine as at least three languages were widely used. In the Byzantine Empire, Greek had its leading position as the language of medicine, but in the Islamic world, where medical sciences were also very developed, the Arabic language was predominant. In Western Europe Latin was established in every scientific field, especially in the 11th century. Several medical works were translated from Greek and Arabic into Latin in that era (Maher 1986).

During the Renaissance, Europe had a major role in the field of medical sciences, thus Latin was used almost exclusively as the language of medicine. In Medical Renaissance (Wear et al. 2009), the period around 1400 to 1750, there was a major progress in medical knowledge and a renewed interest in the ancient ideas of the Greeks and Romans, and most significant medical observations were recorded in Latin, which was the language of university teaching at the time. There were, however, some exceptions, e.g. Paracelsus and Paré taught and published most of their works in German (Fehér 1997: 2685). Medical texts were first translated into national/vernacular European languages in the 14th and 15th centuries (Crossgrove et al. 1998), but Latin retained its firm position as the European language of science. Latin, as the language of printed scientific books until the middle of the 17th century, has left its mark on European scientific discourse. The prestige of Latin, as the language of a dominant culture, can be seen in the adoption and integration of borrowings and switches to Latin on the part of academic authors. The vernacularisation process, which began in the last quarter of the 14th century (Taavitsainen 1994a, 2001), did not undermine completely the use of Latin in scientific writings. The gradual loss of classical patterns and the influence of classical culture can be observed in the adoption of

26 Although, the Russian language used to be the dominant language of mathematics and also other sciences for decades in Hungary and Eastern Europe before the political changes in the 1990s.

Latin expressions, and in the alternating use of both languages. Borrowing from and code-switching to Latin occurs frequently in scientific scholarship even after the 15th century. Latin remained a prerequisite for medical education in most countries of Europe, and to this day the majority of scientific terms are still based on Old-Greek or Latin.

As a consequence of the spreading of French in the 17th century, first in France and then in the whole Europe, Latin was forced to a second place in the medical literature, and French emerged as the language of sciences. The French language became the primary language not only in medicine but in each field of sciences and culture. After the French Revolution, the French language was mostly used by the medical community in Europe, sharing its prominence with German (Navarro 1996).

This role was overtaken by German and English in the 19th century, when journal publication in medicine started to play a part in nationalizing medical communication (Taavitsainen 2006: 644). In the latter part of the 19th century and the early part of the 20th century, the Bismarck era, French remained the language of diplomacy, but German became the dominant language of science. German deserves special attention because it is the immediate predecessor of English as the language of science. At the beginning of the 20th century, German was clearly the language of science, and even US academic surgeons regularly took periods of their education in the great surgical clinics of Europe partially as part of the quest of a working knowledge of German (Benfield and Howard 2000).

At the beginning of the twentieth century, German played the most important role, with a slight temporary setback around World War I, and an abrupt disappearance after World War II (Vandenbroucke 1989: 1462). The 'victory' of the English language in medicine over all other languages (and not only in Europe but worldwide) started during World War II.

After World War II, when political and economic strength was centered in the English speaking nations, English became the language of medicine. The continuing growth of the use of English in medicine is shown in Table 5.

Table 5. Languages used in medical publications cited in Medline[27] *(based on Ammon 1998:152).*

	1980 (%)	1990 (%)	1996 (%)
English	72.2	79.5	88.6
German	5.8	3.9	2.2
Japanese	2.8	2.6	1.8
Spanish	1.3	1.5	1.2

Since much of the science and technology research in the 1950s and 1960s was conducted in English, most of the information was written in English. Swales (1990: 10) claims that:

"the fact that English now occupies an overwhelmingly predominant role in the international world of scholarship and research [...] entails that the coming generation of the world's researchers and scholars need [...] to have more than adequate professional skill in the English language if that generation is to make its way without linguistic disadvantage in its chosen world."

English prevails in medical research writing (cf. Table 6) to an extent that researchers have even noticed register narrowing due to the lack or scarcity of medical writing in national languages (Gunnarson and Backlund 1995).

The International Federation (for Information and) on Documentation (FID) reports that nearly 85% of all the scientific and technological information in the world today is written and/or abstracted in English (Ammon 2001), thus, it has become necessary for the members of the medical community to be able to search scientific literature in English. Researchers must be able to express themselves in this language if they want to be fully accepted members of the international academic community. This has become more and more important over recent years as the pressure to produce work in English and publish internationally has increased. Within academia it has been said that one has to "publish in English or perish" (Bakewell 1992; Viereck 1996). Weinreich highlights that the English language is used as a convenient strategy for coping with an ever-increasing amount of information: everything that is not in English is simply disregarded (1988).

27 Medline, the U.S. National Library of Medicine's bibliographic database, consists of more than 11 million articles from over 4,800 indexed titles.

Table 6. Selected journals that changed from native tongue to English (Benfield and Howard 2000: 645).

Current name	**Same original name**	**When**
The Thoracic and Cardiovascular Surgeon	No	1978
Journal of Experimental Animal Science	No	1991
Annals of Thoracic and Cardiovascular surgery	No	1995
Journal of Cancer Research and Clinical Oncology	No	1997

Publications in major international medical journals are considered more valuable, and these medical journals are almost all in English; in addition, most medical journals published in English refuse to accept contributions in another language (Treanor 1999). In 1995, for example, English was the language of over 95% of publications in the *Science Citation Index*; the remaining percentage was made up of French, German, Russian, and – at about 0.5–0.7% – all other languages (van Leeuwen et al. 2001), and this trend reoccurs in the medical science (Egger et al. 1997). One of the dangers of the increasing use of English in medicine is that it widens the gap between physicians, other health workers and patients: in the worst scenario, physicians will not be able to talk about their subject in their native language (Csedő 2005). This would effectively lead to a breakdown in the communication between medical experts and the public at large, and also physicians working in primary health care still definitely need medical literature to be available in their native language (Fehér 1997).

English is the international language used in both written and oral communication between health professionals involved in research, and it is the language used even at national meetings (Gunnarsson 2001). The following examples are taken from the field of cardiology to describe the recent situation. Both at the European Society of Cardiologists Conference, 2007, (that is, the annual gathering of cardiologists) and at the 27th European Stroke Conference, 2008, English was the only conference language. While English is officially prescribed as the official language at the latter conference (European Stroke Conference 2008 Final Congress Programme, General Information) this is not the case at the European Society of Cardiologists Conference, 2007. At the latter, the dominant position of English seems to be taken for granted, though both conferences took place in officially non-English speaking countries (Vienna, Austria, and Nice, France, respectively).

The use of English as an international language of medicine is described by many scholars. English may be seen as a neutral lingua franca, or it may be seen as a dominating powerful language (Tardy 2004). English may even be seen acting as something of a Tyrannosaurus rex, "a powerful carnivore gobbling up the other denizens of the academic linguistic grazing grounds" (Swales 1997: 374). After a lifetime of work on scientific English, Swales (1997) is so concerned about other languages of scholarship being on the way to extinction that he labels English a *lingua tyrannosaura.* The widespread concern in political and academic circles in Scandinavian countries with domain loss signifies a perception that segments of the national language are at risk from the English monster, hence the national policy to ensure that Danish, Norwegian and Swedish remain fully operational in all domains (Phillipson 2008).

Domains are not 'lost' but are subject to linguistic capital accumulation, and the forces behind an increased use of English may marginalize other languages (Phillipson 2008). This is a gradual, long-term process, and generally unnoticeable, but sometimes the underlying agenda can be seen in operation. Thus, language policies connected to the Bologna process or the creation of a single European higher education and research area are largely concealed, but policy statements imply that 'internationalization' means "English-medium higher education" (Phillipson 2006: 14).

Therefore, non-English speaking physicians, researchers and practicing doctors have no other option but to learn English if they want to be informed of the latest developments in their fields (Alcaraz and Navarro 2006). The trend to use one lingua franca, English, leads to the use of technical terms in English even in daily non-English language conversations of medical experts. Anglicisms are not only present at the lexico-semantic level, they also affect semantic and syntactic levels, but examples of ortho-/typographic changes and new rhetorical patterns can also be identified in the first language of physicians (Salager-Meyer et al. 2003; Alcaraz and Navarro 2006; Keresztes 2006b).

Nevertheless, the former lingua franca of medicine, Latin, has still kept its position in hospital communication between medical doctors and also in written documents: the diagnoses and the anatomical terminology are in Latin, and the rest of the medical report is in the national language. A new feature of the medical language, however, is the appearance of the use of English initialisms[28] and words (e.g. the signs and symptoms) in these documents instead of national language ones (Keresztes 2003; Taavitsainen 2006).

English-speaking nations form a virtual cartel over scientific information (Nylenna et al. 1994), systems organized according to an English-based sociology of knowledge. In non-English speaking countries, scientific

---

28 Initialism is the word in this dissertatation used as a collective term for abbreviations and acronyms. For details see Section 5.1.2.4.

manuscripts submitted in the national language of the country are commonly considered inferior to English-language manuscripts of the same scientific quality (Vandenbroucke 1989). An English version of a manuscript is considered more acceptable than a national language version of the same manuscript (Nylenna et al. 1994). In several non-English speaking countries, publishing in the native tongue has become a handicap to physicians with academic ambitions (Bakewell 1992). On-going discussion shows criticism toward the increasing use of English. It is thought that domain loss is dividing people into two groups: the highly educated and the less educated (Taavitsainen and Pahta 2003). It is clear that the well-educated group knows English well, since English is used in academic studies. This has brought pressure for scholars to write in their native tongue, and, thus, make their thoughts clear also to non-academic audiences which do not have a good command of English, and thus, are deprived of information on health and medicine. It is also a subject of debate whether the change from English as a foreign language to English as a second language is really a step forward (Taavitsainen and Pahta 2003).

Globalization brings on a challenge of preserving national identity. In certain communities, where the use of the national language of minorities is endangered, not by the globalization of English but by the dominance of the official language of the country, the minority language is better preserved even in the field of sciences and medicine (Keresztes 2006a). English in this context functions more like a second or additional language than a foreign language.

Davis (1995, 2006) points out that some countries (such as the UK) have instituted policies about language use and interactions, for example, in the care of the elderly, although such awareness is not widespread. This is crucial, however, because caregivers often engage in 'ghosting' – speaking over the person's head as if they were absent – an interactional phenomenon that is linguistically dehumanizing and debilitating (Ramanathan 2009).

2.3.2. The English language in Medical Hungarian

Medicine is one of the fields which is most affected by the influence of the English language (Kontra 1981; Keresztes 2003). During the 1980s there was a clear opening toward the west in Hungary, which led to an unprecedented boom in the adoption of English words in almost all areas of life, including the field of medicine. The result of the English influence is that Hungarian borrows English loans, adapts them as Anglicisms, and subsequently integrates them into the (medical) vocabulary (Keresztes 2007b).

In the past 50 years, the use of the English language has become predominant in European medicine, and, following this trend, in the last 15–20 years it has become the leading language used by Hungarian physicians as well. At present young medical researchers make fewer grammatical and spelling mistakes in their acquired English than in their native Hungarian. Moreover, a language barrier is created between upper class medical science and lower class medical practice. It is a situation that not only do physicians seem unwilling to change, but one that they actively encourage in the more prestigious section of academia. Nevertheless, doctors working in primary health care and other health workers still definitely need medical literature to be available in Hungarian. However, scientific and technical journals in countries like Sweden and Hungary publish more material in English than they do in their national languages (Gunnarson 2001; Bősze 2004).

In 2004, a new Hungarian journal was launched, Magyar Orvosi Nyelv (Hungarian Language of Medicine). The main aim of the editors is to show the present situation of this specific language, which is 'very dim' according to them, and to purge this language as far as possible mainly of the English effects (Buda 2002; Grétsy 2004; Bősze and Palkovics 2006). They consider most English contact-induced features phenomena to be avoided, and they want to preserve the purity of the Hungarian medical language by giving guidance to medical writers, and spreading newly formed or long forgotten Hungarian terms instead of the 'intruding' English ones.

Recent sociolinguistic studies of the Hungarian language of the medical register are few in number yet (but cf. Gönye 1999; Cselnovszkyné Tarr 1999; Demeter 2005; Keresztes 2007a; Mészáros 2009).

2.3.3. International scientific vocabulary

International scientific vocabulary (ISV) comprises scientific and specialized words whose language of origin may or may not be certain, but which are in current use in several modern languages. The name 'International Scientific Vocabulary' was first used by Philip Gove in Webster's Third New International Dictionary (WTNI) in 1961. According to WTNI most ISV words have been created by taking a word with a rather general meaning from Latin or Old Greek, and conferring upon it a very specific meaning for the purposes of modern scientific discourse. ISV words are typically compound words, and their morphology may vary across languages. Each language pronounces the resulting neo-lexemes within its own phonemic rules, and makes morphological connections using its regular morphological system. McArthur (1998) characterizes ISV words and morphemes as 'translinguistic', as they can operate in many languages that serve as mediums for education, culture, science, and technology. According to McArthur, no other set of words and morphemes is so international.

Medical terminology rests on a fundamentally Latin nomenclature with roots, prefixes and suffixes drawn from Greek and Latin (Dirckx 1983). Most twentieth century additions to the language of medicine are English words built of Latin stems and affixes. New taxonomic coinages, however, are Latin in form even when, as is usual, they are Greek in origin. New names for diseases, e.g. skin diseases are also frequently Latin phrases, in continuation of a pattern established centuries ago. The English language had been receiving slow but steady influx of words from Greek, often via Latin. Some medical terms that look like English (E) words are in fact corruptions of Greek (G) words, cf. E *dropsy* from G *hydrops,* E *palsy* from G *paralysis,* E *pleurisy* from G *pleuritis* going via both Latin and French.

The role of Latin as the lingua franca of Western scholars in the post-Renaissance world was a main reason why the terminologies of the emerging natural sciences consisted chiefly of Latin and Latinized Greek words. But there was a second and not less convincing reason: Latin was a dead language, thus hardly more subject to alteration. Latin afforded a vast fund of words to which specific technical meanings might be arbitrarily assigned without danger of conflict or confusion with vernacular or idiomatic use. Latin and Greek provided a large stock of root words and affixes from which the scientists could coin new terms that, if not altogether self-explanatory, were at least readily understood and remembered by the members of the international scientific discourse community.

New words are built up from existing lexical elements usually by two processes, affixation and compounding. Affixation refers to the attachment of a prefix or suffix to a word root or stem. Compounding is the joining of two or more words or stems, as in pyosalpinx and erythrocyte. In ISV a prefix usually modifies the meaning of the word to which it is attached, and suffix usually changes the grammatical category or function of the word. Thus, the prefixes *a-, non-, un-* generally negate or reverse the idea contained in the word root or stem: *asystole, nonsteroid, unsaturated.*

2.4. Genres in Medicine

Kress highlights that "genres are [...] crucial indicators of the regulation of the domains of public and private in particular instances. [...] Generic forms encode socially and culturally given modes of interrelation and interaction in specific social occasions" (1986: 414).

Variation within modern genres of the professional language is described by Swales (1990) and Bhatia (1993); and assessments of diachronic variation are dealt with by Taavitsainen (1994a, 1994b) and especially in the field of medicine, by Rébék-Nagy (1997). Swales (1981, 1985) defines genre as "a recognizable communicative event characterized by a set of communicative purpose(s) identified and mutually understood by the members of the professional or academic community in which it regularly occurs". Thus, genres do not belong to individuals but are the properties of discourse communities. These discourse communities are "socio-rhetorical networks that form in order to work toward sets of common goals ... [they have] familiarity with the particular genres that are used in the communicative furtherance of those sets of goals" (Swales 1990: 34). Institutional context (including system and methodology) in which the given genre is used and also in which it has a dominant role, and conventions of that institutional setting should be considered when analyzing professional genres (Bhatia 1993).

Corpus-based studies have shown that genres of writing may be very heterogeneous in their linguistic features and that there is variation even within a narrowly defined genre. Bazerman and Paradis (1991) affirm that medical discourse evolves and emerges in relation to scientific practices. Written texts within professions give us insight into how the professions constitute themselves and carry out their work through texts (Bazerman 1998). Professional writing can also be seen as negotiation between text participants, and the social nature of this communication is emphasized in it (Myers 1990; Gunnarsson et al. 1997). Internationalization is an increasingly important factor in medical writing, and the position of English as the lingua franca of medicine has an influence on the writing conventions of medical texts today.

The concept of genre is a key term in medical communication, as all medical communicative events can be classified into specific written or spoken genres (Pique-Angordans and Posteguillo 2006). Editorials, research articles, abstracts, case reports, presentation papers or posters can be found in many other academic disciplines, however, each of them develops a set of peculiarities characteristic of the medical profession alone. Genres change according to changes in sociocultural needs, new genres are created and older ones may cease to exist.

Medical writing is a general label with a great deal of variation across several genres, such as the research article, the experimental article, the review article, the case report, and the handbooks. Some genres of scientific and medical writing have so far received detailed attention, for example, studies of the medical research article, the epistolary article, and the experimental report are discussed by Atkinson (1992, 1996) and Rébék–Nagy (1997), and the experimental article by Bazerman (1988). The most important genres for practising physicians, the patient case notes, the hospital discharge summaries, referral and consultation letters, have not yet been extensively researched (van Naerssen 1985; Yanoff 1988; Warta 2006; Ramanathan 2009).

2.4.1. Physician–patient communication

Sociolinguistics, the study of language differences, varieties and of ways as to how these can be interpreted, has devoted special attention to health professional–patient communication, "where differences in modes of talking, values and knowledge feed into institutional asymmetries" (Roberts 2006: 743). West (1984) explores asymmetrical power relations, while Fisher and Todd (1983) describe the decision-making process and the discursive representation of health and illness. Wodak (1997) examines the institutional order and how it is reflected in routine encounters between patients and health professionals. More thematic discourse studies have been published in the field recently with the publication of a new journal, *Communication and Medicine* (first issue in 2004) edited by Sarangi.

The 'inner life' of doctors (Meier et al. 2001) has an essential role in effective physician–patient interaction: "studies suggested that physicians respond to the patient's expression of needs and emotion during the visit with emotions of their own" (Vegni et al. 2005: 70). However, only few studies have explored this issue from a doctor's perspective. In particular, the difficulties that the physician may experience in a relationship with the patient seem to be an issue that is still understudied (Lowe et al. 1998; Vegni et al. 2001, 2004, 2005). On the other hand, 'voices' of the patient were studied by Cordella (2004), and the multilingual aspects of physician–patient communication from the aspect of the latter participant were discussed by Roberts (2006).

Several theoretical perspectives fostered the early studies of physician–patient communication, and from a sociological perspective, the concept of 'power' was a central issue. The 'medical model' elaborated on by Parsons

(1951, 1958, 1978), and Freidson (1961, 1970, 1975, 1986) defines a hierarchical relationship between doctor and patient. Ten Have (2001) identifies two trends in medical interaction research: one that focuses on physicians' behaviors in the course of performing particular professional communication strategies, and the other focusing on the medical encounter as an activity type or genre. Power, however, remains a significant theme within this tradition.

Psychoanalysis and psychotherapy offer a different point of view. Concepts like therapeutic transference and counter-transference inspired Balint (1957) in his work with small groups of general practitioners. His aim was to make doctors aware of how the complex interaction between them and their patients can be built up over a life-time partnership. Rogers (1957) and his ideas of a therapeutic relationship based on unconditional positive regard required attention for such concepts as empathy and interest, and focused on the importance of non-verbal behavior. These theoretical approaches, formulated between 1940 and 1970, provide the foundations for the purposes of communication in health care as distinguished by Ong et al. (1995), creating a good personal relationship, exchanging information, and making treatment decisions.

Pendleton and Hasler published a collection of 16 papers in 1983 on doctor–patient communication, highlighting various aspects of the consultation with the physician, the behavior of doctors, doctor–patient relationship, medical practice and medical education. Communication between doctors and patients is attracting attention not only in the field of linguistics but within health care studies as well. During the past two decades, descriptive and experimental research has tried to shed light on this communication process. The doctor–patient relation is one of the most complex relations (Figure 7) as it involves interaction between individuals in non-equal positions; however, the issues it involves are of vital importance and require close cooperation (Chaitchik et al. 1992).

From a medical point of view, doctors need information to establish the right diagnosis and treatment plan, whereas from the patient's point of view, two requirements have to be met: the requirement of knowing and understanding, and the requirement of feeling known and understood (Ong 1995). Two types of interaction analysis systems can be identified: 'cure' systems which are meant to capture the instrumental (task focused) behavior, and 'care' systems which are meant to measure affective (socio-emotional) behavior (Sensing 1991). These two types of systems reflect patients' need for cure and care when visiting a doctor: the need to know and understand (cure) and the need to feel known and understood (care). Traditionally, the ideal doctor–patient relationship was paternalistic: the doctor directed care and made decisions about treatment on their own, but during the last two or three decades, this approach has been replaced by the idea of 'shared decision-making' (Beisecker and Beisecker 1990; Brock and Wartman 1990; Chaitchik et al. 1992).

Background variables →	***Actual content of communication*** →	***Patient outcomes***
- culture - doctor–patient relationship - types of patients and doctors - disease characteristics	communicative behaviors: - instrumental behaviors - affective behaviors	short-term and intermediate, e.g.: - satisfaction - compliance - recall and understanding of information long-term, e.g.: - health status - psychiatric morbidity

Figure 7. Theoretical framework of doctor–patient communication (based on Ong et al. 1995: 914).

Despite the substantial body of research describing doctor–patient communication which has accumulated over the past 25 years, relatively little attention has been devoted to the vocabulary adapted during medical consultations. Vocabulary can be seen as an "ingredient" of the communication process, active during all doctor–patient interactions. Physicians can speak their national/vernacular language, but they also speak the medical language, which is mainly influenced by the English language worldwide (Ong 1995). Patients are typically unfamiliar with this medical language (Bourhis et al. 1989), thus, it can be expected that physicians should switch from the medical language to the vernacular language when communicating with their patients. On the other hand, patients may have some basic understanding of the medical language, and might attempt to use it for the sake of communicative effectiveness. When discussing medical issues with their patients, it may be difficult for physicians to clearly differentiate between the two vocabularies (Hadlow and Pitts 1991).

Research on the interactional process of the consultation has been dominated recently by Conversation Analysis. One of the first sociologists to look closely at physician–patient communication was Cicourel (1983), who examined participants' inferential process, and miscommunication between physicians and patients. Other ethnographic studies looking at patterns of medical discourse were prepared by Silverman (1987) and Atkinson (1996), who referred to communication between doctors and other health professionals as being 'backstage talk' when clinical knowledge is reproduced. Much of the literature on medical discourse confines itself to physician–patient interaction in biomedical settings and proposes improvements in communication to biomedical models of the doctor–patient encounter, such as the 'biopsychosocial' approach (Cooper et al. 2003, Demeter 2005). The discoursive events involving physicians interacting with other health worker are discussed through research into grand rounds (Martin 1992; Atkinson 1999), team meetings of occupational therapists (Mattingly 1998) and public health campaigns (Pigg 1996). The issues of medical authority and power from the perspective of conversation analysis are also addressed and "the ways in which local medical interactions reflect the global circulation of discourse forms" (Wilce 2009: 205).

Women's language in medical interviews has been studied by Bonnano (1982, 1995): hedges, euphemisms, vagueness, tag questions and intensifying expressions were described, stressing the extent to which the sex variable in linguistic behavior was causing "a serious communication barrier between physicians and their patients" (1982: 28).

Medical encounters in general were researched by Byrne and Long (1976), ten Have (1989) and Aldrich (1999), examining the structure of routine medical encounters and associating the phases of these encounters with particular interactional sequences. Specialty and subspecialty medical encounters reflecting the complex and ongoing context of specialty care are dealt with by Barton (2000, 2006).

Freidson (1970) challenged the basic assumptions of the Parsonian model of the physician's behavior, that is, its normative basis from a sociological point of view. For Freidson and the approaches that were to follow, the assumption was that the medical profession's power was based on its appeal to its service orientation and scientific expertise that legitimated its mandate and autonomy. Yet the profession was also seen as "a group acting to preserve and confirm this position" (Riska 2001: 146).

The intense phase of research on the American medical profession that followed between 1975 and 1985 may be related to the dramatic change of the American health care system that began during those years. There were two main trends in this research: one approach focused on the extraordinary power that the medical profession had acquired in the American health care system, whereas the other trend projected the end of this power "as a sign of a structural change of American health care characterized by a bureaucratic and consumer challenging structure" (Riska 2001: 147).

British research on health professions and occupations has been less physician–centered than the American research, and has presented a broad view of the division of labor between various health professions, which even included the lay carers as health workers (Abbot and Wallace 1990).

2.4.2. The hospital discharge report[29]

The hospital discharge summary is a standardized genre which has been crystallized as a particular textual construct across various types of organizations. It is a complex genre and the combination of narrative fragments: the 'story' describing what happened to the patient, the medical steps taken, the outcome of these steps and the follow-up (Iedema 2006).

A complete medical record must be kept on every patient. This medical record is a permanent document: it gives a complete history of all that is done for the patients during their hospital stay. Medical records contain both subjective and objective information about the patient's condition, plan for treatment and follow-up. Subjective information is gained from the patient and family members, whereas objective information is obtained from physical examinations and laboratory records (van Naerssen 1985).

The discharge report is a concise summary of hospitalization, written for the primary care provider who will follow the patients after their hospital stay, or for the admitting doctor at next hospitalization. Discharge reports presuppose knowledgeable and entitled readers, "the possibility of understanding is based on a shared, practical and entitled understanding of common tasks between writer and reader" (Garfinkel 1967: 201).

The origin of this genre goes back to the medieval period when the core of medical instruction was based on typical cases of disease, and the genres connected with them were the 'consilia' and the 'practica', whereas 'consilium' was a piece of advice on a particular case offering diagnosis and therapy (French 2003). These Latin medical texts provided the model for the vernacular versions. The discourse of discharge summaries was investigated and described by Cicourel (1974), West (1984) and van Naerssen (1985).

Historically, the discharge summary was used mainly for documentation of acute hospital care, and there was little need for information transfer because the same physician often provided inpatient and outpatient care. The advent of hospital physicians, however, has created a division of labor in the spectrum of patient care and inherent discontinuity between acute hospitalization and community management (Kripalani et al. 2007). In this new model of care, the discharge summary becomes a vital tool for communication and information transfer.

Internationalization is an increasingly important factor in scientific writing, including the hospital discharge summary, and the position of English as the

29 In some medical contexts it is referred to as the "hospital discharge summary" or "final report".

lingua franca in medicine has an influence on the writing conventions of these medical texts as well (Taavitsainen and Pahta 2000).

Most hospitals produce dictated discharge summaries. These documents are considered important in the follow-up care of hospitalized patients and in planning diagnostic and therapeutic interventions for readmitted patients. Ideally, the quality of a discharge summary should be measured by its influence on subsequent patient care. Such a measure should include concepts of the extent and timeliness with which the summary is disseminated (Sackley and Pound 2002).

Discharge summaries serve many purposes, the most important of which is the communication of the information between consultants based in hospitals and family physicians based in the community. High-quality discharge summaries are necessary for the continuity of patient care. Despite their importance, their quality is sometimes shown to be suboptimal with deficiencies in summary content, accuracy, timeliness or use of language (Rao et al. 2005).

2.5. Patients' rights[30]

Patients' rights are a reflection of human rights. The human right movement has gathered importance in the world since 1945, when, in the Charter of the United Nations, member states reaffirmed their faith in fundamental human rights. This was followed in 1948 by the adoption of the Universal Declaration of Human Rights and in 1950 by the signature of the European Convention of Human Rights. The rights of the patients, as specific human rights have become recognized throughout the European region only in the past two decades (Carmi 2002). This has triggered off a positive international trend in the consideration, definition and promotion of patients' rights and led to the development of a movement in Europe to ensure the rights of patients (Leenen et al. 1993).

Until the beginning of 1970s the health professional–patient relationship was primarily defined by the rules of medical ethics. In the following two decades the focus was shifted to legal provisions and the issue started attracting greater international attention.

The first international event with such focus was the European Consultation on the Rights of Patients convened under the auspices of the WHO Regional Office for Europe and hosted by the Government of the Netherlands in 1994. It had a very deliberate purpose – to define principles and strategies for promoting the rights of patients, within the context of the health care reform process

30 Some important documents on WHO and Hungarian patients' rights are given in Appendices 11 and 12.

underway in most countries. The Consultation came at the end of a long preparatory process during which WHO/EURO encouraged the emerging movement in favor of patient's rights by carrying studies and surveys on the development of patients' rights throughout Europe.

The Consultation also formulated for the first time the Principles of patients' rights and presented them in a comprehensive document to help the countries develop comprehensive policies. The following principles were adopted (cf. website http://conventions.coe.int):

- the right to respect as a human being,
- the right to self-determination,
- the right to physical and mental integrity and security,
- the right to respect for privacy,
- the right to respect on moral, cultural and religious values, and
- the right to such protection of health as is afforded by appropriate measures for disease prevention and health care and to the opportunity to pursue the highest attainable level of health.

The document also contains information about health services and how to use them best. The following recommendations are described (cf. website http://conventions.coe.int):

- patients should be informed about their health status, including the medical facts about their condition; about the proposed medical procedures together with the potential risks and benefits of each procedure; about alternatives to the proposed treatment, including the effect of non-treatment; diagnosis, prognosis and progress of treatment;
- information may only be withheld from the patient when there is good reason to believe that this information would cause serious harm;
- information must be communicated to the patient in a way appropriate to his capacity for understanding, minimizing the use of unfamiliar technical terminology;
- patients have the right not to be informed, at their explicit request;
- patients have the right to choose who, if anyone, should be informed on their behalf;
- patients should have the possibility of obtaining a second medical opinion;
- when admitted to a health care establishment patients should be informed of the identity and professional status of the health care

provider taking care of them and of any rules and routines which refer to their stay and care; and

- patients should be able to request and be given a written summary of their diagnosis, treatment and care on discharge from a health care establishment.

An important aspect of the European challenge is how to develop health care systems based on values enclosed in the European Convention on Human Rights and the European Social Charter. Present ongoing reforms in health care are mostly motivated by escalating health costs and increasing demands of the population. The question is how reforms of health care systems should ensure equitable access to health care, which is both adequate and of optimal quality (WHO 2007).

Finland was the first country in the world to establish a special patients' rights law in 1992. The law was preceded by 20 years of discussions in the Finnish Parliament. The law is 'administrative', i.e. it contains directives, which define the provider's duties instead of rights which patients can demand. The second country to present patients' rights law was the Netherlands. This was part of a more comprehensive law reform, the Medical Contract Law, presented in 1995. Since Finland and the Netherlands have shown the way, a few other countries have introduced similar legislation – Israel (1996), Lithuania (1996), Iceland (1997) Hungary (1997) and Denmark (1998). Several other countries in Europe and worldwide have presented patients' rights laws since then. Other countries have chosen to seek different methods to strengthen the patient's position. France introduced a Patient Charter in 1974 and Great Britain in 1991. These Charters contain recommended minimum standards.

The 17th World Congress on Medical Law was held in Beijing in 2008[31], discussed the most pressing ethical issues for the 21st century: legislation on patients' rights and how to implement it, teaching of medical ethics and law, ethics committees, status and rights of patients. The good health of a population is a pre-requisite to the social well-being and economic functioning of a nation. Health promotion and health care are important social goods, raising fundamental questions about social obligations and goals and the protection of human rights as essential for promoting health (Carmi 2002).

31 The 18th World Congress on Medical Law is held in Zagreb August 2010.

2.6. Cardiology

Cardiology is a subspecialty (fellowship[32]) of Internal Medicine. Internal medicine is a special branch of conventional medicine that treats diseases of the internal organs of the body. Qualifications needed to be satisfied to become a doctor of internal medicine include a basic medical degree, internist training, and three or more years of study and practice in an internal medicine specialty. Specialties in internal medicine (in the UK) include allergy, cardiology, endocrinology, gastroenterology, genetics, geriatrics, hematology, immunology, infectious diseases, metabolism, molecular medicine, nephrology, neurology, oncology, pulmonology, and rheumatology.

Cardiology is the branch of medicine concerned with the heart and blood vessels, known as the cardiovascular system. It encompasses a wide variety of disorders related to different parts of the heart and the vascular system. A physician who specializes in cardiology is called a cardiologist. In the Western world, cardiology is an ever-growing field within internal medicine. Extensive studies have identified risk factors for heart diseases, including diabetes mellitus and obesity. Both are on the increase within the general population and this will inevitably lead to increased incidence of heart diseases, even with growing public awareness of these health matters.

Cardiology is one of the most technologically sophisticated, professionalized, institutionalized, and highly invasive medical disciplines. Cardiologists are physicians who specialize in diagnosing and treating heart problems, such as chest pain, irregular heartbeats, high or low blood pressure and clogged arteries. They investigate patients with a suspected heart disease by taking a very careful, extensive history of the patient's condition, and performing a complete physical examination.

The first physician to describe the blood vessels was William Harvey, an English physician in 1628. A French anatomist, Raymond de Vieussens, first characterized the structure of the heart chambers and valves in 1706. These two key contributions allowed a major work, considered to be the true beginning of the field of cardiology, to be written. In 1749, Jean-Baptiste Sénac published *Traité de la structure du coeur, de son action, et de ses maladies* [Treated structure of the heart, of its action, and of its diseases]. The publication discussed the physiology and anatomy of the heart and even discusses some heart diseases that are still present today. When the stethoscope was invented in 1816 by René Laënnec, the art of auscultation, a key tool in the study of the heart, took off.

32 Fellowship is used for a specialty/subspecialty in the UK.

The milestones in Cardiology (Lozsádi and Czuriga 2009) are provided below:

1628 William Harvey, an English Physician, first described blood circulation.

1706 Raymond de Vieussens, a French anatomy professor, first described the structure of the heart's chambers and vessels.

1733 Stephen Hales, an English clergyman and scientist, first measured the blood pressure.

1816 René Laënnec, a French physician, invented the stethoscope.

1903 Willem Einthoven, a Dutch physiologist, developed the electrocardiograph.

1912 James B. Herrick, an American physician, first described heart disease resulting from hardening of the arteries.

1938 Robert E. Gross, an American surgeon, performed the first heart surgery.

1951 Charles Hufnagel, an American surgeon, developed a plastic valve to repair an aortic valve.

1952 F. John Lewis, an American surgeon, performed the first successful open heart surgery.

1953 John H. Gibbon, an American surgeon, first used a mechanical heart and blood purifier.

1961 James R. Jude, an American cardiologist, led a team performing the first external cardiac massage to restart a heart.

1965 Michael DeBakey and Adrian Kantrowitz, American surgeons, implant mechanical devices to help a diseased heart.

1967 Christiaan Barnard, a South African surgeon, performed the first whole heart transplant from one person to another.

1982 Willem DeVries, an American surgeon, implanted a permanent artificial heart, designed by Robert Jarvik, an American physician, into a patient.

2006 Various trials began looking at injecting stem cells into hearts damaged following myocardial infarction (heart attack) to see whether they can repair the damage.

The American College of Chest Physicians (ACCP) is the world's largest clinical cardiopulmonary and critical care medical society with more than 17,000 members in 100 countries. Members include physicians, allied health professionals, and PhDs from the specialties of pulmonology, critical care medicine, thoracic surgery, cardiology, sleep, and other chest-related specialties. Founded in 1935, the ACCP works to promote the prevention and treatment of diseases of the chest through leadership, education, research, and communication.

The American Society of Hypertension (ASH) is the largest US organization dedicated exclusively to hypertension and related cardiovascular disease. The ASH was founded in 1985 as a Society dedicated to clinical and basic research, and education in hypertension, related cardiovascular disease and vascular health. The mission of the Society became 'to organize and conduct educational activities designed to promote and encourage the development, advancement, and exchange of scientific information in all aspects of research, diagnosis, and treatment of hypertension, and related cardiovascular diseases' (cf. website www.ash-us.org).

The history of institutionalized cardiology in Hungary started at the end of the 1940s (Lozsádi and Czuriga 2009), when Imre Zárday endeavored to form the Scientific Society of Cardiology. At the Capital City Consulting Room for Heart Examination, along with Sándor Pelczner and Gyula Szutrély, he organized 'non-official' extension courses which were the basis for the 'new society' founded in 1955 and which started its work under the name of Specialized Cardiological Group of the Medical Division of the Union of Medical Workers (cf. website www.mkardio.hu).

Cardiology was the main subject of the 1963 Congress of Hungarian Internal Specialists organized by the members of the National Institute of Cardiology and those of the specialized group, and chaired by György Gottsegen. This was for the first time after the war that there was an international participation at such a congress.

The Federation of Hungarian Medical Societies (MOTESZ) was set up in the mid-1960s, and in 1966 the Hungarian Society of Cardiology was formed within its framework from the former specialized group (cf. website www.motesz.hu). In the 1990s, the Hungarian Society of Cardiology had already been a well-known scientific society with broad-scale international relations and an active membership of over 1,000 physicians.

The amount of research carried out in the field of cardiology is great, and papers are published in 17 prestigious, cardiology related journals mostly of American and British publishers (e.g. *American Heart Journal, British Journal of Cardiology, European Heart Journal*).

Research results of Hungarian cardiologists can be published in *Cardiologia Hungarica*, the scientific quarterly of the Hungarian Society of Cardiology, both in Hungarian and in English (cf. website www.mkardio.hu/ch). The journal was established in 1972 by Kálmán Ghyczy.

A comprehensive volume of 1,120 pages covering various field of cardiology was published in Hungarian in 2009, *Klinikai szív-elektrofiziológia és aritmológia* [Clinical cardioelectrophysiology and arrhythmology] gaining the

Medical Nivo Prize of the year 2009 from the Hungarian Academy of Sciences. The authors are all members of the University of Szeged, Tamás Fazekas, Gyula Papp, Miklós Csanády, Csaba Lengyel, László Rudas, László Sághy, Róbert Sepp and András Varró.

The number of linguistic studies in the field of Cardiology is low (Hansch and Fleck 2006; Benfield 2007). Further sociolinguistic research is needed to reveal and analyze the language of cardiology, the communicative behavior and language attitude of cardiologists and their patients.

2.7. Overview of methodology

In my research, I used two methods to describe the cardiological subregister of the Hungarian language of medicine, to reveal and analyze the English contact-induced features in this technical language, and to investigate the attitude of various discourse communities affected by it towards the English language. With Method 1, I examined Hungarian hospital discharge report written by cardiologists. English language contact-induced featured were identified in these reports, and the collected features were categorized and analyzed. With Method 2, semi-structured interviews were prepared with physicians and patients to gain information on their attitudes toward the English language as a lingua franca of medicine, and to detect the motives behind the borrowing phenomena identified with Method 1.

2.7.1. Attitude studies

Baker (1992: 10) states that "attitude is a hypothetical construct used to explain the direction and persistence of human behavior". If the definition of language attitude is taken in a broader sense, it can allow all kinds of behavior concerning language to be considered, e.g. attitudes towards language maintenance and planning efforts (Fasold 1984: 148). Attitudes are crucial in the status and importance of a language in the society and for the individual. The attitude is individual, but it has origins in collective behavior. Baker (1992) claims that attitudes are learned predispositions, not inherited, and are likely to be relatively stable. However, attitudes are affected by experience, thus, they can change during the life of the individual. In many discussions in social psychology, the concept of 'attitude' is defined as a tendency to react favorably or unfavorably to a class of objects (Foddy 1993; Edwards 1994). Language attitudes are complex constructs, as both positive and negative feelings can be attached to e.g. the same language situation (Baker 1988).

Studies of language attitudes have been following two theoretical approaches: the behaviorist approach and the mentalist approach. According to Fasold (1984: 147–148), under the behaviorist perspective attitudes are found in the responses people have to social situations. Under the mentalist perspective attitudes are viewed as an internal, mental state, which may give rise to certain forms of behavior. It can be described as "an intervening variable between a stimulus affecting a person and that person's response" (Fasold 1984:147; Appel and Muysken 1987: 16).

In the mentalist approach two methods are primarily employed for exploring language attitudes: the questionnaire/interview and the matched guise technique. One of the methodological debates regarding the study of language attitudes is based on the use of direct vs. indirect methodology (Cooper and Fishman 1974). Some studies, e.g. Gal (1979) employed the direct questioning method to investigate attitudes amongst inhabitants of Oberwart to their languages (German and Hungarian). Indirect methods for obtaining data about language attitudes have also been used by various researchers including Fishman (1971), who examined attitudes among Puerto Ricans.

Various surveys examine language attitudes focusing on individual attitudes toward majority and minority languages and bilingualism (e.g. Fenyvesi 1995a; Lanstyák and Szabómihály 1997; Kontra 2003; Péntek 2004; Bartha 2007; Kontra et al. 2010). Some studies on language attitudes focus on attitudes to second language learning. Perhaps the most influential of these studies is Gardner and Lambert (1959), which suggested that the motivation to learn and use a language is shaped by attitudes; and language attitudes toward the English language in non-English speaking countries have also been investigated by several scholars (e.g. Dürmüller 1989 in Switzerland, Ladegaard 2000 in Denmark, and Dörnyei 2001 in Hungary). The main dimensions along which views about languages can vary are social status and group solidarity. Another dimension, called in-group solidarity or language loyalty, reflects the social pressures to maintain languages/language varieties, even one without social prestige (Edwards 1982:20). Fasold suggests that attitudes towards a language are often the reflection of attitudes towards members of various ethnic groups (1984:148): people's reactions to language varieties reveal much of their perception of the speakers of these varieties (Edwards 1982:20).

When studying language attitudes, the concept of motives is important. The two basic motives in language attitude studies are the instrumental and integrative motives. Gardner and Lambert (1959) suggest that integrative motivation is most powerful, as the individual desires to be part of a group identity, and therefore they will make an effort to learn and use a language.

However, instrumental motivation (for employment, study or immigration) has also been acknowledged as equally important in the learning or maintenance of a language (Gardner and MacIntyre 1991; Baker 1993; McGroarty 1996).

In multilingual communities, the different motivations to learn each language would depend on the perceived usefulness of each, and the functions each fulfils for the individual and the society. Dörnyei (2006) provides data on the components of motivation in language learning in Hungary. Instrumental motivation is particularly important for Hungarian scientists and physicians who perceive English language study as the key to research, self-development and professional success. Baker (1993: 95) writes that language attitudes shape the amount of effort the individuals will make towards maintaining their own language and learning a second one.

The attitude towards Englishisms seems different from country to country: the history of the respective country plays a role, its connections with the Western world or with the United States, and also its size and its closeness of contacts (cf. Juaristi et al. 2008: 47–72). Warnings about future language death due to English influence may also be motivated by strong nationalist feelings in certain contexts. The borrowings arise from language contact causing various linguistic changes, which are accompanied by certain attitudes and state policies (Mesthrie 1995; Fischer 2008).

Over the past 50 years, a substantial amount of research on attitudes to language variation has emerged around the world and across the disciplines beginning with Lambert et al. (1960) and Labov (1966). The study of language attitudes frequently resides at the core of interaction analysis. Social scientists have approached this form of research from the perspective of both the listener and the speaker. While the findings have varied across variables of culture, dialect, accent, and context, scholars have argued that determining the effects of language on social judgment is an integral part of uncovering the communication process (Giles and Billings 2004).

Edwards (1982) points out that there are three broad possibilities for the underlying patterns of speech-style judgments: they may reflect intrinsic linguistic superiorities/inferiorities; intrinsic aesthetic differences; or social convention and preference. It is, however, sociolinguistically unpalatable for languages and language varieties to be reasonably described, as intrinsic linguistic superiorities/inferiorities suggest, as being 'better/worse', 'correct/incorrect', or 'logical/illogical'. Similarly, with intrinsic aesthetic differences, aesthetic judgments of language varieties do not in fact seem to be based on inherent qualities of beauty, "though they may be represented as such by members of speech communities" (Giles and Billings 2004: 191). Therefore, the evaluations of language varieties do not seem to reflect intrinsic linguistic or aesthetic qualities so much as the levels of status and prestige that they are conventionally associated with in particular speech communities.

Language attitude studies in the medical arena are not as frequent. Fielding and Evered showed that 'received pronunciation' speakers are more likely to be perceived as having psychosomatic symptoms than non-standard accented patients, even when they are voicing exactly the same complaints. Moreover, medical student listener-judges in this study perceived lexical and syntactic differences between two supposed patients they heard on audiotape, despite the fact that these features were in fact held constant. Patients' social class has been shown to affect "the frequency of communication difficulties experienced by doctors, with working-class patients being disadvantaged as a consequence" (Fielding and Evered 1980: 193).

Most research in occupational settings has related to employment interviews (cf. Hui and Yam 1987; Cargile and Bradac 2001). Hopper and Williams (1973) showed that speech characteristics (for Standard American, African-American, Mexican-American, and Southern white speakers) were relevant to employment decisions, but decreased in importance when the interviews were for lower status jobs. Language attitudes are sensitive to local conditions and changes in the sociopolitical milieu (cf. Baker 1992; Giles and Pierson 1988; Lippi-Green 1997).

Attitudes and motivation are significant in determining linguistic proficiency and achievement (Gardner 1985; Oxford and Shearin 1994; Oxford 1996; Dörnyei 2001, 2006) and can affect language acquisition favorably or unfavorably depending on the nature of the learner's experiences, family, and culture (Gardner 2004). Hungarian physicians, especially those working in tertiary care, devote much their time and effort to acquiring a high level of English language knowledge, which is a requirement in their profession, but at the same time, they mostly strive for maintaining their professional Hungarian as well. The present study is designed to follow the direct questioning method with the interview technique, which is used to investigate the language attitudes of certain speech communities (physicians and patients) towards the English language.

2.7.2. Semi-structured interviews

Semi-structured interviews (Scheele and Groeben 1988) are conducted on the basis of a loose structure consisting of open-ended questions (Flick 2002) that define the area to be explored, at least initially, and from which both the interviewer and interviewee may diverge in order to pursue an idea in more detail (Britten 1995). They are generally organized around a set of predetermined open-ended questions, with other questions emerging from the dialogue between interviewer and interviewee. Questions encourage the interviewee to share rich descriptions of phenomena while leaving the interpretation or analysis to the investigators. A semi-structured interview combines a highly structured agenda with the flexibility to ask subsequent questions, and an important aspect of the technique is that the interview is tape-recorded.

The goal of the semi-structured interview is, in general, to "reveal existing knowledge in a way that can be expressed in the form of answers and so become accessible to interpretation" (Flick 2002: 87).

Semi-structured interviews are usually scheduled in advance at a designed time and location. Semi-structured interviews can occur either with an individual or in groups. It is necessary for the interviewer to rapidly develop a positive relationship during the interviews, as establishing rapport is an essential component of the interview described in a classic work by Douglas (1985).

The anonymity of the interviewee in relation to the information shared must be maintained. During interviewing, the interviewee may share information that could "jeopardize their position in a system" (di Cicco-Bloom and Crabtree 2006: 319). This information must remain anonymous and protected from those whose interest conflicts with those of the interviewee. Interviews may result in opportunities for individuals to vent their frustrations and share their experiences. It is therefore required that interviewees give their informed consent to participate in the interview (Silverman 2000).

Direct transcripts of semi-structured interviews can be very reliable and interesting provided that they are faithful to the spoken word and the speech thus recorded represents the vernacular. Transcripts of all kinds are more reliable than other types of written records, but even modern transcripts of sociolinguistic interviews are not simple representations of "reality" either. Typically, the transcriber is the only person to have access to the audio-recording itself (cf. Miethaner 2000).

In sociolinguistics, interviews and tape recordings are accepted as direct evidence, but in practice what is published and what many sociolinguists commonly work with is transcripts, and transcribing is not always objective and unambiguous (Miethaner 2000). Some means of *assessing the validity* of individual texts or collections is needed. Schneider proposes the consideration of four hierarchically ordered sets of criteria, with "the higher levels indicating a higher level of validity, respectively" (2004: 85). These are the nature of the texts, the conditions of the recording, the internal consistency and the external fit.

3. Research questions

The main aims of this book are to describe a subregister of the Hungarian language of medicine, the language of cardiology, to reveal and analyze the English contact-induced features in this specific purpose language, and to investigate the attitudes of various discourse communities affected by the language of cardiology toward the English language and toward the changes induced by the English language.

3.1. The guiding research question and its explication

In general, this book focuses on the influence that the English language has on the Hungarian language of medicine/cardiology and on what the attitudes of physicians and their patients are toward this influence.

This complex major question is broken down into the following smaller research questions:

- What English contact-induced features can be revealed in this specific purpose language by analyzing cardiology discharge reports?

- What interference types can be identified, and which are the most frequent contact linguistic features appearing in these documents?

- Have these features become inherent elements of this specific purpose language?

- What are the attitudes of various discourse communities (patients, family/primary care and tertiary/secondary care physicians) towards the fact that English has become the lingua franca of medicine/cardiology?

4. Methodology

In my research two distinct methods are applied to find the answers to the research questions posed in Section 3.2. The research and analysis of English language contact-induced features in one type of medical documents, the cardiological discharge reports, is complemented by semi-structured interviews with members of the medical community (secondary and tertiary care cardiologists and family physicians) and their patients. The combination of data collected with the two methods wishes to compensate readers for the weaknesses and blind spots of each single method, and intends to provide better insight into present day Hungarian for medical, especially for cardiological purposes.

4.1. Method 1: Research of hospital discharge reports

4.1.1. Data collection

Under Method 1, I use the corpus USZCCDR (University of Szeged Corpus of Cardiological Discharge Reports) based on altogether 234 randomly chosen full length hospital discharge reports taken from the field of cardiology. These documents were prepared in 2005, 2007 and 2009, and follow the new style of the hospital discharge reports described in the MEES (Standards of Hungarian Health Care – translation by the author)[33] and KES (Standardized Hospital Care – translation given on the website)[34] in 2001, 2003 and 2007.

The year 2005 was chosen as my starting point of analysis, for the following reasons. First, all these data were available in a computerized form. The first documentation standards concerning hospital care were issued in Hungary in 2001. Reports from previous years, i.e. before the year 2001, are different not only in their format but partially in their content as well. Overall computerization was introduced and the computer program for full patient documentation was launched at the university clinics of Szeged afterwards. Hospital discharge reports from earlier years were prepared in a non-standardized way or were not fully computerized. The subsequent two years were selected randomly to show more recent results, too. My research is a

---

33 Website http://www.eum.hu/egeszsegpolitika/minosegfejlesztes

34 Cf. Appendix 2.

synchronic linguistic investigation, thus, comments on changes from one studied year to the other will not be discussed.

Second, the year 2005 was selected on the basis of personal communication with senior practising cardiologists working at the Department of Cardiology in Szeged, as several medical/cardiological advances that had been achieved by the end of the 1990s and in the first years of the 21st century had been introduced at the Department of Cardiology by that time.

All these reports were written by Hungarian cardiologists working at a university clinic in a municipal town (specifically at the Department of Cardiology, University of Szeged) during the examined period of time.

USZCCDR comprises 216,703 words in 234 printed reports. Personal data such as name, date of birth, address and social security number were removed from each report prior to data analysis. Reports were then numbered (coded) and scanned to a personal computer, and access to the coded files containing USZCCDR was restricted only to the writer of this book.

Data collection was performed manually, first, as English language contact-induced phenomena were identified in the coded reports by looking through each report one by one, and collecting and recording identified contact phenomena in a chart giving the code of the report, the context and the subheading under which the item appeared. Identified data were then categorized, and the statistical analysis of data was performed by a computer program developed for the research. The program counted the occurrences (frequency of each identified item) within the whole corpus, and it also counted the occurrences within a single report. Statistical data were then transported into an Excel data table in MS Excel 2007.

4.1.2. Reliability of data

Reliability gives the extent to which results can be considered consistent or stable. It refers to the "degree of consistency with which instances are assigned to the same category by different observers or the same observer on different occasions" (Hammersley 1992: 67). Reliability usually refers to the degree to which the findings in a study are "independent of accidental circumstances of their production" (Kirk and Miller 1986: 20). It deals with replicability: referring to the extent to which the experiment, the test or measurement yields the same result on repeated trials (Silverman 2000).

In this research, consistency has been kept by using data taken from hospital discharge reports that have been issued at the same institute in a given period of time by the same health personnel. Reliability was also provided by standardized data processing performed by a computer program developed for the research. The word-search and -analyzing program individually read the text files and searched for the required items by importing them from the searched USZCCDR.

4.1.3. Validity of data

Validity means the degree to which a test measures what it claims to be measuring. In data collection, it means that the findings truly represent the phenomenon that is claimed to be measured. Seliger and Shohamy (1989: 95) claim that "any research can be affected by different kinds of factors which, while extraneous to the concerns of the research, can invalidate the findings". Possible factors that can threaten the validity of the research would be controlled in this survey, and each report would be closely looked at, all relevant linguistic data be analyzed, categorized and described.

In my previous research (2003, 2006b and 2007a), I have already studied the influence of the English language on the Hungarian language of medicine. The categories of data (see below) have been set up on the basis of those findings.

Internal validity in this research is also provided by a medical expert (a cardiologist from the University of Szeged) who speaks English at an advanced level, and who is reading through and validating my data, the collection of the most frequent examples of various English language interferences. He called my attention to some English language contact-induced phenomena which are widely used by cardiologists in oral communication, however, they cannot be found in the analyzed written texts, the discharge report. One such an example was the term *tüske* 'thorn/spike' that can be considered a loan meaning, as the English lexeme has a sememe 'a sharp peak in an electronic recording' which has been borrowed and used by Hungarian cardiologists for the same phenomenon in medical recording.

External validity is the extent to which findings can be generalized to a larger group or other contexts. In Hungary there are only four municipal centers providing cardiological care for patients. In my research, data were collected at one of these centers. As members of the medical team, the cardiologists, were not necessarily born and trained in the same area, and since physicians tend to move from one center to the other, we can suppose that results might be generalized to the whole Hungarian discourse community of cardiologists.

4.1.4. Data analysis: categorization

One aim of the research was to identify English contact-induced features in the Hungarian hospital discharge reports. On the basis of Haugen (1950), Weinreich (1953), Kontra (1981), Lanstyák (2000, 2006) and my previous research results (Keresztes 2003, 2006b, 2007a, 2007b) the following categories were set up for data categorization and evaluation:

- borrowing of orthographic features (spelling, capitalization, and punctuation)
- lexical borrowing (loanwords proper, assimilated loans, eponyms, and acronyms)
- semantic borrowing (loan translations, loanblends, and loan creations)
- grammatical features (e.g. use of definite articles, and passive voice)
- other features (e.g. organization of data).

Mostly based on the classification of borrowed items by Haugen (1950), Weinreich (1953), Kontra (1981) and Lanstyák (2000, 2006), during the categorization of data of lexical and semantic borrowings, I followed the subdivision below:

lexical and semantic changes

externally borrowed features (English contact-induced features) | internally borrowed features

External borrowing of lexical and semantic features (lexemes) refers to contact-induced changes between languages, i.e. Hungarian lexemes borrowed from English, e.g. E *flow* > H *flow*, E (to) *trigger* > H *triggerel*(ni), E *peak gradient* > H *csúcsgrádiens*[35].

Internal borrowing of lexemes is used for borrowing between discourse communities of the same language, e.g. E *mapping* (information technology) > E *mapping* (cardiology), H *zörej* (non-technical) 'noise' > H *zörej* (cardiology) '(cardiac) murmur'. Internal borrowings are not discussed in the present book as

35Examples are taken from the analysed corpus to explain why the very categories described were selected for the description and categorization of the discussed data.

it is suspected that no English contact-induced change is involved, however, it has not been examined within the scope of this study.

External borrowing of lexemes is further divided into three categories: borrowing of loanwords, loan substitutions and pseudo-loans.

externally borrowed lexemes

loanwords | loan substitutions (hybrid loans) | pseudo-loans

Loanwords are lexical items that are borrowed from English into the Hungarian language of medicine either undergoing certain orthographic and/or morphological changes (assimilation), (E) *stress* > (H) *stressz*, or remaining unassimilated in these respects, e.g. (E) *stent* > (H) *stent.* Loanwords are further subdivided according to the assimilation of the English language words to the Hungarian language: words without orthographic assimilation (loanwords proper), and orthographically and/or morphologically assimilated words (assimilated loans). Semantic changes (narrowing or shift) are not considered in this classification, they are discussed separately.

loanwords
(lexical borrowings)

loanword proper (without orthographic assimilation) | assimilated loanword (orthographic and/or morphological assimilation)

Loan substitutions (hybrid loans) are semantic borrowings. Semantic borrowing implies the transference of a sememe or unit of meaning, e.g. E *contrast material* > H *kontrasztanyag*. Loan substitutions[36] are semantic borrowings involving four types of language contact-induced change: loan translations, loanblends, loan meaning and loan creation.

36 Substitution is not used here to refer to assimilated loanwords (as Haugen uses it) but as a collective term for semantic borrowings.

loan substitutions
(semantic borrowings)

loan translation | loanblends | loan creation | loan meaning

Loan translations are calques, showing analogy of meaning between English and Hungarian, but their form/orthography is different. They are usually made up of two or more free Hungarian morphemes, and with their combination, a word carrying the semantic features of that of the English item is formed, e.g. E *benefit risk ratio* > H *haszon-kockázat arány*, E *sudden cardiac death* > H *hirtelen szívhalál*. A loan translation is always a polymorphemic unit (although graphically it can be either uni-verbal or multi-verbal).

Loanblends are hybrid calques. Loanblends are formed by 'transfer' and 'reproduction' according to Weinreich's (1967) terms. In this type of borrowing one or more English morphemes are borrowed and one or more Hungarian morphemes are added to them to form a new sememe, e.g. E *peak gradient* > H *csúcsgrádiens*, E *sign of strain* > H *strainjel*.

A loan meaning is a semantic calque, when only a semanteme but not the form of an English word is transferred to a Hungarian word, e.g. E *spike* (medicine) 'a sharp peak in an electronic recording' > H *spike,* and H *tüske* (non-technical) 'thorn' > H *tüske* (cardiology) 'a sharp peak in an electronic recording'.

Pseudo-loans are words or word elements in Hungarian that were borrowed from English but are used in a way that native English speakers would not recognize. Pseudo-Englishisms often take the form of blends, combining elements of multiple English words to create a new word, e.g. E *circulatory (nurse)* + E agentive suffix *-or* > H *cirkulátor*.

In loan creations the translational equivalence is abandoned as it is based on conceptual transmission. It is the creation of a new Hungarian word according to an English conceptual model without any formal relation to this model in terms of lexical structure. It reflects the English model without being formally related to the English term, e.g. E *temporary collapse in (pulmonary and cardiac) circulation* > H *keringésmegingás* 'a swing in circulation', E *achiving HIS bundle pacing* > (H) *HIS pacelés kötegválaszt igazolt* 'HIS pacing justified bundle reaction/answer'.

When I analyzed and categorized data collected from the hospital discharge reports, I compared data identified in USZCCDR with those provided by non-technical and medical dictionaries[37]:

Bakos, Ferenc. 2007. *Idegen szavak és kifejezések szótára* [Dictionary of foreign words and expressions]. 2007. Budapest: Akadémiai Kiadó.

Benjámin, Katalin. 2006. *Brencsán orvosi szótár* [Brencsán medical dictionary]. 4th edition. Budapest: Medicina Könyvkiadó.

Benkő, Loránd. 1967. *A magyar nyelv történeti etimológiai szótára* [Historico-etymological dictionary of the Hungarian language]. Budapest: Akadémiai Kiadó.

Fábián, Pál and Magasi, Péter. 1992. *Orvosi helyesírási szótár* [Medical orthographic dictionary]. Budapest: Akadémiai Kiadó.

Lozsádi, Károly. 2006. *Etymologia medica* [Medical etymology]. Budapest: Medicina Kiadó.

Merriam–Webster's Advanced Learner's English Dictionary (see website http://www.merriam-webster.com).

Mosby's Medical Dictionary. 8th edition. 2009. Amsterdam: Elsevier.

Országh, László and Magay, Tamás. 1998. *Angol-magyar nagyszótár* [English–Hungarian dictionary]. Budapest: Akadémiai Kiadó.

Pusztai, Ferenc (ed.) 2003. *Magyar értelmező kéziszótár* [The concise dictionary of the Hungarian language]. Budapest: Akadémiai Kiadó.

Zaicz, Gábor. 2006. *Etimológiai szótár* [Etymological dictionary]. Budapest: Tinta Kiadó.

In certain cases, when no data were included in the above listed Hungarian sources for the searched item, I also refer to data found at websites www.pirula.net and www.hazipatika.com, and other medical, especially cardiological websites (e.g. websites http://www.doktorinfo.hu, www.informed.hu, and http://www.mkardio.hu).

I used the *Magyar irodalmi és köznyelv nagyszótárának korpusza/Magyar történeti korpusz* [Corpus of the academic dictionary of Hungarian/Hungarian historical corpus] (see website http://www.nytud.hu/adatb/index.html) for reference to compare the prevalence of data in USZCCDR with a non-technical corpus.

During the morphological and grammatical analysis of data, I mainly relied on Kenesei et al. (1998), É. Kiss et al. (2003) and Korchmáros (2006).

---

37 Unfortunately, there are only two English–Hungarian/Hungarian–English medical dictionaries available at present, which are either relatively outdated (Véghelyi and Csink 1971) or having been translated from German and giving only wordlists (Unseld 2006).

Statistical analysis of data was performed by a computer program developed for the research. The word-search and -analyzing program was created in the Microsoft Visual Studio Professional Development Environment written in C#. The software individually reads the text files (.DOC and .TXT) and searches for the required words by importing them from the searched words database. Then the program counts the frequency of each required word and stores it in its database. After that, the program prepares an Excel data table in MS Excel 2007 from each searched document.

The program reads the documents through the COM interface and the results are also written directly into the Excel table through COM according to the previous arrangements. The program was developed to be able to work with both .DOC(X) and .TXT files, and it can be dynamically extended or modified.

Further processing of MS Excel 2007 database was performed by the use of SPSS 15.0 for Windows program. The development of the program was performed by Zoltán Domokos program developer.

4.1.5. Ethical issues

Data contained in hospital discharge reports are of confidential nature, thus, access to them is limited to the "subjects" of the report, i.e. the patient, and to entitled health personnel. Therefore, I had handed in an application to the head of the university clinic (officially classified as the Department of Cardiology) to authorize access for me to these documents. From each document the personal data of the patient were removed by an attendant of the clinic, thus, the individual patient cannot be identified, and confidentiality of patient data is kept.

4.2. Method 2: Research of language attitude

4.2.1. Subjects

In the second phase of the survey, interviews were carried out with speakers of the investigated speech communities. 11 cardiologists working in tertiary and secondary care, i.e. at the cardiology department of the university clinic and at outpatient clinics in the same town, were interviewed on their attitude towards the fact that English has become the lingua franca of medicine and cardiology. 6

family physicians working in primary care at the same settlement, and referring patients with cardiological problems to secondary and tertiary care institutes, were also interviewed on the above mentioned issue. Finally, I interviewed 8 cardiological patients who had undergone cardiological management at the same university clinic about their attitudes towards the spread of the English language in health care, and especially in the Hungarian special purpose language of cardiology.

4.2.2. Interviews

Patton claims that good questions in qualitative interviews should be open ended, neutral, sensitive, and clear to the interviewee (Patton 1987). He lists six types of questions that can be asked: those based on behavior or experience, on opinion or value, on feeling, on knowledge, and on sensory experience and those asking about demographic or background details. It is usually best to start with questions that the interviewee can answer easily and then proceed to more difficult or sensitive topics. Most interviewees are willing to provide the kind of information the researcher wants, but they need to be given clear guidance about the amount of detail required. It is possible to collect data even in stressful circumstances (Cannon 1989; Britten 1995).

In semi-structured interviews the questions are not fully determined and standardized before the interview occurs but the interviewer has a list of core questions that define the areas to be covered and the order in which questions are asked may vary. Wordings cannot be standardized as the interviewer tries to use the interviewed person's own vocabulary when framing supplementary questions. Also, during the course of an interview, the interviewer may introduce further questions as he/she becomes more familiar with the topic being discussed.

For examining the language attitude of members of the above-mentioned speech communities, the semi-structured interview has been conducted. This type of interview has been selected as it combines a highly structured agenda with the flexibility to ask subsequent open-ended questions from the interviewees. The main goal of the interview has been to reveal the interviewees' attitude towards a linguistic phenomenon, the presence and dominance of the English language in a Hungarian special purpose language, the language of cardiology in a way that can be expressed in the form of answers, which can be interpreted and described.

The interviews have been divided into four main parts. After recording the interviewee's demographic data (age, sex, occupation), the questions in the first part have been aimed as a warm-up, asking the speakers about their knowledge of languages, especially of the English language.

The second part is concerned with the presence and use of the English language in their professional life. One aim of the interview has been to measure how dominant a role the English language plays in the activities of the participants: for what and how they use English in their daily routine at the clinic/office and in their scientific life. In this section, interviewees have been asked to give examples of English contact-induced features (loanwords, initialisms, grammatical structures, etc.) that they can identify in their own speech or writing, and which they use regularly.

In the third part of the interview, the attitudes of the participants to different aspects of the English language dominance have been revealed. Interviewees have been also asked to describe situations when either their patients or their colleagues did not understand something from the discharge report written by them. As the maintenance of good atmosphere in the conversation has been essential, this part has been handled with special care. Distribution of power, turn-taking and management of the topic have been delicate issues throughout the interview. Thus, the rhetoric of argumentation has been carefully considered and elaborated prior to the conversation. During the interview some *ad hoc questions* have also been asked to reflect on personal remarks of the interviewees depending on the direction of their train of thoughts.

In the fourth part, interviewees have been given a cardiological discharge report and asked to read it and underline in the text everything they would write differently. The questions designed for physicians' interviews can be seen in Appendices 5 and 6.[38]

Fulfilling the criterion of depth, ad hoc decisions have also been made and necessary priorities established in the interview situation. Immediately after the end of the interview, I noted my impressions of the communication, of the interviewee as a person, of his/her behavior in the situation, possible external influences etc. Thus, context information has been documented and used as instructive.

Patients have been interviewed in the same way on the same topic, but their questions have slightly been modified according to their role played in the physician–patient interaction. The questions designed for patients' interviews can be seen in Appendix 7.

Each interview has been recorded by an Olympus W-10 digital voice recorder. The recordings have been copied to a computer voice file, and given a number 1 to 25. The interviews have been transcripted and then saved in separate computer files and coded by the appropriate number.

4.2.3. Data evaluation

In analyzing the recorded data of interviews, the coding of procedures (noting the presence and the use of the English language in the researched discourse community's life, and their attitude towards the English language) and analysis of the content was carried out.

Interview questions were referred to by numbers, which can be identified in Appendices 5–10 containing both the English and the Hungarian versions of the interview questions. In analyzing the content, categories that were derived from the theoretical model set up during the planning phase of the research were used. These categories were brought to the empirical material and not developed from it; however, they were repeatedly assessed and modified when necessary.

In the analysis, the procedures offered by Fairclough (1995) were followed, i.e. the method based on three components: description, interpretation and explanation.

The analysis of the recorded and transcribed data had three main phases. The first phase of data analysis involved transcribing and coding the data. Coding was done by adding comments to the transcript. Then data were grouped according to the four main aspects described in 4.2.2, and interpreted focusing on the major questions. And then an explanation for the interpreted data was formulated.

4.2.4. Validity of interview data

Validity of interview data is defined by "the extent to which an account accurately represents the social phenomena to which it refers" (Hammersley 1990: 57). Interviews are based on self-reports of participants, on what and how they do things in their professional life, and cannot examine what they actually do. However, the aim of the study is only to investigate to what extent the English language is used in the Hungarian language of cardiology, and what contact-induced features can be identified in the language of the cardiologists' discourse community, and that is revealed not only through the interviews but is documented in the hospital discharge reports as well.

---

38 In Appendices 5–10 both the English and the Hungarian versions of the interview are available.

The number of participants was low; however, results can be considered comparable and representative, thus meaningful and balanced considering the characteristics of the participants, as various age groups were involved, especially concerning the main target population: cardiologists. As far as the physicians' and their patients' attitudes are concerned, attitudes that are expressed through self-assessment were investigated, thus, the question of validity in this respect is irrelevant.

4.2.5. Ethical issues

Four ethical issues should be considered in the interview process: reducing the risk of unanticipated harm to the interviewee, protecting the interviewee's information, effectively informing interviewees about the nature of the study, and reducing the risk of their exploitation.

Interviewees have been informed about the main aims of the research, and have given their prior consent to the recording of the interview, and to the publishing of the data that were gained from the interview and evaluated by the researcher. The Consent Form can be found in Appendix 3.

The anonymity of the interviewees in relation to the information shared must be maintained, as during interviewing, the some of the interviewees shared information that could jeopardize their position in the health care system. This information must remain anonymous and protected from those whose interest conflicts with those of the interviewees.

After the interview, recordings have been saved to a personal computer accessible only to the researcher. A code number has been given to each interviewee for identification. Interview data is available only to the author of this book, and the interviewees' confidentiality is kept by publishing only such data on the basis of which interviewees cannot be identified.

The consent of the head of the Department of Cardiology has been asked for to perform the interviews with the physicians working at that department and with the patients having been discharged from that department, and consent has also been asked for from the heads of the secondary care cardiology units for the same reason. As family physicians run a private practice no further consent has been asked for their interviews, only their own consent was obtained.

4.3. Complex evaluation of data collected by Methods 1 and 2

In the last phase of my research, I assessed the results found in the hospital discharge reports and described in the interviews, and deepened, generalized and formulated the findings (Figure 8). Analyzing both types of data made it available for me to evaluate my findings in a more comprehensive way and to arrive at more complex conclusions. The original questions could be answered from different perspectives, thus, leading towards a more appropriate and extensive solution of the issue.

1. Data collection ⟶ 2. Data analysis ⟶ 3. Interviews ⟶ 4. Data analysis
(from hospital discharge reports)

⟶ 5. Complex analysis and interpretation of data
(collected through both methods)

Figure 8. Study design.

After the collection and evaluation of data from the written hospital documents, data gained during the semi-structured interviews helped me interpret the results achieved in the 1st phase of the research, and highlight the human factors behind the written data. There is interest in subjective viewpoints of all the three parties, physicians from primary, secondary/tertiary care, and patients, and a better understanding of the object of the research is aimed at. In this phase of the research I attempted to identify complex relations from the distinct data to increase the complexity of the examined issue by including context. The results of the two analyses were compared and to the extent possible, integrated (cf. Creswell 2005). Results gained with Method 1 provide the opportunity for generalizability, while result collected with Method 2 provide a better understanding of the context and meaning.

4.4. Delimitations and limitations of the study

The scope of this study would not allow for an investigation of medical Hungarian as a whole, only one subspecialty is focused on in the investigation, the Hungarian language of cardiology. The selection of the field was done by the author of this book proposal for various reasons such as the availability of cardiologists and their documents for her, the innovativeness of this subspecialty, and a general interest towards the discipline.

Although the author intends to interview physicians working at a university clinic, at an outpatient clinic and in family practices, the results of the research might not give a comprehensive picture of the professional language used by cardiologists in Hungary in general.

All data are collected in a municipal town of Hungary, and different data might be collected in different settlements. However, it can still give good insight into the language of this discourse community.

There is also a limitation imposed on the number of available discharge summaries. Some examples of summaries from the 1980s[39] are also offered to the author to compare present data with previous documents, but the study is not designed to deal with longitudinal changes. That can be the aim of a further survey.

Tremendous help was offered to the author by both linguistic and medical experts to perform this multidisciplinary research, to reveal the scope of English interferences present in the language of Hungarian cardiologists. Linguistic experts, who are acknowledged at the beginning of this book, helped in providing literature and setting up the linguistic categories used in describing the English language contact-induced features found in the analyzed USZCCDR. Medical experts supported the research by reading through and validating data identified as contact-induced features, and also by explaining the processes behind certain medical procedures or management options. Nevertheless, the above mentioned questions might not be investigated and answered fully according to the expectations of both parties. Therefore, further investigations might be relevant to give an even more complex and detailed description of the Hungarian language for cardiological purposes.

39 These summaries were hand written, much shorter than the recent ones and their format, the lay-out and also to some extent their content was also different.

5. Results and discussion

5.1. Results and discussion of data obtained by Method 1

Following the tradition established by Weinreich (1953) on languages in contact and their speakers, I studied hospital discharge reports written in Hungarian by Hungarian/English bilingual physicians and analyzed the micro-linguistic level of the results of contact-induced language change, i.e. borrowing. Borrowing is the "incorporation of foreign features into a group's native language by speakers of that language" (Thomason and Kaufman 1988: 37) including both lexical and structural (orthographical and grammatical/syntactic) borrowing.

This study deals with contact-induced changes that are due to borrowing, where native speakers of Hungarian adopt vocabulary and structural features from English. Any feature that can be code-switched from one language to another can turn into a permanent interference feature (a borrowing) in the recipient language. More generally, "any feature that can appear in a single bilingual person's speech or writing at any time can turn into a permanent change in the entire language" (Thomason 2003: 694). Although in section 2.1 above various universal linguistic constraints on linguistic interference are listed, these constraints are possibly not absolute concerning the kinds and degrees of linguistic inference that can occur in the language of sciences dominated by the English language, and we should, therefore, follow the assumption of Thomason's that "everything appears to be possible, although some things are improbable" (2003: 695) in the speech (and writing) of bilingual physicians.

"Bilinguals rarely deactivate the other language totally" (Grosjean and Soares 1986:146), therefore, unconscious and involuntary incorporation of almost any foreign structural feature into one of the bilingual's languages can occur when bilinguals speak or write. Thomason highlights that "deactivation of entrenched non-salient elements of speech (most syntactic elements) is probably much harder to do" (2003: 698). The phonetic and phonological elements are also likely to be non-salient and entrenched, whereas the lexicon is more likely to be salient.

With Method 1 (Section 4.1), I researched 234 hospital discharge reports written by Hungarian cardiologists at a Hungarian university clinic between 2005 and 2009. On the basis of previous linguistic research described mainly by Haugen (1950), Weinreich (1953), Kontra (1981), and Lanstyák (2000, 2006), and my own previous results (Keresztes 2003, 2006b, 2007a, 2007b), I identified borrowed[40] elements according to five categories: orthographic (Section 5.1.1), lexical (Section 5.1.2), semantic (Section 5.1.3.), grammatical/syntactic (Section 5.1.4) and other features (Section 5.1.5). Each section is closed by discussion on the described language contact-induced feature and conclusions derived from the results, whereas Section 5.1.6 provides an overall conclusion on the results obtained with Method 1.

Nevertheless, the results gained through Method 1 do not aim to exhaust the problem of borrowing in the Hungarian language of medicine, not even in the language of cardiology. Selected problems are delineated, and the actual cases of interference forms that have been cited were selected out of a multitude of others for their illustrative value to highlight the tendencies of English language contact-induced changes in Hungarian cardiology discharge reports, and based on these results to draw further conclusions on the current Hungarian language of cardiology and medicine.

When analyzing and categorizing data collected from USZCCDR, I compared and cross-checked the data from USZCCDR with dictionary entries (lexemes[41]) provided by English and Hungarian medical and Hungarian general dictionaries. The dictionaries were selected on the basis of three factors: most widely used ones (based on the number of copies sold or number of visitors at their website), most prestigious dictionaries (based on the opinions given by members of the discourse community, personal communication) and finally, their availability during the research (each English monolingual dictionary is available both at the University of Szeged Library and at the http://www.thefreedictionary.com and at http://www.merriam-webster.com, and the Hungarian monolingual dictionaries are available in the University of Szeged Library).

The abbreviations below are used in the Results and discussion section (5.1) to refer to dictionaries or the dictionaries' websites and other works checked for reference.

List of abbreviations for the reference dictionaries:

AHMD: *American heritage medical dictionary*. 2007. Philadelphia: Houghton Mifflin Company.

40 I use the term "borrowing" in situations of "full bilingualism" (in the sense Thomason 2005 describes it), and not for cases of imperfect learning (which is interference through language shift).

BISZ: Bakos, Ferenc. 2007. *Idegen szavak és kifejezések szótára* [Dictionary of foreign words and expressions]. 2007. Budapest: Akadémiai Kiadó.

BOSZ: Benjámin, Katalin. (ed.) 2006. *Brencsán orvosi szótár* [Brencsán medical dictionary]. Budapest: Medicina Könyvkiadó.

DMD: *Dorland's medical dictionary for health consumers*. 2007. Saunders.

EKSZ: Pusztai, Ferenc (ed.) 2003. *Magyar értelmező kéziszótár* [The concise dictionary of the Hungarian language]. Budapest: Akadémiai Kiadó.

LEM: Lozsádi, Károly. 2006. *Etymologia medica* [Medical etymology]. Budapest: Medicina Kiadó.

MMD: Mosby's medical dictionary. 2009. Elsevier.

MW: Merriam–Webster's Advanced Learner's English Dictionary. (see website http://www.merriam-webster.com)

OHSZ: Fábián, Pál and Magasi, Péter. 1992. *Orvosi helyesírási szótár* [Medical orthographic dictionary]. Budapest: Akadémiai Kiadó.

TESZ: Benkő, Loránd. 1967. *A magyar nyelv történeti etimológiai szótára* [Historico-etymological dictionary of the Hungarian language]. Budapest: Akadémiai Kiadó.

ZESZ: Zaicz, Gábor. 2006. *Etimológiai szótár* [Etymological dictionary]. Budapest: Tinta Kiadó.

List of abbreviations for other works used as a reference with Method 1:

MIK: Magyar irodalmi és köznyelv nagyszótárának korpusza/Magyar történeti korpusz [Corpus of the academic dictionary of Hungarian/Hungarian historical corpus] (see website http://www.nytud.hu/adatb/index.html)

UMN: É. Kiss, Katalin, Kiefer, Ferenc and Siptár, Péter. 2003. *Új magyar nyelvtan* [New Hungarian grammar]. Budapest: Osiris Kiadó.

In certain cases, when no data are available in the above listed Hungarian resources for the searched item, I also refer to data found at www.pirula.net, www.hazipatika.com, and other medical, especially cardiological websites (e.g. www.informed.hu, http://www.doktorinfo.hu, http://www.mkardio.hu).

41 Lexemes are the units listed in a dictionary. A lexeme is used in my book with the definition of a set of related meanings associated with a set of related word forms (cf. Cruse 2003).

5.1.1. Contact-induced changes in orthography

As Method 1 involved the research of written documents, the orthographic results of language contact such as spelling (Section 5.1.1.1), capitalization (Section 5.1.1.2), and punctuation (5.1.1.3) are described in this section, but not phonemic interference. However, in case of English–Hungarian language contact, the study of orthographic features can partially be helpful to draw certain conclusions also about phonemic interference, since Hungarian has a near-phonemic (shallow) orthography, i.e. written graphemes mostly correspond to phonemes.

Both the English and the Hungarian language uses the Latin alphabet, which makes the assimilation of borrowings easier, but the English language has relatively complicated spelling rules (i.e. deep orthography) compared to Hungarian. Thus, despite the similar pronunciation of the borrowed words, the Hungarian orthography of assimilated English loanwords is, in most cases, different from the English orthography.

The orthographic form of a borrowing depends not only on the degree of conventionalization, i.e. earlier English loanwords are usually assimilated to the Hungarian language (e.g. *diszkomfort, rezidens*) but also on the homogeneity/heterogeneity of the contacting languages. When we deal with a homogeneous alphabetical pair of languages (English–Hungarian, for example), the transplantation of lexical units can occur mechanically, without any changes; the units of one language can be easily transferred into the other language (Kabakchi 1998).

5.1.1.1. Re-Englishization of spelling

The vast majority of English terms in Hungarian reveal themselves as foreign because of their spelling pattern, they are graphically unassimilated (e.g. *bypass, flow*) or there is a lack of relation between pronunciation and spelling (e.g. *pace, mapping*). In some cases, the borrowed word acquires a native status by the adaptation it undergoes. This adaptation allows the loanword to be adjusted to the phonetic or spelling norms of the borrowing language.

In the field of medicine (and sciences in general), however, there is a kind of reverse tendency toward the use of unassimilated orthography, i.e. Hungarian physicians tend to use the English spelling of the previously assimilated (mainly international) loanwords, re-foreignizing them, or return to the English orthography, re-Englishizing them. Re-Englishization[42] is the term used in this book (for which I am grateful to Balázs Sinkovics, personal communication in 2009) to describe a contact linguistic phenomenon that is relatively common in written medical texts: the original international (I) or assimilated Hungarian (H) orthography is changed either into the English (E) orthography (e.g. E *shunt* > H *sönt* > H *shunt*) or into an assumed English orthography that actually does not exist, thus leading to the development of a pseudo-English spelling (e.g. E/I *plaque* > H *plakk* > H *plack*).

Examples of this phenomenon (re-Englishization) collected from USZCCDR belong to the core vocabulary of cardiology (e.g. *block, plaque, shock, shunt, test*), or they denote certain chemical elements and compounds (e.g. *cholesterol, levothyroxine*).

A short etymological description of both the English and the Hungarian terms, where feasible (based on data in the dictionaries mentioned above), the meaning of these words in both languages, their prevalence in MIK (for a comparison with a large corpus of non-technical Hungarian language), and examples of the graphic forms of these words taken from USZCCDR are given below.

a. attak/attack:

MW (the reference dictionary on general English) traces back the word *attack* to 1562 and defines it as being a Middle French or Old Italian loanword in English with 7 major meanings, out of which the medical meaning of the lexeme is defined in this dictionary in **3a:** *a fit of sickness; especially: an active episode of a chronic or recurrent disease* and in **3b**: *a period of being strongly affected by something (as a desire or mood).*

MMD (one of the reference dictionaries on medical English) defines it as *an episode in the course of an illness, usually characterized by acute and distressing symptoms.*

This word (*attak*) is listed in TESZ (the reference general Hungarian etymological dictionary published in 1967) and it is derived from the German language in the meaning of *roham, támadás* 'attack' or 'assault' used in the army. It appeared first in the written literature in 1787 according to this dictionary. The word is not listed in ZESZ (the reference general Hungarian etymological dictionary published in 2006). EKSZ (the reference dictionary on the Hungarian language) gives the medical meaning of *attak* as *roham* 'attack'. According to BISZ (the reference dictionary on Hungarian loanwords) *attak* is

42 Englishization is a term used to refer to the linguistic influence of English on another language (Kachru 1979).

derived from French but was borrowed via German, and it has two meanings. The second one is the medical meaning: *roham (a betegség hirtelen fellépő tünete)* 'attack (sudden onset of the symptom of the disease).

According to LEM (the etymological dictionary of medical Hungarian words) *attak* is the assimilated Hungarian word derived from the French *attaquer,* and it is defined as *támadás, roham.* BOSZ (the reference dictionary on medical Hungarian) gives both orthographies, *attak/attack,* and defines the meaning as *roham*. OHSZ (the reference dictionary on the spelling of Hungarian medical words) lists only *attak*.

No match was found on this term with either spelling in MIK (the reference corpus on non-technical Hungarian texts). When I searched www.informed.hu for *attack* 87 results were found, and only 21 for the assimilated form *attak*.

In the discharge reports under investigation *attak* was used in only 3 reports (e.g. *ischaemias attak*), and *attack*, with the re-Englishized orthography, was used in 11 reports (e.g. *regisztrált attack, transiens ischaemias attack*).

While the reference dictionary on Hungarian loanwords, the medical etymological dictionary and the dictionary on Hungarian medical spelling (published in 1992) give only the assimilated form (*attak*), both the referred medical website and USZCCDR show that the re-Englishized orthography is used more frequently.

In USZCCDR, both *attak* and the re-Englishized *attack* are used only as root words, no prefixes or suffixes are added to them, thus morphological assimilation of neither word can be proved. *Attak/attack* is usually used with medical adjectives e.g. *ischaemias* 'ischemic' being the noun in the attributive construction.

b. blokk/block:

MW traces back the etymology of *block* to the 14th century from Middle English *blok,* from Middle French *bloc* and from Middle Dutch *blok;* akin to Old High German *bloh* with 8 meanings. The medical meaning is described **2c(1)***: interruption of normal physiological function (as of a tissue or organ); especially***:** *heart block,* **2c(2):** *local anesthesia (as by injection) produced by interruption of the flow of impulses along a nerve* **and 2d***: interruption or cessation especially of train of thought by competing thoughts or psychological suppression.*

MMD refers to the Old French *bloc* as the origin of the word, and defines the word as **1:** *a disruption in the conduction of a nerve impulse. The term may apply to stoppage of nerve conduction as produced by local anesthetics, inhibition of beta receptors by beta-blocker drugs, or prevention of* *neuromuscular transmission by blockade of nicotinic receptors by muscle-relaxant drugs.* **2:** *a device to maintain separation of the teeth, such as a bite block.*

Blokk is a German loanword (from *Block*) that appeared first in a written Hungarian text in 1796 (TESZ and ZESZ) with the meaning *őrhely* 'post' (TESZ), *jegyzettömb, árcédula* 'writing pad, price tag', and was first used as a verb as *blokkol* in writing in 1959 (ZESZ). BISZ also defines *blokk* as a German word that was borrowed via French, and has 12 different meanings, the 10th and 11th being of medical origin: **10:** *helyi érzéketlenség; ennek előidézése* 'local anesthesia; the causing of it' and **11:** *valamely szerv hirtelen megállása, súlyos zavara, elzáródása* 'sudden cessation in the function of an organ, severe disorder, obstruction'. EKSZ provides many meanings of *blokk* none of which is medical.

BOSZ defines *block/blokk* as *megállás, elzáródás, akadály; helyi érzéstelenség* 'cessation in function, obstruction, blockage; local anesthesia'. LEM does not contain this word, and OHSZ gives only *blokk.*

MIK provides 28 matches for *blokk* and 6 for *block*. USZCCDR contains 47 matches for *blokk* and 196 matches for *block*.

It is one of the most frequently used words in cardiology discharge reports as it is used to refer both to common pathological conditions in the cardiovascular system (e.g. *inkomplett szárblock, hemiblock* 'incomplete branch block, hemiblock') and a type of medication (*beta blockoló* 'beta blocker'). Although the loanword *blokk* is widely used in Hungarian in other, general meanings listed in BISZ, due to the intensive contact of researching physicians with the English language, they tend to use the unassimilated English orthography instead of the assimilated Hungarian form in several cases.

The re-Englishized noun, *block*, is used as a root word in the reports in attributive constructions (e.g. *bal/jobb Tawara-szár block*, *teljes/másodfokú pitvar-kamrai block*, *AV block*, *pitvar-kamrai block*, *bifascicularis block* or *centroseptalis block*), as well as a noun with Hungarian case endings and suffixes (e.g. *bidirectionalis isthmus blockot igazoltunk, functionalis blockkal járó*, *beta blockoló* and *blockolású*). The latter examples demonstrate that regardless of being orthographically unassimilated (or having turned back to an unassimilated form), it is morphologically assimilated to the Hungarian case endings and suffixes. From a morphological point of view, the re-Englishized word (*block*) is productive: both adjectival and nominal derivational suffixes can be added to the word root (as *blockoló* and *blockolás*, respectively).

c. diffúz/diffuse

In MW the etymology of this word is defined as Middle English from Latin *diffuses,* and 2 meanings are given for it: **1:** *being at once verbose and ill-organized* **2:** *not concentrated or localized.* The second meaning can be related to medicine.

In MMD the etymology of this word is derived from the Latin *diffundere,* and the meanings are: **1:** *to spread out* **2:** *becoming widely spread, such as through a membrane or fluid.*

The Hungarian word *diffúz* comes from the Latin word *diffundere* or *diffuses,* and according to BISZ it is used in sciences to mean *szétszórt, rendezettség nélküli* 'disintegrated, without organization'. EKSZ gives the meaning *rendezetlenül szétszórt* 'diffusely scattered' for *diffúz*. It is not listed in LEM or TESZ.

Diffusus/diffúz is given in BOSZ with the meaning *szétszórt, kiterjedt, elmosódott határú* 'disintegrated, spread, without sharp contour' but *diffuse* is not listed. None of the three variants (assimilated Hungarian, Latin or re-Englishized) are listed in LEM. Two orthographic forms are listed in OHSZ (*diffusus/diffúz*) but not the re-Englishized orthography.

In www.pirula.net the English orthography *diffuse* is also given as a possible variant. MIK gives 12 instances for *diffúz* but none for *diffuse*.

In scientific texts (as well as in hospital discharge reports) physicians sometimes stick to the original (i.e. Latin) spelling *diffus(us)* (e.g. *diffus hepar laesio*). In the hospital discharge reports under investigation, all three forms (*diffúz, diffus* and *diffuse*) are used by physicians (e.g. *diffúz hypokinezis* 'diffuse hypokinesis', *diffus myocardium laesio* 'diffuse myocardiac leasion', *az RCA diffuse kaliberingadozó* 'the RCA is with diffuse caliber fluctuation'), but *diffúz* is the most frequently used orthographic variant.

No derivational suffixes were added to the re-Englishized *diffuse*, it is only used as an adjective in USZCCDR.

d. plakk/plaque

The etymology of the English word *plaque* (1845) according to MW leads us back to Middle French *plaquer,* Middle Dutch *placken* and akin to Middle Dutch *placke* and Middle High German *placke.* 3 meanings are defined in MW the second and third ones of which are related to medicine: **2a:** *a localized abnormal patch on a body part or surface* **2b:** *a sticky usually colorless film on teeth that is formed by and harbors bacteria* **2c:** *an atherosclerotic lesion* **2d:** *a histopathologic lesion of brain tissue that is characteristic of Alzheimer's disease* *and consists of a dense proteinaceous core composed primarily of beta-amyloid that is often surrounded and infiltrated by a cluster of degenerating axons and dendrites*, **3:** *a clear area in a bacterial culture produced by viral destruction of cells.*

MMD also describes the French origin of the medical term, and two meanings of it are given: **1:** *a flat, often raised patch on the skin or any other organ of the body*, **2:** *a patch of atherosclerosis.* AHMD, however, gives a more specific medical meaning that can be related to cardiology: *a deposit of material in a bodily tissue or organ, especially one of the fatty deposits that collect on the inner lining of an artery wall in atherosclerosis.* Whereas the McGraw-Hill Concise Dictionary of Modern Medicine (2002) gives the specific meaning of *plaque* used in cardiology: *an early lesion of ASHD* (Arteriosclerotic Heart Disease) *found in persons of any age in larger vessels.*

The Hungarian term *plakk* was most probably borrowed from French (*plaquer*), it is not listed in EKSZ, TESZ or ZESZ but in BISZ describing that it is a medical word meaning: *a környezettől világosan elváló folt* 'a patch being unambiguously separated from its surroundings'.

BOSZ gives the meaning of *plakk/plaque* as **1:** *körülírtan kiemelkedő folt* 'a circumscribed, elevated patch', **2:** *egybefüggő sejtrétegen kialakuló, kerekded világos terület, amely több vírusszaporodási ciklus során az összefüggő sejtek elpusztulása vagy feloldódása révén keletkezik* 'a rounded, light area developing on a confluent cell layer, which was formed during several viral proliferation cycles by the destruction or dissolvation of confluent cells'. No match was found for either spelling in LEM, but OHSZ gives both *plakk* and *plaque* but the entry of the second orthographic form redirects the reader to the first one.

MIK provides 1 match for *plakk* and none for *plaque*.

As this term is mostly used in medicine (especially in cardiology, dermatology and dentistry), I also checked some Hungarian medical websites for further information on the meaning, use and spelling of the word. The website www.hazipatika.com uses the spelling *plakk*, and defines the phenomenon as *a vérből az artériák belső falára lerakódó mész és zsírnemű anyagok, amelyek az érfal megkeményedéséhez és az erek beszűküléséhez vezetnek* 'calcification and fatty substance deposited on the inner wall of the arteries from the blood, which leads to the hardening and narrowing of the arteries' and www.informed.hu explains the term (*plakk*) as *koleszterinnel átitatott foltok* 'patches impregnated by cholesterol'. On the other hand, www.pirula.net uses the spelling *plaque*, and defines it as *lepedék* 'coating'.

In the discharge reports both spelling variants can be found *meszes plaque* 'calcified plaque' and *erythemás papulák-plakkok* 'erythematous papules and plaques'. The word with the re-Englishized spelling (*plaque*) is used not only in its root form but in some cases suffixes are also added to it, e.g. the plural suffix in *echodús meszes plaqueok* 'echodense calcified plaques'. A certain type of hypercorrection/pseudo-Englishizm[43] (or overfulfilment of the norm if Englishized forms are considered to be more prestigious) was also identified concerning the spelling of this word when in some discharge reports the orthography *plack* was used to describe the same phenomenon.

e. sokk, shock

If we trace back the etymology of the English word *shock*, we find (in MW) that it comes from Middle French *choc,* from *choquer* to strike against, from Old French *choquier,* probably of Germanic origin; akin to Middle Dutch *schocken* to jolt (date: 1565). 5 meanings are given in MW the last 3 of which are related to medicine: **3a(1):** *a disturbance in the equilibrium or permanence of something* **3a(2):** *a sudden or violent mental or emotional disturbance* **3b:** *something that causes such disturbance* **c:** *a state of being so disturbed,* **4:** *a state of profound depression of the vital processes associated with reduced blood volume and pressure and caused usually by severe especially crushing injuries, hemorrhage, or burns,* **5:** *sudden stimulation of the nerves and convulsive contraction of the muscles caused by the discharge of electricity through the animal body.*

MDD, focusing only on the meaning related to medicine, also designates the word as French origin, and defines the term as: *an abnormal condition of inadequate blood flow to the body's tissues, with life-threatening cellular dysfunction.*

The Hungarian word *sokk* has an international origin as it comes from the German word *Schock*, or the French word *choc*, or the English word *shock.* It first appeared in written literature in 1865 according to TESZ and ZESZ, and it is an international word meaning *ütközés* 'collision' and in medical sense *megrázkódtatás* 'shock' (also in EKSZ). According to BISZ, *sokk* has a French and English origin, and it is used in medicine to mean *a szervezetet ért heveny megrázkódtatás kiváltotta súlyos működési (keringési) zavarokkal járó állapot* 'a condition accompanied by severe functional (circulatory) disturbances triggered by an acute shock to the body'. It can also be used in the meaning of *idegsokk* 'neural shock'. The spelling *shock* is also listed in BISZ, but only to direct[44] the

43 In this book the term pseudo-Englishism is used for the linguistic phenomenon when elements of a borrowed item are substituted by other elements which themselves do not conform to the native structures of the borrowing language.

44 I use the term direct the reader when the word that is considered the norm/standard by the dictionary comes alphabetically later in the dictionary (cf. shock – sokk), and redirect is

reader to *sokk*. BOSZ, however, gives *shock* as the main entry (directing from *sokk* to *shock*) describing that it is an English loanword meaning *az egész szervezetre kiterjedő működési elégtelenség* 'functional failure affecting the whole body'. OHSZ gives both entries, but *shock* only to direct us to *sokk*. In MIK, there were 37 matches for *sokk* and 4 matches for *shock*.

In the discharge reports *shock* is used several times as a root word e.g. *cardiogen shock* 'cardiogenic shock' or *DC shock* 'DC shock', and as a compound *shockelektróda* 'shock electrode', *shock terápia* 'shock therapy'. In some instances Hungarian physicians handle *shock* as a foreign word either italicizing it in the text, or putting a hyphen between the root and the Hungarian suffix (signaling its unassimilation with the hyphen): hyphenated Hungarian accusative case suffix (*-t*) is added in e.g. *SR 200 J-os shock-ot* 'an SR 200 J shock', but also unhyphenated suffixes are used: *shockkal* 'via shock', *DC-shockkal szüntették meg* 'it was ceased via DC shock'. These instances show total morphological and partial orthographical assimilation of the loanword.

f. sönt/shunt

According to MW *shunt* is an English word that is derived from Middle English, and it gives 2 meanings of the noun, the first of which also carries a medical connotation: **1c:** *a surgical passage created to divert a bodily fluid (as blood) from one vessel or part to another; also:* *a device (as a narrow tube) used to establish a similar passage.*

In DMD *shunt* is defined as **1:** *a passage or anastomosis between two natural channels, especially between blood vessels, formed physiologically or anomalously,* and **2:** *a surgically created anastomosis; also, the operation of forming a shunt.*

BISZ contains both orthographies (*shunt* and *sönt*), but the main entry is *sönt*, where the reader is directed from *shunt*. 3 meanings are given with the last 2 being related to medicine: **2:** *2 ér közötti kóros vagy mesterségesen létesített összeköttetés,* **3:** *a vér visszafelé áramlása a szívben.* TESZ and ZESZ does not contain an entry on either form. EKSZ gives the word with assimilated Hungarian orthography (*sönt*) with the same meaning as BISZ (see above).

BOSZ sayes that *shunt* is the same as *sönt* and describes that the word has an English origin. Two meanings are given: **1**: *mellékáramlás* 'paraflow', **2:** *megkerülő út egy szervrendszeren belül* 'a bypass within a system'. LEM does not have an entry for this word.

MIK does not give any match for either *sönt* or *shunt*. USZCCDR gave no match for *sönt,* and *shunt* was used only in 3 discharge reports (*bal jobb shunt*

---

used when the standard word comes alphabetically earlier in the same dictionary (cf. plaque – plakk).

'left right shunt', *shunt műtét* 'shunt implantation'). The phenomenon designated by *shunt/sönt* has recently rarely been used by cardiologists, and the word *bypass* is used instead (Gábor Marton, M.D., cardiology resident, personal communication in 2010).

g. teszt/test

According to MW the English word *test* in its original meaning (*a vessel in which metals were assayed*) comes from Anglo–French *test, tees* and Latin *testum*. Currently it has 4 meanings, three of which are related to medicine: **1(1)**: *a critical examination, observation, or evaluation: trial, the procedure of submitting a statement to such conditions or operations as will lead to its proof or disproof or to its acceptance or rejection,* **1(2):** *a basis for evaluation: criterion* **c:** *an ordeal or oath required as proof of conformity with a set of beliefs,* **2a**: *a means of testing: as* **2a(1):** *a procedure, reaction, or reagent used to identify or characterize a substance or constituent* **2a(2):** *something (as a series of questions or exercises) for measuring the skill, knowledge, intelligence, capacities, or aptitudes of an individual or group* **2b:** *a positive result in such a test,* **3:** *a result or value determined by testing.*

DMD defines *test* as **1:** *an examination or trial,* **2:** *a significant chemical reaction,* **3:** *a reagent.*

EKSZ, TESZ and ZESZ write that *teszt* is an international word that appeared first in a Hungarian written text in 1913 with the meaning: *próbatétel, kísérlet, vizsgálat* 'trial, experiment, examination'. It was borrowed into the Hungarian language mainly via English as an international word. BISZ describes that *teszt* is an English loanword, and it gives 2 meanings, both of which are related to medicine: **1:** *próba, működési próba* 'trial, functional trial', **2:** *képesség, tudás vagy személyi vonások vizsgálatára alkalmas, meghatározott feladatsorból álló próba* 'a test made up of a series of defined tasks to examine a skill, knowledge or personal characteristics'.

BOSZ defines *teszt* as *próba, jellemző reakció kiváltására irányuló vizsgáló módszer* 'test, a method to examine a triggered characteristic reaction', but has a separate entry for *test* saying that it comes from English and it means *próba* 'test'. LEM does not contain either *test* or *teszt.* OHSZ gives both forms but directs from *test* to *teszt.*

MIK gives 189 matches for *teszt* but none for *test* in the above meaning.

In the studied medical discharge reports the unassimilated test is used only when a specific test is described in the name of which unassimilated English word(s) can be found, e.g. predischarge test. In other cases the assimilated form, teszt is used, e.g. pitvari extrastimulus teszt 'atrial extrastimulus test', vércukormérő tesztcsík 'test paper for measuring blood glucose'.

5.1.1.1.1. Re-Englishization of the names of chemical elements and compounds

The reverse tendency in orthography was found in the discharge reports not only in case of the above listed frequently used nouns and adjectives but also in some less frequently used chemical names.

a. acetylsalicylic acid/acetilszalicilsav

DMD gives a very short definition for *acetylsalicylic acid* by defining it as *aspirin*, and if we look up the entry of *aspirin*, it gives that *it is a medicine that relieves pain and reduces fever.*

BISZ has an entry only for *acetil-szalicilsav*, BOSZ contains *acetilszalicilsav* (unhyphenated) and also gives the Latin form of the term: *acidum acetylsalicylicum*. OHSZ contains only *acetilszalicilsav*.

MIK does not have any match for this term. The assimilated Hungarian form was used in only 3 discharge summaries but the Re-Englishized variant was used in more than 60 reports. This word appeared mainly in the Recommended therapy section of the reports with giving the trade name: *Aspirin Protect* in parentheses afterward.

b. enoxaparin/ enoxaparol

DMD defines *enoxaparin sodium* as *a low molecular weight heparin used as the sodium salt as an antithrombotic. Enoxaparin* is not entered in any of the Hungarian dictionaries I reviewed. Therefore, I turned to further sources and found a Hungarian definition for *enoxaparin* at website http://www.ogyi.hu: *az enoxaparin nátrium egy olyan kis molekulatömegű heparin nátriumsója, amelyet sertés bélnyálkahártyából nyert heparin benzil-észter származékának lúgos depolimerizációjával állítanak elő* 'enoxaparin sodium is a low moleculecular weight heparin that is gained via basic depolimerization of a derivative of benzo-esther heparin from the mucosa of the pig' .

Enoxaparol (sodium) is used in two discharge reports. The orthography *enoxaparol* is a case of hypercorrection, an element of a borrowed item is substituted by another element which itself does not conform to the native structures of the borrowing language. It can also be categorized as an example of pseudo-Englishism based on the English morphology of certain chemicals ending in *-ol* (cf. *cholesterol, mannitol, xylitol*). The international orthography of *enoxaparin* is changed into the assumed English orthography *enoxaparol,* which does not exist in English. This phenomenon may reinforce the assumption that the effect of the English language (dominance and prestige) is so strong among cardiologists that due to the intensive written contact it can lead to the development of pseudo-Englishisms as well.

c. klorid/chloride

MW says that chloride has a German etymology (Chlorid) and dates from 1812. It has 2 meanings: **1:** a compound of chlorine with another element or group; especially**:** a salt or ester of hydrochloric acid, **2:** a monovalent anion consisting of one atom of chlorine.

DMD defines chloride as a salt of hydrochloric acid; any binary compound of chlorine in which the latter is the negative element.

The assimilated Hungarian word klorid is given in BISZ and EKSZ (and *chloride*, the unassimilated or re-Englishized orthography is not) with a Greek and Latin etymology, and the meaning: *fémnek vagy szerves gyöknek klórral alkotott vegyülete* 'a compound of a metal or an organic radical with chlorine'. TESZ and ZESZ do not have an entry for either *klorid* or *chloride*, but they say that the word *klór* 'chlorine' appeared first in written documents in 1829 (ZESZ) or 1831 (TESZ), and it is an international word from the German *Chlor*, French *Chlore* and Italian *cloro. Klorid* 'chloride' is a derived form of this assimilated loanword.

BOSZ does not have an entry for either orthography, it only contains *klór* with the meaning: *a 17. rendszámú elem* (*chlorum*) 'element No. 17 (chlorine)'. OHSZ lists only *klorid* but not *chloride.*

MIK gives 2 matches for *klorid* and none for *chloride.* This form (*klorid*) was, however, not used in any of the discharge reports under investigation, as in each case the unassimilated form, *chloride* was used (e.g. *potassium chloride*).

d. koleszterin/cholesterol

In MW *cholesterol* is said to be as a member of the International Scientific Vocabulary derived from *chol-* and Greek *stereos* meaning *solid.* It appeared first in written documents in 1894. The meaning given for cholesterol is *a steroid alcohol* $C_{27}H_{45}OH$ *that is present in animal cells and body fluids, regulates membrane fluidity, and functions as a precursor molecule in various metabolic pathways and as a constituent of LDL may cause arteriosclerosis.*

DMD says that *cholesterol* is *a sterol found in all animal tissues, blood, bile, and animal fats: a precursor of other body steroids. A high level of cholesterol in the blood is implicated in some cases of atherosclerosis, leading to heart disease. Formula:* $C_{27}H_{45}OH$. *Former name cholesterin.*

The standard, assimilated Hungarian word for *cholesterol* is *koleszterin.* BISZ also gives the Greek derived orthography of the word, *cholesterin*, directing the reader to *koleszterin,* but it does not list cholesterol as an orthographic option. *Koleszterin* is give by EKSZ with the meaning *az ember és az állatok szervezetének sejtjeiben található kristályos vegyület* 'chrystal compound found in human and animal cells'.

BOSZ defines *koleszterin* as *állati szterin (a zsírokban kis mennyiségben található aromás alcohol)* 'an animal sterol (aromatic alcohol found in lipid in a small amount)'. It also gives *cholesterin* (but not *cholesterol*) directing us to *koleszterin.* There is no entry in ZESZ on *koleszterin.* The same is found in OHSZ (*cholesterin* and *koleszterin* but not *cholesterol*).

MIK gives 1 match for *koleszterin* and none for the re-Englishized orthography, *cholesterol.* In medical writings physicians frequently use the Greek derived orthography of the word: *cholesterin.* In USZCCDR, the term is written both with Greek derived, unassimilated orthography *cholesterin* and with the English spelling *cholesterol* (e.g. *cholesterinszegény étrend* 'low cholesterol diet', *hypercholesterinaemia* but *cholesterol polipok* 'cholesterol polyps').

e. levotiroxin/levothyroxine

Levothyroxine is not given in any of the English monolingual reference dictionaries. DMD gives a definition, however, of -thyroxine as obtained from the thyroid gland of domesticated food animals or prepared synthetically; used as the sodium salt in the treatment of hypothyroidism, and the treatment and prophylaxis of goiter and thyroid carcinoma.

Neither orthographies are given in any of the referenced Hungarian dictionaries. BOSZ, similarly to DMD, gives the word tiroxin, in the assimilated form with the meaning anyagcsere-szabályozó pajzsmirigy hormone 'a thyroid hormone regulating the metabolism'. The website www.hazipatika.com contains both levotiroxin and levothyroxine, not only tiroxin/thyroxine, and describes it as a szintetikus levotiroxin (levothyroxine) hatása azonos a pajzsmirigy fő hormonjáéval, a tiroxinnal 'the effect of synthetic levothyroxine is the same as that of thyroxine, the major hormone of the thyroid gland'. The re-Englishized orthography is also given as a means of identification of the chemical agent.

MIK contains no match for either word. In USZCCDR only the re-Englishized orthography was used (e.g. l*evothyroxine sodium*).

5.1.1.2. Capitalization

Capitalization is writing a word with its first letter as an upper-case letter. Proper names, the first word of each sentence, and titles, acronyms and some initialisms are capitalized in Hungarian.

5.1.1.2.1. The abbreviation of liter

The International System of Units (SI) is the standard system of measurements used by many scientists all over the world. The litre (UK) or liter (US) is a metric unit of volume. The liter is not an SI unit, but it is accepted for use with the International System. The symbol for the liter is the lowercase letter *l* or the uppercase letter *L*. A cursive or script small letter *l (ℓ)* is also used but is not accepted by the BIPM (Bureau International des Poids et Mesures). The symbol for liter was originally l (lowercase letter *l*). In order to reduce confusion with the Arabic numeral 1, L (uppercase letter *L*) was accepted as an alternative symbol in 1979. The United States National Institute of Standards and Technology recommends the use of the uppercase letter *L* (cf. website http://www.economicexpert.com/a/Litre.htm).

In Hungarian, however, liter is still abbreviated by the lowercase *l.* In the cardiology discharge reports physicians seem to follow the recommendations, as in most cases liter is abbreviated by *L,* e.g. *Giga/L, L/L, mmol/L.*

As the measurement liter is mostly used in the "Results of laboratory findings" section of discharge reports, we may also explain the almost exclusive use of the uppercase *L* by the fact that standardized programs for describing the laboratory findings are used at the Department of Cardiology following the recommendations and guidelines issued by the Hungarian Ministry of Health in accordance with European guidelines and WHO recommendations. The programs are in English offering English initialisms (e.g. *MCHC, prothrombin INR*) for laboratory examinations and for their measurements. Physicians, who wrote the studied discharge reports, however, use the uppercase *L* not only in the Results section but also in other non-program generated sections of these reports.

5.1.1.2. Punctuation

The appearance and usage of punctuation marks varies between languages, but they have a common function, they clarify the meaning of the written text. Punctuation marks are symbols that indicate the structure and organization of a written language (e.g. colon, comma, question mark, brackets, hyphen, or quotation marks). Punctuation is placed in the text to make meaning clear and to make reading easier. The various punctuation marks perform four functions: they separate, group or enclose, connect and impart meaning. The function of a punctuation mark is the basis for the rules governing its use and should be the basis for determining whether or not it is needed. The cardiology discharge report is a text type that involves little comprehensive text and is built up mainly of sentence fragments, references, initialisms, but few complete, complex sentences can be found in it. Very little punctuation is used, and when it is, the punctuation marks that occur are mainly commas, periods, parentheses and slashes.

Generally, English uses fewer punctuation marks, especially fewer commas than Hungarian, and the use of the colon and the semi-colon is also slightly different (Klaudy 1997). Hospital discharge reports are, however, not appropriate texts for detecting the changes in the use of these punctuation marks due to their specific characteristics. Only certain punctuation marks and the difference in their use compared to the standard Hungarian punctuation rules can be distinguished. I will discuss only changes in the use of the decimal separator and the quotation marks.

Punctuation marks themselves are mainly discussed within grammatical features of a language, but I follow the line of certain contact linguists (e.g. Ammon 1998, Görlach 2001 and Alcaraz and Navarro 2006) and discuss them among orthographic features.

5.1.1.2.1. The decimal separator

The symbol used to separate the integral part of a decimal number from its fractional part is called the decimal point. A decimal comma is used not only in continental Europe (www.mathworld.wolfram.com) but in most of North and South America (with the exception of the United States and Canada), and also in most of Africa (Wells 1986). The decimal comma is the standard variant for describing decimal values in Hungary. However, we must mention that it is a relatively new variant that was introduced only in the 1950s, most probably as the result of German language contact (Deme 1956; Náray-Szabó and Sztáray 2001).

Physicians almost exclusively use the decimal point in Hungarian cardiology discharge reports instead of the decimal comma, e.g. *triglicerid 1.16, glükóz 5.2.*

As most decimal fractions are mentioned in the "Results of laboratory findings" section of the discharge report, we may explain the exclusive use of the decimal point with the fact that certain standardized programs for describing the laboratory findings are used at the department of cardiology (see 5.1.1.2.1). The programs are in English offering English initialisms (e.g. *MCHC, prothrombin INR*) for laboratory examinations and the decimal point in figures for normal ranges. However, physicians who write these discharge reports use the English orthography for expressing the decimal separator in other sections of the discharge report as well, e.g. in the Physical examination section: *testsúly: 83.5 kg*, or in the Past medical history section: *1-1.5 mm-es ST-depressio mutatkozott* 'a 1-1.5 mm ST depression was recorded', *kb. 1.5 éve* 'approximately 1.5 year ago'.

5.1.1.2.2. Quotation marks

Quotation marks are punctuation marks used in pairs to set off speech, a quotation, a phrase, or a word. According to current recommendation by the Hungarian Academy of Sciences (A magyar helyesírás szabályai 2000) the main Hungarian quotation marks are comma-shaped double quotation marks set on the base-line at the beginning of the quote and at apostrophe-height at the end of it for first level: „…". In English, however, they come as a pair of opening and closing marks in either of two styles: single '. . .' or double ". . .".

Some instances of the use of the English type of quotation marks are found in the Hungarian cardiology discharge reports, almost exclusively when determining the blood group: *Vércsoport:"A" Rh pozitív* 'Blood group: "A" Rh positive' but also in some other cases when the physician wants to indicate that he/she uses a'foreign' term, e.g. *"Sheperd's crook" anatómiával* 'with "Shepherd's crook" anatomy'.

5.1.1.3. Discussion on the change of orthographic features

Interference features can be found in all linguistic subsystems: phonetics, phonology, orthography, morphology, syntax, lexical semantics, discourse and even narrative structure. The more intense the contact, the more kinds of linguistic features can turn up as interference features. Features that are deeply embedded in interlocking structures are in general less likely to be borrowed, because they are less likely to fit into the recipient language's structures; that is why inflectional morphology tends to be borrowed last (Thomason 2003).

There is an increasing, very intense language contact between non-English speaking scientists and the English speaking scientific world (mainly through reading), and as English is the medium of international communication in the medical sciences with a very high prestige among researching physicians, several English language contact-induced features can be seen even at the level of orthography in international medical writing (Ammon 1994).

Several types of Englishisms are used in the Hungarian cardiology discharge reports I analyze showing the desire of the writers of these reports to satisfy the requirements of the profession in view of language use as well. Pseudo-Englishisms or hypercorrections can also be found (*enoxaparol, plack*) that might be the compensatory technique for the lack of high English proficiency. Lanstyák and Szabómihály (2005), however, claim that hypercorrect forms (like these) are not cases of borrowing, but rather by-products of the borrowing process.

Re-Englishizations are common linguistic phenomena in the discharge reports, the phenomena denoted by *attack, block, diffuse, shock* and *test* are very frequently referred to and described in cardiology. They may be assimilated to the Hungarian morphological system, i.e. they may act as root words in accordance with Hungarian syntactic rules, or as roots taking over Hungarian suffixes (cf. *blockoló* 'blocker'). Complete morphological assimilation of English loanwords, which still remain unassimilated orthographically, is a special feature of scientific writing, where the writers of the texts are bilingual in Hungarian and English, and widespread borrowing has become common in their institutional language use.

When a term has been encountered (read or heard) and learned in English first, the meaning is more directly accessible in English, even if there is an available Hungarian equivalent (assimilated borrowing or calque). This may be particularly true in case of complex professional and academic terms (e.g. *heads-up tilt table test, overdrive pace*). But the terms above (cf. *attack, block, diffuse, shock* and *test*) do not belong to this very technical vocabulary, they are used in more than one meaning also in the non-technical Hungarian language, as well as in several fields of science, e.g. *attak* is used in the language of the army, the media or industry, *plakk* is used in dentistry and in the chemical industry, and the term *teszt* is used in each field of sciences as well as various domains of education, industry, management or catering. Re-Englishizations should be, therefore, explained by other factors, the most important of which can be the social factors, especially the scientific dominance and prestige of the English language over the Hungarian language of medicine with all the scientific achievements, research, and publications behind it.

The influence of these social factors has been increasing in recent years, which may be proved by the appearance of these words in the Hungarian dictionaries: *attack, block, diffuse, plaque, shock* are given as accepted variants of *attak, blokk, diffúz, plakk* and *sokk* in BISZ (2006) and BOSZ (2006) but OHSZ (1992), however, gives both variants, always directing/redirecting the reader to the assimilated variant of the word, and TESZ (1967) gives only the assimilated forms of *attak*, *blokk* and *sokk.* Instances of morphological hypercorrection or the appearance of morphological pseudo-Englishisms can also support the idea of the strong prestige of the English language.

Changes in punctuation are also due to intense written language contact between English and Hungarian. The contact-induced use of English punctuation marks is quite common among translators when translating from English into their native tongue (personal teaching experience). It can be considered as a case of code-switching. But among physicians it does not seem to be a random phenomenon, as the changes in the use of the decimal separator and the quotation marks detailed above are among the most frequently identified English language contact-induced changes in the cardiology discharge reports.

Seeing the English orthography regularly during analyzing laboratory findings, physicians may be under a heavy influence of the English language (close written contact and the prestige factor) that leads them to use the English orthography both in certain cases of capitalization (uppercase letter L for *liter*) and in punctuation. As Hungarian medical texts (textbooks, reference books or research articles) are seen by them less frequently than English texts, they may consider the English orthography to be the requirement and to be the only acceptable variant.

5.1.2. Contact-induced changes in the lexicon

There has been wide-scale technological innovation and scientific progress in the field of cardiology since the last decade of the 20th century; therefore, the results of medical advances – new investigational and surgical techniques, therapeutic options and even recently identified abnormal conditions – should be given an appropriate technical name. Untermann (1978) identifies seven ways of coining new terms for new phenomena in the language of medicine:

- borrowing,
- the use of proper nouns (eponyms and trade names),
- non-technical words becoming established in technical usage,
- compounding and suffixal derivation,
- the formation of free compounds: noun and determiner,
- Greek and Latin based neologisms, and
- the use of abbreviations and acronyms or formulae.

Based on the results of my research into Hungarian cardiology discharge reports I concluded that examples for each type of 'term formation' can be found in the Hungarian language of cardiology. When I studied the Hungarian lexicon of cardiology through the discharge reports, I focused on only those instances of term formation which were induced by English language contact.

Lexical borrowings form the largest group of all language contact-induced features. Borrowed lexical features involve various English morphemes. In close contact situations both free and bound morphemes are borrowed (Thomason 2003). In USZCCDR, the majority of borrowed morphemes are, however, free morphemes.

As the language of medicine is based on Latin (and Greek), several medical words have Latin origin and they are composed of Latin or Latinate elements. These words, however, cannot be considered Latin borrowings, they are rather the members of the international scientific vocabulary (ISV). ISV words in the Hungarian language of medicine involve words such as *hormon* 'hormone' and *vitamin* 'vitamin', etc. Other Latin origin words were borrowed into Hungarian earlier, but recently they have become more widely and frequently used as an indirect effect of their frequent use in the English language of medicine, e.g. *detektál* 'detect', *elongál* 'elongate', *pozicionál* 'position'. The spread of Latinisms or Re-Latinization can be attributed to the renaissance of the Latin culture, and the increasing intercultural exchange of terms. Latin can be used as a common source language for borrowing and term formation, especially in technical languages, thus, national languages share and mutually encourage the use of Latinisms that are described as internationalisms. Recent linguistic research highlights that the Latinate words are in fact borrowed via scientific English (Fábián 1991; Taavitsainen 2001; Nádasdy 2002). Latinisms/internationalisms make international communication easier and are vitally used in national technical languages (Pogarell and Schröder 1999). However, not every linguist shares this concept (Skutnabb-Kangas 1984, 1996; Phillipson 2003) thinking of it as a form of linguistic globalization, and purists also consider it another form of English language globalization, i.e. hidden Englishization (Zimányi 2003; Bősze 2009).

Lexical morphemes may be introduced into Hungarian directly via code-switching from English, and then changing from code-switches to borrowings through increasingly frequent usage by the code-switching speakers (in our case, by Hungarian cardiologists). As not all members of the discourse community engage in code-switching (e.g. family physicians are not necessarily fluent speakers of English beside Hungarian), borrowings are adopted by them and other non-bilingual speakers (cf. Thomason 2003). It is a very common way of the incorporation of English words into the Hungarian language of medicine.

The level of integration in phonology is determined by the degree of similarity and dissimilarity between the phonological systems of the source and recipient languages. Filipović (1996) provides three terms to account for the changes that can occur when integrating an English loanword on phonological level: zero transphonemisation, partial or compromise transphonemisation, and free transphonemisation. When there is no difference between the phonological systems (zero transphonemisation), the Englishism is pronounced according to the Hungarian language pronunciation. In 'partial' or 'compromise transphonemisation' some elements of the Hungarian language differ in phonological description from the English, the pronunciation of the borrowed item is only partially the same as the English source word. In 'free transphonemisation', when elements of the English source word do not have any equivalents in the Hungarian language, the substitution is free.

Hungarian is a language in which orthography is dominantly based on pronunciation, so the spelling rules of morphemes are determined by the pronunciation used by speakers of 'standard' Hungarian. Whereas in the case of English, there is a certain lack of correspondence between graphemes and phonemes, morphemes sometimes have several phonetic forms, depending on the context in which they occur.

No phonological examination was undertaken in the present study, as Method 1 is based on the analysis of written corpora and Method 2 focuses on attitudes toward language contact-induced change. Thus, no further description of literature on phonological changes is discussed here.

The majority of borrowed English terms reveal themselves as foreign because of their orthography. Some of the 'older layers' of English borrowings are both orthographically and morphologically fully assimilated loanwords, e.g. *koktél* 'coctail', *meccs* 'match', *penicillin* 'penicillin' or *teszt* 'test'. They are identified by *A magyar nyelv történeti-etimológiai szótára* (TESZ) [Historico-etymological dictionary of the Hungarian language] as English loanwords that were borrowed in 1822, 1879, 1929 and 1912, respectively. More recent borrowings are mostly not fully assimilated in both aspects, i.e. both orthographically and morphologically.

On the orthographical level, the borrowed item can be formed on the basis of the pronunciation of the corresponding source word, it may follow the orthography of the source word without any change, follow partly the pronunciation and partly the spelling of the borrowed source item in either order, or it can be formed under the influence of an intermediary language through which the English source word has passed on its way to the receiving language (Filipović 1996).

Hungarian (H) uses the Latin script, thus, it has many items in which the Latin graphemes correlate with phonemes corresponding closely to their English (E) equivalents. Such words are taken over without changes. However, certain English graphemes are missing or at least are extremely rare in Hungarian, thus, grapheme replacement (e.g. of *ch, q, th, x, y* or *w*) may occur.

Integration of loanwords on the morphological level can be described similarly to phonological changes by three processes according to Filipović (1996):

'zero transmorphemisation', when there is no morphological assimilation,

'partial transmorphemisation', when the English word retains the English suffix of the source word, or

'complete transmorphemisation', where the original suffix of the English word is completely replaced by a corresponding native suffix

Hungarian is a Finno-Ugric language with typical Uralic morphology in most respects. It makes extensive use of morphological processes. It is agglutinative, as it tends to use a separate affix for each morpheme. Hungarian is almost exclusively suffixing, and suffixes are used both in derivation and in the elaborate inflectional systems for nouns and verbs (Fenyvesi 2005). Being an Indo-European language, English, however, has flexional morphology, but it does not hinder the adoption of English words by Hungarian speakers.

Hungarian nominals inflect for number, case and person – the person of the possessor. The Hungarian case system is very rich with several semantically diverse cases such as the comitative and 9 different locative (e.g. inessive, elative, illative and suppressive) cases – altogether between 17 and 27 cases, depending on how case is defined (Kenesei et al. 1998). In English, however, there is limited noun inflection (cf. possessive *'s* and plural *-s*). The Hungarian language entirely lacks gender, and English has gender distinction in only 3rd person singular personal pronouns.

Hungarian verbs inflect through the grammatical dimensions of person, number, tense and mood, and Hungarian makes more use of morphological derivation, whereas, English uses more analytic constructions in expressing similar distinctions (Thomason 2005).

Thus, adoption and adaptation of morphemes from English into Hungarian is salient, but due to the morphological differences between the two languages certain features are not transferred at all or only with much restriction.

Considering the process of lexical borrowing, I am mostly following the categorization set up by Haugen (1950), Weinreich (1953), Kontra (1981) and Lanstyák (2006). Contact-induced lexical and semantic changes are classified as external borrowings, i.e. borrowings from English or from other languages via English, and internal borrowings (this particular type of borrowing is not analyzed in the present study as it does not involve the English language). External borrowings are further divided into three categories: the borrowing of loanwords (see Section 5.1.1), loan substitutions/hybrid loans, i.e. semantic loans (see Section 5.1.2), and pseudo-loans. Pseudo-loans are not discussed in details as I have found only two borrowings of this category: *enoxiparol* and *plack*. They are described in Orthographic changes in Section 5.1.1.

Considering the process of borrowing, loanwords are subcategorized based on the assimilation of the English word into the Hungarian language: loanwords proper (see Section 5.2.1) and assimilated loans (see Section 5.2.2).

English language contact-induced lexical features from USZCCDR are discussed according to the above described classification:

loanwords

loanword proper — assimilated loanword

Poplack and Meechan highlight that lexical borrowing involves mainly "major-class content words such as nouns, verbs, and adjectives" (1998: 127). USZCCDR also supported their claim. In the next three sections I analyze nouns (Section 5.1.2.1.), adjectives (Section 5.1.2.2.) and verbs (Section 5.1.2.3) that have been identified as being English loanwords in the Hungarian cardiology discharge reports I have studied. Considering the word class of the identified items in USZCCDR, loanwords proper involve nouns and adjectives, and assimilated loanwords involve nouns, adjectives and verbs.

5.1.2.1. Loanwords proper

In this book the discussed loanwords proper are words and phrases that are transferred from the English language (of medicine) to the Hungarian language of cardiology with no orthographic or morphemic substitution. 57 loanwords proper have been identified in the discharge reports which are nouns (n= 47) and adjectives (n=10). Verbs appear only in the form of assimilated loans in USZCCDR.

Most borrowed English terms can be identified as loanwords due to their orthography. Therefore, at least in theory, we have to distinguish between the 'borrowing process', i.e. when the borrowed term enters the recipient language, and 'consecutive process', i.e. when the borrowed term undergoes phonological, orthographic, morphological and semantic changes. Phonological changes are not discussed in this book. English loanwords proper have not undergone orthographic changes (yet) but some of them are affected by morphological and semantic changes (see Table 9 below).

5.1.2.1.1. Noun loanwords proper

Generally nouns form the largest class of loanwords in borrowing, commonly over 80 per cent (Görlach 2002b). Medical language has been dominated by nouns both in ancient and in modern times (Langslow 2004). According to my results based on the corpus of 234 Hungarian cardiology discharge reports (total number of words: 216,703) the number of borrowed noun loanwords proper compared to all borrowed items (except for acronyms and abbreviations)[45] is around 80 per cent.

My data show that nouns clearly outnumber the other two categories, which could be explained in two different ways. First, as Bernsten (1990: 76) reports "nouns are typically most common, reflecting the high percentage of signifiers for new objects and concepts". This could be the case in the studied medical text type, the hospital discharge report, since the register/text type is directly related to the naming of diseases, medical interventions, findings and management. Second, as Sager et al. (1980) claim, nouns are typically found in those pieces of discourse in which not actions but the transmission of ideas is intended (as is again the case of the reports under investigation). In this respect, individual

45 Borrowed acronyms and abbreviations are discussed in Section 5.1.2.2. Numerically they constitute the largest group of English borrowed items in my corpus. But counting their percentage here would be misleading.

lexical items may become register markers in a topically-restricted register (Biber 1995).

Noun loanwords proper from the reports are given in Table 7 with the source language they were borrowed from (English proper borrowings, members of the international scientific vocabulary (ISV) or originating in other languages but having been borrowed into the Hungarian medical vocabulary via English), examples taken from USZCCDR, and if they are listed in BISZ, EKSZ, TESZ, ZESZ, BOSZ, LEM and OHSZ, and their prevalence in MIK (for the abbreviations see Section 5.1).

Table 7. English noun loanwords proper in the studied corpus

Borrowed term	**Source language**	**Examples from the studied corpus**	**BISZ**	**EKSZ**	**TESZ**	**ZESZ**	**BOSZ**	**LEM**	**OHSZ**	**MIK (n)**
(acetyl-salicylic) acid*	E	*acetylsalicylic acid*	Ø	Ø	Ø	Ø	Ø	Ø	Ø	Ø
arrest	L via E	*sinus arrest*	(+)	Ø	Ø	Ø	Ø	Ø	Ø	Ø
attack*	E	*transiens ischaemias attack* 'transient ischemic attack'	(+)	+	(+)	Ø	+	(+)	(+)	Ø [in 1799]
beat	E	*beat to beat, fusion beat*	(+)	(+)	Ø	Ø	Ø	Ø	Ø	(347)
block*	E	*pitvar-kamrai block* 'atrio-ventricular block'	(+)	+	(+)	(+)	+	Ø	(+)	6
branch	E	*postbranch szűkület* 'postbranch stricture'	(+)	+	(+)	Ø	Ø	Ø	Ø	Ø
burst	E	*extrastimulá-ció illetve burst során* 'during extra-stimulation or burst'	Ø	Ø	Ø	Ø	Ø	Ø	Ø	Ø
bypass	E	*bypass operáció* 'bypass operation', *aorto-coronalis bypass műtét* 'aorto-coronary bypass operation'	+	Ø	Ø	Ø	+	Ø	+	Ø
chloride*	E	*potassium chloride*	(+)	+	(+)	Ø	Ø	Ø	Ø	Ø
cholesterol*	E	*cholesterol polipok* 'cholesterol polyps'	(+)	Ø	Ø	Ø	(+)	Ø	(+)	Ø
end stage	E	*end stage ishaemiás cardio-myopathia* 'end stage ischemic	Ø	Ø	Ø	Ø	(+)	Ø	(+)	Ø

		cardio-myopathy'								
enoxaparin*	ISV	*enoxaparin (Clexane) 2xl ml sc.*	Ø	Ø	Ø	Ø	Ø	Ø	Ø	Ø
enoxaparol*	(pseudo-)E	*Enoxaparol sodium*	Ø	Ø	Ø	Ø	Ø	Ø	Ø	Ø
entrainment	Fr via E	*entrainment mapping alapján* 'on the basis of entrainment mapping', *entrainmentet sikerült elérni* 'we managed to perform entrainment'	Ø	Ø	Ø	Ø	Ø	Ø	Ø	Ø
flow	E	*TIMI 1-2 flow látható* 'TIMI 1-2 flow can be seen, *lassult flow-t láttak* 'slowed flow was visualized', *a flowt nem limitálja* 'flow is not limited'	Ø	Ø	Ø	Ø	(+)	Ø	Ø	Ø
follow up	E	*follow up során* 'during follow up'	Ø	Ø	Ø	Ø	Ø	Ø	Ø	Ø
graft	E	*véna graft* 'vein graft', *grafttal* 'with graft', *homografton keresztül*'via homograft'	+	Ø	Ø	Ø	+	Ø	+	Ø
kinking	E	*kinking a jobb carotis internán* 'kinking in the right internal carotid artery'	Ø	Ø	Ø	Ø	+	Ø	Ø	Ø
levo-thyroxine*	E	*levothyroxine sodium*	Ø	Ø	Ø	Ø	Ø	Ø	Ø	Ø
mapping	E	*entrainment mapping alapján* 'on the basis of entrainment mapping'	+	Ø	Ø	Ø	+	Ø	Ø	Ø
monitor	L via E 1865 TESZ	*ABPM monitor, többparamé-teres monitorizálás* 'multi-parameter monitoring', *Holter monitorizálása* 'Holter monitoring'	+	+	(+)	+	Ø	Ø	+	40 [in 1877/ 1979]
pace	E	*kamrai pace szünteti* 'it is ceased by ventricular pace, *Overdrive paceléssel* 'with Overdrive pacing', *intracardialis*	Ø	Ø	Ø	Ø	Ø	Ø	Ø	Ø

		high rate pacelést követően 'after intracardiac high rate pacing'								
pacemaker	E	*pacemaker beültetés* 'pacemeker implantation', *pacemakerek* 'pacemakers'	+	+	Ø	Ø	+	Ø	+	2 [in 1976]
penicillin	ISV 1948 TESZ	*gyógyszerei: penicillin* 'Medications: penicillin', *cave penicillin* 'penicillin allergy'	+	+	+	+	+	+	+	12 [in 1961]
plack*	E	*vastag plack látható* 'a thick plaque is visible'	(+)	Ø	Ø	Ø	(+)	Ø	(+)	Ø
plaque*	E	*rajta egy-egy meszes plaque* 'with one or two plaques on it'	(+)	Ø	Ø	Ø	+	Ø	+	Ø
potassium	ISV	*potassium, potassium chloride*	+	Ø	Ø	Ø	+	+	+	1 [in 1795]
puff	E	*3x1 puff Atrovent, Nitrát puff hatására* 'due to a Nitrate puff'	+	(+)	(+)	(+)	+	Ø	Ø	(376)
pull-back	E	*pull-back során* 'during pull-back'	(+)	Ø	Ø	Ø	Ø	Ø	Ø	Ø
recovery	E	*recovery során* 'during recovery', *eseménytelen recovery* 'uneventful recovery'	Ø	Ø	Ø	Ø	Ø	Ø	Ø	(2)
reentry	E	*AV-csomó reentry indult* 'AV-node reentry was initiated', *macroreentry*	(+)	Ø	Ø	Ø	Ø	Ø	Ø	(3)
scan	E	*natív scanek készültek* 'plain scans were performed', *scaneken* 'in the scans'	(+)	Ø	Ø	Ø	(+)	Ø	(+)	Ø
sense / oversensing	E	*jó sense mellett* 'with good sense', *átmeneti T hullám oversensing miatt* 'due to temporary T wave oversensing'	Ø	Ø	Ø	Ø	Ø	Ø	Ø	10 [in 1943]
shock*	E	*shock terápia* 'shock therapy'	(+)	(+)	(+)	(+)	+	Ø	+	4 [in 1979]
shunt*	Re-Englishization	*shunt műtét* 'shunting operation'	+	(+)	Ø	Ø	+	Ø	(+)	Ø

sludge	E	*sludgeképződés látható* 'sludge formation can be visualized'	Ø	Ø	Ø	Ø	Ø	Ø	Ø	Ø
sodium	ISV	*Enoxaparol sodium, Levothyroxine sodium*	+	Ø	Ø	Ø	+	+	(+)	Ø
spike	E	*pacemaker spike-ok* 'pacemaker spikes', *inefectiv spikeokat láttak* 'we have seen inefective spikes'	Ø	Ø	Ø	Ø	Ø	Ø	(+)	1 [in 1984]
spray	E	*nitrolingual spray, sprayre szűnt* 'was ceased by spray'	+	+	Ø	Ø	+	Ø	+	7 [in 1973]
stent	E	*stent beültetés* 'stent implantation', *Lekton motion stent vezetődrótttal* 'with Lekton motion stent guidewire', *a stentben* 'in the stent', *stenttől* 'from the stent', *stentet* 'stent (accusative)', *stentelést végeztünk* 'we have performed stenting'	Ø	Ø	Ø	Ø	+	Ø	Ø	(11)
stroke	E	*minor stroke, iscaemias stroke* 'ischemic stroke'	+	+	Ø	Ø	Ø	Ø	Ø	(1)
study	E	*kamrai study* 'ventricular study', *studyt végeztünk* 'a study was performed'	Ø	Ø	Ø	Ø	Ø	Ø	Ø	8 [in 1991]
tamponade	Fr via E	*tamponade jelek nem észlelhetőek* 'no tamponade signs are visible'	(+)	(+)	Ø	Ø	(+)	Ø	Ø	Ø
team	E	*gastroenteroló gus-sebész-onkológus team* 'gastro-enterologist-surgical-oncological team', *onkoteam* 'oncoteam'	+	Ø	Ø	Ø	Ø	Ø	Ø	6 [in 1986]
test*		*predischarge test*	(+)	(+)	(+)	(+)	(+)	Ø	(+)	Ø
upgrade	E	*upgrade céljából* 'to perform an upgrade',	(+)	Ø	Ø	Ø	Ø	Ø	Ø	Ø

		biventricularis upgrade 'biventricular upgrade'								
vitamin	ISV 1922 TESZ	*vitamin B complex, vitamin C*	+	+	+	+	+	+	+	151 [in 1933]

Abbreviations and symbols used: E: English, F: French, G: German, ISV: international scientific vocabulary, L: Latin, +: the morpheme is listed in the given reference dictionary with the same orthography, (+): the morpheme is listed in the given reference dictionary/corpus with different orthography/with different sememe, Ø: the morpheme is not listed in the given reference dictionary/corpus, [] first written datum.
*marked items are discussed in 5.1.1.

Arrest is listed in BISZ giving Latin as the source of borrowing in the form of *arrestál* with the meaning *letartóztat* 'arrest'. The other Hungarian reference dictionaries contained no data on this item, and there was no match found for *arrest* in MIK. MMD defines the term only in a verbal meaning: *to withstand, to inhibit, restrain, or stop (the course of a disease).* DMD gives a nominal meaning of the term as well: *cessation or stoppage, as of a function or a disease process,* and it specifies the meaning of *arrest* for cardiology as well: *Sinus arrest: a pause in the normal cardiac rhythm due to a momentary failure of the sinus node to initiate an impulse, lasting for an interval that is not an exact multiple of the normal cardiac cycle.* In USZCCDR, the word is used in only one context: *sinus arrest.*

Beat is listed in BISZ and EKSZ in the form of *beat* with giving English as the source of borrowing, used in one meaning *beatzene* 'beat music'. The other Hungarian reference dictionaries contained no data on this item, MIK gives 347 matches for *beat* but all in the meaning *beatzene.* MMD defines *beat* as *the mechanical contraction or electrical activity of the heart muscle, which may be detected and recorded as the pulse or on the electrocardiogram, respectively.* The loanword is used in cardiology in the same meaning (e.g. website www.noise.physx.u-szeged.hu: *beat to beat: folyamatos ütésenkénti analízis* 'beat to beat: continuous analysis during each beat').

Branch is listed in BISZ in the form of *branch* with giving English as the source of borrowing, used in one meaning: *elágazás* 'branch', a word used in informatics, and in TESZ (1848) it is derived from French in the meaning of *faág, elágazás* 'branch of a tree, branching' and EKSZ gives the word as *brancs* (*érdekcsoport*) 'syndicate'. The other Hungarian reference dictionaries contained no data on this item, MIK gives 10 matches for *branch* but these are not relevant as they are all fragments of a different word. MMD defines *branch* as *an offshoot arising from the main trunk of a nerve or blood vessel.* The loanword is also used in this meaning (cf. website www.pirula.net: *branch: ág, ramus*). USZCCDR contained the word as a compound: *postbranch*, which is composed of a Latin prefix (*post-*) and the English word root.

Burst is not listed in any of the referred Hungarian dictionaries, and no match was found for it in MIK. MMD defines *burst* in a verbal meaning: *to break suddenly while under tension or expansion. Burst* is used in the Hungarian language of cardiology for *sorozatos külső ingerület* 'serial external stimuli' (Gábor Marton, M.D. personal communication in 2010), as *antitachycardia-ingerlés típusa* 'a type of antitachycardiac stimulus' (see website www.portal.tmkorhaz.hu). *Burst* has undergone a semantic change (narrowing) compared to the English lexeme.

Bypass is listed in BISZ as an English borrowing and the entry directs us to the 2nd meaning of *sönt* (2 ér között kóros vagy mesterségesen létesített összeköttetés 'abnormal or artificial connection between two vessels'). BOSZ gives that it is an English borrowing see *shunt* (cf. *sönt* is not listed), in the meaning of *műtéttípus, áthidalás* 'a type of operation, bypass'. DMD defines bypass as *an auxiliary flow; a shunt; a surgically created pathway circumventing the normal anatomical pathway, such as in an artery or the intestine*. It has a separate entry for *(coronary artery) bypass* that is *a section of vein or other conduit grafted between the aorta and a coronary artery distal to an obstructive lesion in the latter.* In Hungarian bypass is used to mean *érprotézis, áthidaló, elkerülő műtét* 'vessel prosthesis, shunting, bypass operation (cf. website www.hazipatika.com). Both the orthographic form and the semantic fields are kept during the borrowing process, as there is no semantic change compared to the medical meaning of the word.

End stage is not listed in any of the referred Hungarian dictionaries, and no match was found for it in MIK. However, BOSZ and OHSZ have an entry for *end-to-end anastomosis* containing the first morpheme of the borrowed compound. AMHD has an entry for *end stage* meaning *the final phase of a terminal disease.* The compound is used in the same meaning in cardiology: *végső állapot* 'end stage' (cf. website www.pirula.net *end stage – végső állapot pl. betegségnél* 'e.g. of a disease').

Entrainment is not listed in any of the referred Hungarian dictionaries, and no match was found for it in MIK. Entrainment is a French loanword in English. DMD gives two sememes: **1.** *a technique for identifying the slowest pacing necessary to terminate an arrhythmia, particularly atrial flutter.* **2.** *the synchronization and control of cardiac rhythm by an external stimulus.* In Hungarian it is used to describe *a re-entry tachycardiák (anatómiai hátterének) felderítése-térképezése elektromos ingerek/ingersorok leadásával és az erre adott válasz vizsgálatával* 'mapping of (the anatomical background of) reentry tachycardia by stimulus/series of stimulus and examining the reactions' (Gábor Marton, M.D., personal communication in 2010).

Flow is not listed in any of the referred Hungarian dictionaries, and no match was found for it in MIK. BOSZ, however, has an entry for *flowmetria* meaning *adott érszakaszon átáramló vérmennyiség mérése* 'measuring the amount of blood flowing through a certain vessel segment' giving that it is an English (flow) and Latin (-metria) compound. DMD gives two sememes for *flow*: **1.** *the movement of a liquid or gas,* **2.** *the rate at which a fluid passes through an organ or part, expressed as volume per unit of time.* In Hungarian it is used to mean *áramlás* but only for the *flow of the blood.* Thus there is semantic narrowing of Hungarian *flow.* This is one of the most frequently used lexical borrowing in cardiology discharge reports. There is no orthographic assimilation but the borrowed word underwent morphological assimilation (cf. *flow-t láttak* 'flow was seen', *meglassult flow-val* 'with slowed flow', *a flowt nem limitálja* 'flow is not limited') The suffix is added either hyphenated or unhyphenated.

Follow up is not listed in any of the referred Hungarian dictionaries, and no match was found for it in MIK. *Follow up* is entered by Collins English Dictionary (Complete and Unabridged 6th Edition 2003) with two meanings, the second of which is defined as being medical **2.** *(Medicine) a routine examination of a patient at various intervals after medical or surgical treatment.* In Hungarian it is used in the meaning of *folyamatos ellenőrzés* 'on-going control', cf. website http://webio.hu folyamatos ellenőrzés (follow-up). The sememe used in medicine is borrowed without changes in the semantic field.

Graft is listed in BISZ as an English loanword with the meaning *átültetett szövet* 'transplanted tissue'. BOSZ defines it as *átültetett szerv vagy szövet, transzplantátum* 'transplanted organ or tissue, a transplant'. MIK provides no matches for *graft*. DMD contains *graft* with two meanings (nominal and verbal meaning): **1.** *any tissue or organ for implantation or transplantation,* **2.** *to implant or transplant such tissues*. In USZCCDR, *graftol* was not used, thus only the nominal sememe was borrowed. *Graft* is also used in a compound: *autograft*, *homograft*, and morphological assimilation (the Hungarian suffix was added unhyphenated) is also found: *grafttal* 'with graft'.

Kinking is listed only in BOSZ, in the meaning *kanyargós, spirális lefutás (pl. éré)* 'twisted, spiral course (e.g. of a vessel)'. It is not listed in the other referred Hungarian dictionaries, and no match was found for it in MIK. MMD defines *kinking* as a *bending or twisting*. In Hungarian this loanword is used with the same meaning.

Mapping is listed in BISZ in the form *map*, which is an English loanword used in informatics: *leképzett egységek elrendezése* 'arrangement of mapped units'. BOSZ lists only *brain mapping*. MMD defines *mapping* as *the process of locating the relative position of genes on a chromosome through the analysis of genetic recombination. Distances between genes in a linkage group are expressed in map units or organs.* In Hungarian the word *mapping* is used in the same meaning.

Monitor is a borrowing taken over from Latin via English. BISZ gives three different sememes, the third of which is related to the medical meaning: *képernyő* 'screen'. ZESZ gives that it was first printed in a Hungarian document is 1869, and defines it as an international word that was spread via American English in the meaning *kis csatahajó* 'a smaller battleship' and in 1958 in telecommunications, and recently with the meaning *számítógépek képernyője* 'monitor of a computer' (also in EKSZ). TESZ gives another meaning of the word: *figyelmeztető, intő* 'warning'. BOSZ gives no match for monitor, but website http://webio.hu says that *monitoring* means *betegkövetés* 'follow up of the patient's state of health'. DMD gives only verbal meanings of monitor, but it also gives a specialized meaning: *Holter monitor* is a *portable continuous electrocardiographic recorder used to detect the frequency and duration of rhythm disturbances*. Monitor is used in USZCCDR as a noun, e.g. *ABPM monitor,* and as a morphologically assimilated suffixed noun: *monitorizálás* 'monitoring' (cf. *többparaméteres monitorizálás* 'multiparameter monitoring', *Holter monitorizálása* 'Holter monitoring').

Pace is not listed in any of the referred Hungarian dictionaries, and no match was found for it in MIK. DMD gives a specialized meaning of pace: *cardiac pacing is the regulation of the rate of contraction of the heart muscle by an artificial cardiac pacemaker.*

In English the word form *pacing* is used for the sememe of the Hungarian *pace*. Pace is very frequently used in Hungarian cardiology discharge reports, e.g *60/min kamrai fr.-jú pace ritmus* '60/min frequency ventricular pacing', *kamrai pace szünteti* 'ceased by ventricular pacing', *effektív kamrai pace* 'effective ventricular pacing'. It was morphologically assimilated: *pacelés* 'pacing', *pacelési* 'of pacing', and used as a noun after the word root *pace* was added to the thematizing verbal suffix *-(e)l* and the nominalizing suffix *-és*.

Pacemaker is listed in BISZ with the meaning *ütemszabályozó* 'pacemaker' as a medical word borrowed from the English language. BOSZ also gives the meaning *ütemszabályozó* but adds *a szív (esetleg más szerv) ingerképzését szabályozó, az emberi testbe beültethető készülék* 'human implantable device that regulates the rhythm of the heart (or another organ)' (also in EKSZ). MIK give two matches for *pacemaker*. DMD defines *(artificial cardiac) pacemaker* as a *device designed to reproduce or regulate the rhythm of the heart.* This word is a compound of two English word roots, *pace* and *maker,* the first of which was also borrowed into Hungarian (see above) as such. Pacemaker is the most frequently used English loanword in the Hungarian cardiology discharge reports. It was morphologically assimilated as it is used in the plural: *pacemakerek* 'pacemakers'.

Penicillin is a Latin word that was borrowed via English, and BISZ defines it as *egyes ecsetpenész-gombafajok által termelt, fertőzőbetegségek* *kórokozójának szaporodását gátló antibiotikum* 'an antibiotic produced by certain penicillium fungi that inhibits the proliferation of infectious pathogens'. TESZ and ZESZ give that penicillin is an international scientific term that was borrowed from English. BOSZ and EKSZ give that *penicillin* is *a Penicillium notatum gomba által termelt bakteriosztatikus hatású antibiotikum* 'penicillin is a bacteriostatic antibiotic produced by the fungus Penicillum notatum'. MIK gives 12 matches for *penicillin*. DMD gives a longer definition by stating that it is *any of a large group of natural (p. G, p.V) or semisynthetic antibacterial antibiotics derived directly or indirectly from strains of fungi of the genus Penicillum and other soil-inhabiting fungi, which exert a bactericidal as well as a bacteriostatic effect on susceptible bacteria by interfering with the final stages of the synthesis of peptidoglycan, a substance in the bacterial cell wall.* This word is used in the "Drug allergies" and the "Medications" sections of the Hungarian cardiology discharge reports.

Potassium according to BISZ is the French and English name of *kálium*. BOSZ also gives that *potassium* is equivalent with *kálium*. LOZS has an entry for potassium explaining that it originates in Latin meaning *kálium*. In MIK there was one match for *potassium*. MMD gives that *potassium is the chemical element, at. no. 19.* Kálium, the Hungarian proper word is more frequently used in the discharge reports. There were 5 matches for *potassium* and 84 matches for *kálium* in USZCCDR.

Puff is given with 4 sememes in BISZ, EKSZ and TESZ (1834 but non-medical meaning) the third of which is a medical meaning (genetics) (in BISZ) but even that is different from the English meaning of *puff*. ZESZ gives the same sememes as BISZ. The second meaning given in BOSZ is *inhalációs adagolószerkezetből egy adag* 'one dose from an inhaler'. MIK gives 376 matches for *puff* but none in the meaning given by BOSZ. DMD gives that *puff* is *a brief sudden emission of air, vapor, or smoke*. In the Hungarian cardiology discharge reports *puff* is used in the Medications section to describe the administration of the medicine, e.g. *3x1 puff Atrovent.*

Pull-back is not listed in any of the referred Hungarian dictionaries, and no match was found for it in MIK, though BISZ contains the word *pull* that is a sport term borrowed from English. AHMD has an entry on *pull back: to use a surgical instrument to hold open (the edges of a wound or an organ). To prevent any cold spot at ends, active source length can be elongated inside the vessel with application of one after the other. This technique is named pull back. In this technique, at first, distal part of the injured vessel is irradiated. Inflating a balloon in the main vessel before stenting the side branch (stent pull-back technique).*

In Hungarian it is used only as a noun: see website http://web.dote.hu *a szűkületen át visszahúzzuk az eszközt (pull back) a betegnek tartott érszakaszon* 'we pull back the device through the narrowed vessel segment', and no suffixes were added to it in the researced reports (e.g. *pull-back során* 'during pull back').

Recovery is not listed in any of the referred Hungarian dictionaries, but two matches were found for it in MIK with a different meaning. MMD gives two nominal meanings for *recovery*: **1.** *the return to a healthy state,* **2.** *the self-regulation and life force of a patient being returned to a normal balanced status. The patient is considered healthy again.*

In the Hungarian cardiology reports only the first sememe is borrowed, thus there is semantic narrowing, e.g. *recovery során* 'during recovery', *eseménytelen recovery* 'unevetful recovery'.

Reentry is not listed in any of the referred Hungarian dictionaries, except for BISZ where *entry point* is given as a word used in informatics. Three matches were found for it in MIK but in a different meaning. DMD defines it as *reexcitation of a region of cardiac tissue by a single impulse, continuing for one or more cycles and sometimes resulting in ectopic beats or tachyarrhythmias; it also requires refractoriness of the tissue to stimulation and an area of unidirectional block to conduction.* In Hungarian it is used for *rövidzárlatszerű visszacsatolási kör* 'short-circuitlike feedback' (Gábor Marton, M.D., personal communication in 2009). The term is frequently used in the researched corpus, e.g. *AV-csomó reentry indult* 'AV-node reentry was initiated', *macroreentry,* but no Hungarian suffixes are added to the word root.

Scan is not listed in any of the referred Hungarian dictionaries, only in the form of *scanner* and *scanning,* and no match was found for it in MIK. However, scan is a frequently used noun in the cardiology reports referring to the images performed at the department of cardiology. DMD gives both a verbal and a nominal meaning for *scan*: **1**. *to examine or map the body, or one or more organs or regions of it, by gathering information with a sensing device,* **2.** *the data or image so obtained.* In USZCCDR, *scan* is used only as a noun, but taking the Hungarian plural and superessive nominal suffixes, e.g. *natív scanek készültek* 'plain scans were performed', *scaneken* 'in the scans'.

Sense and ***oversensing*** are not listed in any of the referred Hungarian dictionaries, but MIK gives 10 matches for sense, 9 of which are related to a medical meaning. DMD gives two sememes for *sense*: **1.** *any of the physical processes by which stimuli are received, transduced, and conducted as impulses to be interpreted to the brain,* **2.** in molecular genetics, *referring to the strand of a nucleic acid that directly specifies the product.* In cardiology only the first sememe is used in USZCCDR (semantic narrowing). Website www.pirula.net says that *sense* is *érzék, sensus.* For *oversensing* DMD gives the definition: *the sensation of stimuli, such as magnetism or static electricity that are not normally detected by the sense organs.* Website http://www.lam.hu defines *oversensing* as *a pacemaker elektromos hibája/érzékelési zavar/túlérzékelés* 'electric fault/sensing problem/oversensing of the pacemaker'.

Sludge is not listed in any of the referred Hungarian dictionaries, and no match was found for it in MIK. DMD defines *sludge* as *a suspension of solid or semisolid particles in a fluid which itself may or may not be a truly viscous fluid.* In Hungarian there is semantic narrowing of this term, as it refers to *salakképződés (epehólyagban)* 'production of sludge (in the gall bladder)' according to the website www.mgyt.hu or *(epehólyagban található) üledék/sár/iszap* ' sediment/mud (found in the gall bladder)' (cf. website www.pirula.net). In USZCCDR, it was used to refer to this phenomenon in the gallbladder, e.g. *Cholecysta: benne sludgeképződés látható* 'cholecyst: sludge formation is visible'. *Sludge* is not used as a single morpheme but as a word root in a compound, where the second morpheme is a Hungarian word root.

Sodium is listed in BISZ with a Latin origin word meaning *nátrium*. BOSZ gives that it is *natrium*, as well as LOZS: Latin *natrium*.OHSZ has an entry only for *sodium excreting factor*, but not for *sodium* itself. DMD gives that *sodium* is *a chemical element, at. no. 11, symbol Na; the chief cation of extracellular body fluids.* Sodium is an example of Re-Englishization, like potassium, which is a relatively common phenomenon in the Hungarian language of medicine in case of chemical elements and compounds (see Section 5.1.1.1). In USZCCDR *sodium* is used only in the "Medications" section of the discharge reports (*natrium* n=57; sodium=9)

Spike is not listed in any of the referred Hungarian dictionaries, and no match was found for it in MIK. However, OHSZ has an entry for *spike and wave*. DMD describes *spike* in medicine as *a sharp upward deflection in a curve or tracing, as on the encephalogram*. The website www.medlist.com describes spike as *a pacemaker elektromos ingere* 'an electrical stimulus of the pacemaker'. In Hungarian *tüske* 'thorn/spike' is also used in cardiology (Gábor Marton, M.D., personal communication in 2009) to describe the same phenomenon, i.e. a calque for *spike*, but in USZCCDR I found no match for *tüske*. Morphological assimilation (partial and total) of spike is shown: *pacemaker spike-ok* 'pacemaker spikes'and *inefectiv spikeokat láttak* 'ineffective spikes were visible'.

Spray is entered in BISZ and EKSZ with two meanings, the second of which is the medical sememe: **2.** *porlasztócsomagolásban forgalomba hozott orvosi készítmény, permet* 'medicinal product distributed in a spray form, spray'. BOSZ describes that spray is an English borrowing with the meaning *permet, porlasztott anyag* 'spray, vaporized substance'. MIK gives 7 matches for *spray*. MMD defines *spray* as *a liquid divided into smaller streams, as by a jet of air or steam. Spray* was found in USZCCDR both as a word root (*Nitrolingual spray*) and as a suffixed noun (*sprayre szűnt/oldódtak* 'it was ceased with spray/decreased with spray'). The latter example shows that there is not only morphological assimilation of this word in Hungarian but phonemic assimilation as well.

Stent was given only by BOSZ with the meaning: *üreges szervek (erek, epevezeték) nyitvatartására, megtámasztására alkalmazott eszköz* 'a device used for keeping hollow organs open/support them'. No match was found for stent in this meaning in MIK. DMD gives two sememes for stent: 1. *a device or mold of a suitable material, used to hold a skin graft in place.* 2. *a slender rodlike or threadlike device used to provide support for tubular structures that are being anastomosed, or to induce or maintain their patency*. In USZCCDR *stent* is used only in the second meaning (semantic narrowing). *Stent* is one of the most frequently used medical terms in USZCCDR. *Stent* is used both as word root and as suffixed noun in USZCCDR, e.g. *coronaria stent* 'coronary stent', *stent beültetés* 'stent implantation', *stentben* 'in the stent', *stenttől* 'from the stent', *stentet* 'accusative case of stent'*;* it is also used with the English prefix *in-*, e.g. *RCA in-stent stenosisa igazolódott* 'his/her in-stent restenosis was revealed'*;* it is used in trade names, e.g. *Lekton motion stent, Driver stent;* and it was also verbalizes and further monimalized, *stentelést végeztünk* 'stenting was performed'.

Stroke is given by BISZ and EKSZ. BISZ gives 2 meanings for it: the first is connected to sports and the second is the medical sememe: 2. *roham, (szél)hűdés* "attack, stroke' (also given by EKSZ). MIK gave no match for *stroke,* and ZESZ, which gives only *sztrók*, the assimilated form, describing that it is an English loanword meaning *agyvérzés, agyszélhűdés* 'cerebral hemorrhage, stroke'. DMD gives a broad meaning for stroke: *a sudden and severe attack*. In Hungarian it is used in a much narrower sense (semantic narrowing) referring to *gutaütés, agyvérzés, szélütés (vérzés, vagy isémia okozta)* 'stroke, cerebral hemorrhage (caused by bleeding or ischemia), cf. website www.pirula.net. In USZCCDR *stroke* is always used with adjectives modifying its meaning, e.g *minor stroke* 'minor stroke', *iscaemias stroke* 'ischemic stroke', and a Hungarian loan creation for this phenomenon was also identified*: agyi akut katasztrófa* 'acute cerebral accident'.

Study is not listed in any of the referred Hungarian dictionaries, and 8 matches were found for it in MIK, 7 of which had a non-medical/non-scientific meaning. MMD defines study as *the pursuance of education; analysis*. In the Hungarian dicharge reports study is used with the sememe *vizsgálat* 'examination' (semantic narrowing), e.g. *kamrai study* 'ventricular examination'. *Study* is morphologically assimilated, the accusative case ending *-t* is used unhyphenated with the word root: *kamrai studyt végeztünk* 'we performed a ventricular examination'.

Tamponade is given both in BISZ (*gézdugasz* 'gauze roll') and in BOSZ (*tamponálás* 'swabbing'), but with different meanings. DMD gives 2 meaning of the word **1.** *surgical use of a tampon,* **2.** *pathologic compression of a part.* It also defines *(cardiac) tamponade*: *compression of the heart caused by increased intrapericardial pressure due to collection of blood or fluid in the pericardium.* Tamponade is used in the latter meaning in USZCCDR, e.g *tamponade jelek nem észlelhetőek* 'no tamponade sign are visible'.

Team is defined only in BISZ with 2 meanins: **1.** *csapat* 'team', **2.** *valamely munkát együttesen végző csoport* 'a group of people working together'. MIK gives 6 matches for *team.* McGraw-Hill Concise Dictionary of Modern Medicine gives the meaning for a (medical) *team* that is used in the Hunagrian discharge reports *the group of physicians and health care workers who are responsible for a patient's medical needs.* In USZCCDR *team* is used both as a word root (*gastroenterológus-sebész-onkológus team* 'gastroenterologist-surgeon-oncologist team') and as member of an assimilated compound word (*onkoteam* 'oncoteam').

Upgrade is given only by BISZ with a meaning used in information sciences *korszerűsítés, bővítés, újabbra cserélés* 'modernizing, expanding, replacement for a new one'. BISZ gives that *upgrade* is an English loanword. No match was found in MIK for *upgrade.* The same meaning is given by McGraw-Hill Concise Dictionary of Modern Medicine (*technology*) *Replacement of older equipment, software, services. Upgrade* is relatively frequently used in the cardiology report mostly in connection with the pacemaker of the patient, e.g. *PM telep upgrade céljából* 'to upgrade pacemaker battery'; but also in other contexts: *biventricularis upgrade szóba jön* 'biventricular upgrade is discussed'.

Vitamin is an international word that has a Latin and an English element. This is the only lexeme beside *potassium* that is given by each Hungarian reference dictionary. BISZ describes *vitamin* as *a szervezet működéséhez nélkülözhetelen olyan szerves vegyület, amelyet az nem tud előállítani és amelyet a táplálékkal kell felvennie* 'an organic compound that is essential for the functioning of the body, and which the body is unable to produce, and has to take up through diet'. According to TESZ (1922) and ZESZ vitamin is an international word that was borrowed English and German. BOSZ and EKSZ give a longer definition for *vitamin*: *a szervezet életéhez, növekedéséhez, a sejtek működéséhez elengedhetetlenül szükséges, a szervezetben nem kielégítő mértékben képződő szerves anyag, hiánya jellgzetes tüneteket vált ki* 'vitamin: essential for the living, development of the body and for the functioning of the cells, it is not produced by the body in an appropriate amount, vitamin deficiency causes typical symptoms' According to MMD *vitamin* is *any of a group of unrelated organic substances occurring in many foods in small amounts and necessary in trace amounts for the normal metabolic functioning of* *the body; they may be water- or fat-soluble. Vitamin* is used in several discharge reports in the "Medications" section, e.g. *D3 vitamin* 'Vitamin D3', *vitamin C* 'Vitamin C'.

5.1.2.1.2. Adjective loanwords proper

Nouns form the largest class of loanwords in borrowing and adjectives are the second most frequently borrowed items. Contrary to the findings of Sager et al. (1980), who argue that loan verbs are normally second in frequency after loan nouns, my survey of medical texts revealed that adjectives occupy the second position. In fact, no verbal loanwords proper were identified in the studied corpus, only assimilated verbs were found. The descriptive nature of scientific texts could account for this relatively abundant presence of nouns and the moderate use of adjectives and verbs.

Adjective loanwords proper are given in Table 8 with the source language they were borrowed from (English proper borrowings, members of the international scientific vocabulary (ISV) or originating in other languages but having been borrowed into the Hungarian medical vocabulary via English), examples taken for their appearance in USZCCDR, and if they are listed in BISZ, EKSZ, TESZ, ZESZ, BOSZ, LEM and OHSZ, and their prevalence in MIK.

Table 8. Adjective loanwords proper

Borrowed term	**Source languag e**	**Examples from the studied corpus**	**BISZ**	**EKSZ**	**TESZ**	**ZESZ**	**BOSZ**	**LEM**	**OHSZ**	**MIK (n)**
diffuse*	E	*az RCA diffuse kaliberingadozó* 'the RCA is with diffuse caliber fluctuation'	(+)	+	Ø	Ø	(+)	Ø	(+)	Ø
guided/ guiding	E	*LM-RDA IVUS guided angioplasztika* 'LM-RDA IVUS guided angioplasty', *Launcher guiding katéter*'Launcher guiding catheter'	(+)	Ø	Ø	Ø	Ø	Ø	Ø	Ø
high (rate)	E	*Intracardialis high rate pacelést követően* 'after intracardiac high rate pacing'	+	Ø	Ø	Ø	+	Ø	+	(44)
left (main)	E	*Left main: hosszú, ép* 'Left main: long and intact'	Ø	Ø	Ø	Ø	Ø	Ø	Ø	(3)
low(volta ge)	E	*Standard elvezetésekben low voltage* 'low	(+)	Ø	Ø	Ø	+	Ø	+	(9)

		voltage in standard leads'								
non-sustained	E	*Non-sustained kamrai ritmuszavar* 'non-sustained ventricular arrhythmia', *Non-sustained pitvari tachycardia* 'non-sustained atrial tachycardia'	Ø	Ø	Ø	Ø	Ø	Ø	Ø	Ø
sick (sinus syndroma)	E	*sick sinus syndrome* 'sick sinus syndrome'	Ø	Ø	Ø	Ø	+	Ø	Ø	Ø
slow-fast	E	*slow-fast típusú AVnRT* 'slow-fast AVnRT'	(+)	Ø	Ø	Ø	Ø	Ø	(+)	Ø
standard	E	*Standard elvezetésekben* 'in standard leads', *standard négykatéteres vizsgálat* 'standard four-catheter examination'	+	+	Ø	Ø	+	Ø	+	93 [in 1880]
tilt	E	*tilt table teszt* 'tilt table test', *tilt table vizsgálatra* 'for a tilt table test'	Ø	Ø	Ø	Ø	Ø	Ø	Ø	Ø

* marked item is discussed in 5.1.1.

Guided/guiding is given only by BISZ in the form of *guide* but not with medical meaning (**1.** *idegenvezető* 'tourist guide', **2.** *útikönyv* 'guidebook', **3.** *kézikönyv* 'handbook'). The other Hungarian reference dictionaries do not have an entry for either *guide(d)* or *guiding.* MIK has 3 matches for *guide/guidelines*, but none for *guided/guiding.* MMD describes only the nominal sememe (*a guide* or *guidewire*: *a device used to position an IV catheter, endotracheal tube, central venous line, or gastric feeding tube or to localize a tumor during open breast biopsy.* From the perspective of my study, a more appropriate definition is provided by http://www.medtronic.com/physician/vascular/gc_launcher_warnings.html: the *Medtronic Guiding Catheter is designed to provide a pathway through which therapeutic devices are introduced. The guiding catheter is intended to be used in the coronary or peripheral vascular system.* In USZCCDR *guided/guiding* is used as a member of an attributive adjective in an adjectival structure preceded by a trade name, e.g. *Launcher guiding katéter* 'Launcher guiding catheter', an eponym, e.g. *JR* (Judkins right) *guiding*, or the name of the anatomical structure, e.g. *LM-RDA IVUS guided angioplasztika* 'left main ramus descendens anterior intravascular ultrasonographic guided angioplasty'.

High is listed in BISZ in various compounds (e.g. *high-fidelity, high life, high-tech*) but not as a word root. BOSZ only gives *high voltage* as well as OHSZ. MIK provides 44 matches for high in various contexts, but in each case high is followed by an English loanword (e.g. *highchurch, high school, high tory*). In USZCCDR *high* is always followed by *rate* (pacelés) that was found at http://europace.oxfordjournals.org/cgi/reprint/4/4/427.pdf: *high rate pacing is a failure in the functioning of the implanted pacemaker*. High rate is used in Hungarian to mean *magas frekvenciájú* 'high frequency' (Gábor Marton, M.D., personal communication in 2009), cf. *intracardialis high rate pacelést követően* 'after intracardiac high rate pacing'.

Left (main) is not listed in any of the referred Hungarian dictionaries, and 3 matches were found for *left* in MIK. MMD gives the definition of *left main*: *one of a pair of branches from the ascending aorta, arising in the left posterior aortic sinus, dividing into the left interventricular artery and the circumflex branch, and supplying both ventricles and the left atrium*. It is used to refer to the arteria coronaria sinistra (*bal közös törzs* 'left common branch'). Left is used in USZCCDR only in this context, always preceding *main* (e.g. *left main: hosszú, ép* 'left main: long and intact').

Low (voltage) is given by BISZ only in different phrase (Low Church). BOSZ contains *low voltage* with the meaning *alacsony feszültség* 'low voltage'. OHSZ also has an entry for *low voltage*. MIK gives 9 matches for *low*, but none for *low voltage*.

The website http://encyclopedia.thefreedictionary.com defines *low voltage* as it *is an electrical engineering term that broadly identifies safety considerations of an electricity supply system based on the voltage used*. The website http://www.cvphysiology.com defines it as *the wave of atrial repolarization with relatively small in amplitude*. In Hungarian it used in cardiology to mean *az EKG alacsony R hulláma* 'low R wave in ECG' (cf. http://prof-congress.hu/2007/mont/poszter_abst.pdf) and *alacsony amplitúdójú QRS komplexusok* 'low amplitude QRS complexes' (cf. website http://www.humanelettan.usn.hu/).

Non-sustained is not listed in any of the referred Hungarian dictionaries, and no match was found for it in MIK. *Non-sustained* is defined as a condition *that persists for an arbitrary period of time in the absence of intervention* at website http://www.aic.cuhk.edu.hk and *non-sustained VT* is defined as *a run of tachycardia of less than 30 seconds duration* (cf. website http://www.patient.co.uk/doctor). In Hungarian it is used in the meaning of *nem hosszantartó* (cf. website www.pirula.net). In USZCCDR *non-sustained* was used as an adjective describing two pathological conditions (tachycardia), e.g. *non-sustained VT* (ventricular tachycardia), or *non-sustained kamrai ritmuszavar*'non-sustained ventricular arrhythmia', and *non-sustained pitvari tachycardia* 'non-sustained atrial tachycardia'.

Sick (sinus syndroma) is not given in BISZ, but there is an entry for *sick sinus syndroma* in BOSZ: *a sinuscsomóról a pitvarra történő ingerületvezetés* *zavara* 'conducting disorder affecting the sinus node and atrial conduction'. DMD defines *sick sinus syndrome* as an *intermittent bradycardia, sometimes with episodes of atrial tachyarrhythmias or periods of sinus arrest, due to malfunction originating in the supraventricular portion of the cardiac conducting system.* In Hungarian it is used to mean *sinuscsomó-diszfunkció* 'sinus node dysfunction', *szinuszcsomó-betegség* 'sinus node disease' (cf. website http://www.drdiag.hu) and *a beteg sinus csomó instabil működéséből adódó ingerképzési zavar* 'malfunction in the stimulus formation due to the instable function of the sich sinus node' (cf. website http://www.medlist.com). In USZCCDR the adjective sick was used only in this phrase.

Slow-fast is not contained in any of the referred Hungarian dictionaries; however, BISZ contains *slowfox* and OHSZ entries *slow-virus*. In both cases slow is used to mean *reduced speed of action*, so the general sememe has been borrowed with the orthography. *Slow-fast ANVRT* is described in cardiology as the typical or common ANVRT: *the impulse travels over the slow pathway towards the ventricles and returns via the fast pathway to the atria* (cf. website http://en.ecgpedia.org). In Hungarian it is also used as *lassú pálya–gyors pálya* (Gábor Marton, M.D., personal communication in 2010).

Standard is given in BISZ as *sztenderd* with the adjectival meaning: *előírásos, szabványos, megkívánt színvonalnak megfelelő* 'prescribed, standard, appropriate for the required level'. EKSZ gives *standard* in the meaning *előírásos, szabványos* 'prescribed, standard'. BOSZ gives only the nominal meaning of it: *minta, alap, mérték, szabvány* 'sample, basis, measurement, standard'. MIK: gives 93 matches for standard and 34 for sztenderd. The AHMD gives two definitions for standard (adj.): **1.** *serving as or conforming to a standard of measurement or value,* **2.** *widely recognized as a model of authority or excellence.* Standard is the most frequently used adjective in USZCCDR (n=10), e.g. *standard elvezetésekben* 'in standard leads', *standard négykatéteres vizsgálat* 'standard four-catheter examination'. The assimilated orthography, *sztenderd,* is not used in any discharge reports.

Tilt (table) is not listed in any of the referred Hungarian dictionaries, and no match was found for it in MIK. MMD defines *tilt* as *unsteady*; and *tilt table* as *an examining table that allows a patient to be raised to an approximate 60-degree angle during study of the response of the patient's circulatory system to gravitational forces. A tilt table is also used to assist recovery from orthostatic hypotension after prolonged immobility.* A *heads-up tilt table test* is a *method of evaluating patients with neurocardiac syncope.* A Hungarian definition was found for *heads-up tilt table test* at website www.lam.hu/folyoiratok/lam/0306/8.htm: *ferde helyzetben elvégzett orthostaticus stressz teszt* orthostatic stress test performed in a tilt postion', and at website www.eum.hu: *billenőasztalon történő ortosztatikus terheléses teszt* 'orthostatic stress test performed on a tilt table'. In USZCCDR *tilt* is always used preceding *table*, e.g. *tilt table teszt* 'tilt table test', *head up tilt table vizsgálatra* 'for a head up tilt table test'.

The morphological assimilation and semantic changes of the above discussed loanwords proper are shown in Table 9 in a summarized form.

Table 9. Morphological and semantic assimilation of loanwords proper

Loanword proper	Morphological assimilation	Semantic change
(acetylsalicylic) acid	Ø	Ø
arrest	Ø	narrowing (only N)
attack	Ø	Ø
beat	Ø	narrowing (only N)
block	+ *-ot* '(accusative)', *-oló* '-er', *-olás* '-ing'	Ø
branch	Ø	narrowing (only N)
burst	Ø	narrowing/shift
bypass	Ø	narrowing (only N)
chloride	Ø	Ø
cholesterol	Ø	Ø
diffuse	Ø	Ø
end stage	Ø	Ø
enoxaparin/ enoxaparol	Ø	Ø
entrainment	Ø	Ø
flow	+ *-val* 'with', *-t* '(accusative)'	narrowing (only N)
follow up	Ø	narrowing (only N)
graft	+ *-t* '(accusative)'	narrowing (only N)
guided/guiding	Ø	Ø
high (rate)	Ø	Ø
kinking	Ø	Ø
left (main)	Ø	Ø
levothyroxine	Ø	Ø
low (voltage)	Ø	Ø
mapping	Ø	Ø
monitor	+ *-izálás* '-ing'	narrowing/shift
non-sustained	Ø	Ø
pace	+ *-el* 'to pace', *-elés* '-ing'	Ø
pacemaker	+*-ek* '-s'	Ø
penicillin	Ø	Ø
plaque/plack	+ *-ok* '-s'	narrowing
potassium	Ø	Ø
puff	Ø	narrowing
pull-back	Ø	Ø
recovery	Ø	Ø
reentry	Ø	Ø
scan	+ *-ek* '-s', *-eken* 'in scans'	narrowing (only N)
sense / oversensing	Ø	Ø
shock/sokk	Ø	Ø
shunt	Ø	narrowing (only N)
sick (sinus syndroma)	Ø	Ø
slow-fast	Ø	Ø
sludge	Ø	narrowing

sodium	Ø	Ø
spike	+ *-ok* '-s', *-okat* 'spikes (accusative)'	Ø
spray	+ *-re* 'due to'	narrowing (only N)
standard	Ø	Ø
stent	+ *-ben* 'in', *-től* 'from', *-elést* 'stenting (accusative)'	Ø
stroke	Ø	Ø
study	+ *-t* '(accusative)'	narrowing (only N)
tamponade	Ø	Ø
team	Ø	Ø
test	Ø	narrowing (only N)
tilt	Ø	Ø
upgrade	Ø	Ø
vitamin	Ø	Ø

Abbreviations and symbols used: N: noun, Ø: no morphological assimilation/semantic change.

5.1.2.2. Assimilated loanwords

In this book assimilated loanwords are words and phrases that are transferred from the English language to the Hungarian language of cardiology with orthographic/morphemic adaptation and/or with morphological substitution. Most of the terms below have an international or Latin origin, but, according to the referenced dictionaries, they were borrowed via English, or their use in national technical languages (cf. Pogarell and Schröder 1999; Taaivitsainen 2001) among them in the Hungarian language (cf. Buvári 2001; Zimányi 2003; Bősze 2009) has increased due to their intensive use in medical English. Several pseudo-Latin and pseudo-Greek words have been coined in English to denote modern concepts that did not exist in Greek and Roman times (Országh 1968). These neologisms are then borrowed by national languages. Latinisms are also spreading in Hungarian due to the morphological characteristics of the language; derivational suffixes are used to widen the medical vocabulary as well. Mainly verbs and adjectives are formed on the basis of earlier Latin loan nouns. In some cases existing but rarely used Latin lexemes are revived mostly due to the extensive English language contact, where these words (based on Latinate elements) are widely used.

On the orthographical level, assimilated loanwords are formed on the basis of the pronunciation of the corresponding English word, or the assimilated orthography may follow partly the pronunciation of the English language source word and partly accommodating to the Hungarian spelling rules. Changes in spelling include that the English grapheme <c> is usually changed to <k> or <s> is changed to <sz>.

On the morphological level, assimilated loanwords are made up of the combination of the English (assimilated) word root and a Hungarian nominal, adjectival or verbal suffix.

32 assimilated loanwords – nouns (n=15), adjectives (n=6) and verbs (n=11) were identified in the studied discharge reports.

5.1.2.2.1. Assimilated noun loanwords

Assimilated loan nouns are given in Table 10 with the source language they were borrowed from (English proper borrowings, members of the international scientific vocabulary (ISV), or originating in other languages but having been borrowed into the Hungarian medical vocabulary via English), examples taken for their appearance in USZCCDR, and if they are listed in BISZ, EKSZ, TESZ, ZESZ, BOSZ, LEM and OHSZ, and their prevalence in MIK.

Table 10. Assimilated loan nouns from the studied corpus

Assimilated term	**Source language**	**Examples from the studied corpus**	**BISZ**	**EKSZ**	**TESZ**	**ZESZ**	**BOSZ**	**LEM**	**OHSZ**	**MIK (n)**
defibrillátor	L via E	*defibrillator csere* 'exchange of the defibrillator'	(+)	Ø	Ø	Ø	+	(+)	+	Ø
diszkomfort	E (1883 TESZ)	*mellkasi diszkomfortot érez* '[the patient] feels discomfort in the chest'	(+)	Ø	Ø	(+)	Ø	Ø	Ø	Ø
flattern/ fluttern	E	*flatternt* 'flutter (accusative)', *fluttern-re* 'due to flutter'	Ø	Ø	Ø	Ø	(+)	Ø	Ø	Ø
hormon	ISV 1911 TESZ/ ZESZ	*hormonhatás* 'hormonal effect'	+	+	+	+	+	+	+	204 [in 1931]
hospitalize-ció	L via E	*hospitalizációja* '[the patient's] hospitalization'	(+)	Ø	Ø	Ø	Ø	Ø	+	1 [in 1984]
klipp	E	*(fém)klippek* '(metal) clips'	(+)	(+)	Ø	Ø	Ø	Ø	Ø	(9)
koleszterin*	ISV	*koleszterin* 'cholesterol'	+	+	Ø	Ø	+	Ø	+	4 [in 1976]
komplience	Fr via E	*complience-ra* 'on compliance'	Ø	Ø	Ø	Ø	Ø	(+)	Ø	Ø
mobilizáció/ mobilizálás	L via E	*mobilizációt azonnal megkezdtük* 'mobilization was immediately initiated'	(+)	(+)	Ø	(+)	+	Ø	+	7 [in 1921
rezidens	L via E	*rezidens orvos* 'resident doctor'	(+)	(+)	Ø	Ø	Ø	Ø	Ø	(6)
sheat	E	*femoralis sheatjét eltávolítottuk* '(the patient's) femoral sheath was removed'	Ø	Ø	Ø	Ø	Ø	Ø	Ø	Ø

stentelés	E	*stentelést végeztünk* 'stenting was performed'	Ø	Ø	Ø	Ø	Ø	Ø	Ø	Ø
stressz/ sztressz	E	*stressz helyzet* 'stress situation', *sztressz szituációk* 'stress situations'	+	+	Ø	Ø	+	Ø	+	121 [in 1973]
szupport	L back transfor mation	*ballon szupporttal* 'with balloon support'	(+)	Ø	Ø	Ø	(+)	Ø	Ø	Ø
teszt*	ISV 1913 TESZ	*pitvari extrastimulus teszt* 'atrial extrastimulation test'	+	+	+	+	+	Ø	+	57 [1975]

Defibrillátor (E defibrillator) is not listed directly in BISZ, which gives a definition only for defibrilláció 'defibrillation'. BOSZ defines defibrillátor as a szívizom ritmus nélküli fibrillációját elektromos áramütésekkel megszüntető készülék 'a device ceasing the arrhythmic fibrillation of the myocardium with electrical impulses'. LEM contains only L/H fibrillation 'fibrillation': az izomrostok remegésszerű rángása 'shivering jerking of the muscle fibers'. MIK does not provide any match for the word. AHMD gives that defibrillator is an electrical device used to counteract fibrillation of the heart muscle and restore normal heartbeat by applying a brief electric shock. The English defibrillator is orthographically assimilated to Hungarian only by the addition of the diacritical mark above the a (i.e. E <a> > H <á>).

Diszkomfort (E discomfort) is not listed directly in BISZ, which gives a definition only for komfort 'comfort'. ZESZ contains only komfort, and gives that it is an English loan. The other 3 dictionaries and MIK do not give any data for diszkomfort. AHD gives two meanings of discomfort: **1.** mental or bodily distress, **2.** something that disturbs one's comfort; an annoyance. In Hungarian it is used to mean kellemetlenség, kényelmetlenség 'unpleasant, inconvenient feeling' according to website www.pirula.net. In USZCCDR this loanword is always used in a nominal phrase: mellkasi diszkomfort, e.g. bizonytalan mellkasi diszkomfort érzése van 'he/she has an uncertain chest discomfort', mellkasi diszkomfortot érez 'he/she feels chest discomfort'. The latter example shows that the word has also been morphologically assimilated to Hungarian by taking the accusative case ending -t.

Flattern/fluttern (E flutter) is one of the most frequently used assimilated loanwords in USZCCDR, e.g. pitvari flatternt dokumentált 'atrial flutter is documented', EKG-n látható fluttern 'flutter visible in the ECG'. However, the phenomenon is more often referred to by the unassimilated flutter, e.g. pitvari fibrillációs flutter 'atrial fibrilloflutter', pitvari flutter miatt 'because of atrial flutter'. I have 63 matches in USZCCDR for the orthographic form flutter, 30 matches for fluttern and 7 matches for flattern. None of the referenced dictionaries have an entry for either flattern or fluttern. BOSZ, however, gives flutter with an English etymology meaning: szapora pitvaösszehúzódás pitvarlebegésben 'fast atrial contraction in atrial fibrillation'. DMD defines flutter as a rapid vibration or pulsation. There seems to be inconsistency in the spelling of this word as both website http://egeszseg.origo.hu/kislexikon and http://www.doktorinfo.hu give the spelling as flatter. Nevertheless, USZCCDR does not give any match for flatter. Both flutter (with this orthographic form) and fluttern have undergone morphological assimilation, Hungarian suffixes are used with them either hyphenated or unhyphenated: flutter-nel is rendelkező 'also having flutter', fluttert észleltek 'flutter was revealed', pitvari fluttern-re 'for the atrial flutter', pitvar fluttern-je volt 'he/she had atrial flutter'.

Hormon (E hormone) is an international word. BISZ, EKSZ and TESZ give that it is an English word made up of Greek elements, and it means: belsőelválasztású mirigyek által termelt biológiai hatóanyag 'biological substance produced by endocrine glands'. BOSZ gives a very similar meaning by describing that it is belsőelválasztású mirigyek terméke, amelyet a testnedvek továbbítanak 'the production of endocrine glands which is carried by body fluids'. DMD defines hormone as a chemical substance produced in the body which has a specific regulatory effect on the activity of certain cells or a certain organ or organs. No suffixes were added to hormon in USZCCDR, and the word itself was rarely used (n= 2) most probably due to the specificities of the studied medical field, namely that hormones are not central to cardiology.

Hospitalizáció (E hospitalisation/hospitalization) is given only by OHSZ in the form of hospitalisatio/hospitalizáció. BISZ gives the verbal form hospitalizál with the meaning beteget kórházba felvesz, ill. ott kezel 'admit the patient to hospital or treat him/her there'. MIK provides one match for hospitalizáció. DMD gives two sememes for hospitalization: **1.** the placing of a patient in a hospital for treatment, **2.** the term of confinement in a hospital. Hospitalizáció is used both with and without Hungarian suffixes in USZCCDR: angina esetén azonnali hospitalizáció 'immediate hospitalization in case of an angina', hospitalizációja elengedhetetlen 'his/her hospitalization is indispensable'. During the assimilation the Hungarian nominal suffix -áció was added to the word.

Klipp (E clip) is not given by any of the referenced dictionaries, however, BISZ and EKSZ contain videoklip 'videoclip' and MIK give 9 matches for klip but with a different sememe. DMD defines clip as a metallic device for approximating the edges of a wound or for the prevention of bleeding from small individual blood vessels. In USZCCDR it is used with the plural Hungarian suffix -(e)k (klippek) and in a compound (*fémklippek* 'metal clips'), where the first word in the compound is redundant as a *clip* is a metallic device (semantic widening). During the assimilation English <c> became <k>, and the stem-final consonant <p> was doubled (cf. Nádasdy 1989).

Komplience (E compliance) is not given by any of the Hungarian referenced dictionaries. However, BOSZ gives compliance but with a different meaning: egységnyi nyomásváltozáshoz tartozó térfogatváltozás 'change in volume pertaining to a unit of pressure change'. MMD defines compliance with two meanings: **1.** fulfillment by a patient of a caregiver's prescribed course of treatment, **2.** also called pulmonary compliance (in respiratory physiology) a measure of distensibility of the lung volume produced by a unit pressure change. The latter sememe is given by BOSZ, but in USZCCDR komplience, e.g. komplience hiányában 'due to lack of compliance' is used in the first meaning defined by MMD. I also found one match in USZCCDR for the unassimilated English orthography: compliance. It is used hyphenated with a Hungarian suffix: tekintettel a rossz compliance-ra 'considering poor compliance'. The orthographic assimilation probably tries to reflect an English pronunciation of the word.

Mobilizáció/mobilizálás (E mobilization, mobilizing) DMD defines mobilization as the rendering of a fixed part movable. BISZ gives 4 meanings, the third of which is the medical one szabaddá tétel 'making free/mobile'. BOSZ gives 2 meanings of the word: **1.** valamely szerv műtéti úton való szabaddá tevése 'making an organ free/mobile surgically', **2.** a szervezetben raktározott anyag felszabadítása 'mobilization of a substance stored in the body'. EKSZ gives only the verbal meaning of the word. Comparing the English and the Hungarian sememes, we can identify slightly different meanings (i.e. semantic distribution), as in the Hungarian language of medicine it also means that the patient is made to get out of bed and move around.

Rezidens (E resident) is given only by BISZ and EKSZ, which give two different sememes of rezidens: **1.** helytartó, kormányzó, **2.** ügyvivő. MIK provides six matches for rezidens but with the sememes given in BISZ and EKSZ. MMD gives two sememes of resident: **1.** a physician in one of the postgraduate years of clinical training after the first, or internship, year, **2.** a person who receives inpatient care in a long-term care facility. In USZCCDR rezidens is used in the first meaning, cf. website http://rezidens.hu: általános orvosi diplomát szerzett, pályakezdőként dolgozó orvos 'a working junior doctor who has graduated from the medical university'. It is a recently introduced post/training program in the Hungarian health care. So there was no match for rezidens in the discharge reports written in 2005 but it appeared in most discharge reports written in 2007 and 2009. In each case it appeared at the end of the discharge report as Rezidens orvos under a line provided for signature. During orthographic assimilation VCV -s- has become -z-, and word final -t has turned into -s.

Sheat (E sheath) is not given by any of the referred Hungarian dictionaries and MIK does not give any match for it. MMD defines sheath as: a tubular case or envelope. It also gives femoral sheath, which is the investing fascia of the proximal portion of the femoral vessels. Sheat differs only slightly from the English sheath; as Hungarian lacks interdental fricatives, most probably it is spelt <t>, thus the final English letter is lost in the Hungarian spelling.

Stentelés (E inserting a stent) is not given by any of the referred Hungarian dictionaries and MIK does not give any match for it. Stentelés is a noun derived from H stent (noun) (see Section 5.1.1.1.1) > H stentel 'to insert a stent' (verb) (no match found in USZCCDR for it) > H stentelés 'inserting a stent' (noun).

Stressz/sztressz (E stress) is given in BISZ with the orthography stressz meaning: védekező jellegű, huzamosabb fennállása esetén szervi elváltozással járó állapot az állati vagy emberi szervezetben 'a defensive state, which can lead to the development of organic abnormalities in animals and humans if the state is permanent'. EKSZ give the meaning a szervezet vagy a pszichikum megterhelésének hatására létrejött állapot 'a state developed by exertion expressed on the body or mind'. BOSZ lists stressz with a similar meaning: a szervezet védekezőreakciókban megnyilvánuló állapota az őt ért káros ingerekkel szemben 'a state of the body with defensive reactions as a result of harmful stimuli'. OHSZ provides both the original English and the assimilated Hungarian orthography (stress/stressz). None of the dictionaries give the orthography sztressz. MIK provides 118 matches for *stressz*, 251 matches for *stress*, and 3 for *sztressz*. MMD defines *stress* as any emotional, physical, social, economic, or other factor that requires a response or change. The sememe of the English word is much wider (semantic narrowing). Both stressz (*stressz helyzet* 'stress situation') and sztressz (*sztressz szituációk* 'stress situations') were used in the discharge reports under research but not stress. During the assimilation of the word stress > stressz, the word final consonant -s has changed to -sz following the English pronunciation. In the other case (i.e. sztressz) the word opening consonant has been assimilated s- > sz-.

Szupport (E support) is not given by any of the Hungarian reference dictionaries. However, BISZ has an entry for *szupportál* in the meaning: elvisel, tűr 'to bear, to put up with', and BOSZ gives *supportiv* with the meaning: *támogató* 'supportive'. DMD gives three sememes of the word *support*: **1.** *to prevent weakening or failing*, **2.** *a structure that bears the weight of something else*, **3.** *a mechanism or arrangement that helps keep something else functioning*. In USZCCDR *szupport* is used with the third sememe given by DMD. The word is not only orthographically assimilated but morphologically as well, as the Hungarian suffix *-val* is also added to it (cf. *ballon szupporttal* 'with balloon support').

5.1.2.2.2. Assimilated adjective loanwords

Assimilated loan adjectives are given in Table 11 with the source language they were borrowed from (English proper borrowings, members of ISV, or originating in other languages but having been borrowed into the Hungarian medical vocabulary via English), examples taken for their appearance in USZCCDR, and if they are listed in BISZ, EKSZ, TESZ, ZESZ, BOSZ, LEM and OHSZ, and their prevalence in MIK.

Table 11. Assimilated loan adjectives from the studied corpus

Assimilated term	Source language	Examples from the studied corpus	BISZ	EKSZ	TESZ	ZESZ	BOSZ	LEM	OHSZ	MIK (n)
diffúz*	L	*diffúz hypokinezis* 'diffuse hypokinesis'	+	+	Ø	Ø	+	(+)	+	12 [in 1933]
effektív /ineffektív	L	*effektív kamrai pace* 'effective ventricular pace', *ineffektív pacemaker spike-ok* 'ineffective pacemaker spikes'	+	+	Ø	Ø	(+)	(+)	+	13 [in 1943]
elongált	L	*az elongált a. sublclaviaból* 'from the elongated subclavian artery'	(+)	Ø	Ø	Ø	(+)	(+)	+	Ø
intenzív/ intenzifikált	L	*Belgyógyászat Intenzív Osztályról* 'from the Intensive Care Unit of the Department of Internal Medicine', *tekintettel az intenzifikált insulin kezelésre* 'considering the intensified insulin therapy'	+	+	Ø	Ø	+	Ø	+	309 [in 1814]
invazív	L	*invazív javaslat szerint* 'according to the invasive recommendation'	+	Ø	Ø	Ø	+	Ø	+	Ø
triggerelt	E	*triggerelt jobb kamrai PM ritmus* 'triggered right ventricular pacemaker rhythm'	Ø	Ø	Ø	Ø	Ø	Ø	Ø	Ø

Effektív/ineffektív (E effective/ineffective) is given as a Latin origin word with four sememes in BISZ, the third of which is related to medicine: *hatásos* 'effective'. EKSZ gives two sememes: **1.** *valóságos* 'real' and **2.** *hatékony* 'effective'. BOSZ gives only the nominal form of the word: *effektus/effectus* 'effect' but not the adjectival form. LOZS gives that *effectus* is a noun with the meaning *hatás* 'effect'. MIK provides 13 matches for *effektív*. MMD gives the meaning of *effective* as *exerting a measurable effect.* In USZCCDR *effektív/ineffektív* was used with the assimilated spelling and morphological assimilation was also identified, the addition of the Hungarian suffix *-nek*: *effektívnek bizonyult* 'it was proved to be effective'. *Ineffektív* is made up by the addition of the negative prefix *in-*, e.g. *ineffektív lCD shockterápia* 'ineffective ICD shock therapy'.

Elongált (E elongated) is not given in any of the referenced Hungarian dictionaries. But both BISZ and BOSZ give the nominal form *elongáció/elongatio* 'elongation' that is used in medicine for *megnyúlás* 'elongation'. AHD gives the meaning of *elongated* as: **1.** made *longer; extended,* **2.** *having more length than width; slender.* In USZCCDR *elongált* is used to describe the aorta and other arteries: *aorta elongált* 'the aorta is elongated', *elongált a. subclaviaból* 'from the elongated subclavian artery'.

Intenzív (E intensive/intense) is a word built up of Latinate elements. BISZ gives four sememes of *intenzív*, the first of which is related to medicine: **1.** *fokozott, megfeszített (munka), feszült (figyelem)* 'increased, intense (work), close (attention)'. EKSZ gives two sememes of *intenzív*: **1.** *erős összpontosítással végzett* 'performed with high level of concentration' and **2.** *élénk* 'brisk'. It also gives a medical meaning: *speciális ellátást igénylők osztálya* 'a unit for those who require special care'. In BOSZ *intenzív* is given parallel to *intensivus* and defined as *hathatós, beható, nagyfokú, nagymértékű* 'efficacious, intensive, high degree, large'. MIK provides 309 matches for *intenzív*. MMD defines *intensive* as: *of great force or intensity or concentration.* It also provides a definition for the *intensive care unit* (ICU): *a hospital unit in which there is concentrated special equipment and specially trained personnel for the care of seriously ill patients requiring immediate and continuous attention.*

In USZCCDR *intenzív* is used in this latter meaning, *intenzív terápia* 'intensive care'. *Intenzív* is not only orthographically assimilated but morphologically as well, it is used as an adverb, *intenzíven alkalmazott terápia* 'intensively applied therapy' by the addition of the Hungarian adjectival suffix *-en*.

Intenzifikált (E intensified) is not listed in any of the referenced Hungarian dictionaries. No match was found for it in MIK. AMHD gives that *intensified* means *made more intense.* In *intenzifikált insulin kezelésre* 'for intensified insulin therapy' was found.

Invazív (E invasive) is a medical word built up of Latinate elements defined by BISZ as *a szervezetbe erővel, művi úton behatoló* 'forcefully, artificially entering the body'. BOSZ gives the assimilated morpheme as well as the Latinate orthography *invasiv*, and gives the definition *behatolás, beáramlás (kórokozók beáramlása a szervezetbe)* '(pathogens) entering, penetrating (the body). MIK gives no match for either *invazív* or *invasiv*. DMD provides two meanings of the word: **1.** *having the quality of invasiveness,* **2.** *involving puncture of the skin or insertion of an instrument or foreign material into the body; said of diagnostic techniques*. In USZCCDR *invazív* is very frequently used both to refer to a hospital unit: *Invazív Kardiológiai Részleg* 'Invasive Cardiology Unit' or to specify the suggested investigation: *panaszainak invasiv kivizsgálására* 'to investigate his/her complaints invasively'.

Triggerelt (E triggered) is not given by any of the referred Hungarian dictionaries and MIK does not give any match for it. *Triggerelt* is a noun derived from H *trigger* (noun) (see Section 5.1.1.1.1) > H *triggerel* (verb) (no match found in USZCCDR for it) > H *triggerelt* (adjective).

5.1.2.2.3. Assimilated verb loanwords

Verbs compared to nouns and adjectives are relatively rarely used in discharge reports due to the generic features of this text type. Verbs are mainly used in the "Presenting symptoms" and "Past medical history" sections. But the presence of verbs is very low even in these sections; mostly copular sentences are used with nominal and adjectival complements.

No loan verbs proper were found in the researched corpus, and the assimilated loan verbs are mostly of Latinate origin.

Assimilated loan verbs are given in Table 12 with the source language they were borrowed from (English proper borrowings, members of ISV, or originating in other languages but having been borrowed into the Hungarian medical vocabulary via English), examples taken for their appearance in USZCCDR, and if they are listed in BISZ, EKSZ, TESZ, ZESZ, BOSZ, LEM and OHSZ, and their prevalence in MIK.

Table 12. Assimilated loan verbs from the studied corpus

Assimilated term	Source language	Examples from the studied corpus	BISZ	EKSZ	TESZ	ZESZ	BOSZ	LEM	OHSZ	MIK (n)
detektál	L via E	*áramlás*	(+)	(+)	(+)	Ø	Ø	Ø	(+)	5

		detektálható 'flow can be detected', *ép epicardialis coronariakat detektáltunk* 'intact epicardiac coronary arteries have been detected'								[in 1982]
disz-konnektál	E	*az elektródát diszkonnektáltuk* 'the electrode was disconnected'	Ø	Ø	Ø	Ø	Ø	Ø	Ø	Ø
diszlokál	L	*a. carotis communisokat diszlokálja* 'it dislocated the common carotid arteries'	(+)	Ø	Ø	Ø	(+)	Ø	(+)	Ø
hospitalizál	L/G	*stroke miatt hospitalizálták* '[the patient] was hospitalized with stroke	+	(+)	(+)	Ø	Ø	Ø	+	3 [in 1965]
lokalizál	L/ISV 1865 TESZ	*a jobb pitvari posterior-posteroseptalis részre lokalizáltuk* 'it was localized to the postero-posteroseptal area of the right atrium'right	+	+	+	Ø	(+)	Ø	(+)	31 [in 1879]
mobilizál	L	*mobilizáltuk [a beteget]* '[the patient] was mobilized/was made to get out of bed'	+	(+)	Ø	Ø	(+)	Ø	(+)	21 [in 1921]
pozicionál	L	*stentet pozicionálunk* ' astent was positioned'	(+)	(+)	(+)	Ø	Ø	Ø	Ø	(4)
preparál	L 1789 TESZ	*zsebet preparáltunk* 'a pocket was prepared'	+	+	+	Ø	(+)	Ø	(+)	28 [in 1882]
provokál	L 1763 TESZ	*előre dőlés provokálja* 'it is provoked by leaning forward'	+	+	+	Ø	(+)	Ø	(+)	145 [in 1793]
tesztel	ISV	*tesztelni nem sikerült* 'we did not manage to test it'	+	+	+	Ø	(+)	Ø	+	21 [in 1984]
vizualizál	L	*az eltérést vizualizáltuk* 'the abnormality was visualized'	(+)	(+)	Ø	Ø	Ø	Ø	Ø	2 [in 1970]

Detektál (E detect) is not listed in any of the referenced Hungarian dictionaries. BISZ gives a meaning that is used in informatics. EKSZ and TESZ (1923) give the noun form *detektor* 'detector'. MIK gives 5 matches for *detektál.* AHD gives 4 sememes of the word, the first of which is used in USZCCDR: **1.** *to discover or ascertain the existence, presence, or fact of.* This verb was used in USZCCDR several times, e.g. *ép epicardialis coronariakat detektáltunk* 'we detected/found intact epicardiac coronary arteries'. In other cases the adjectival form of *detektál* was used, i.e. *detektálható* 'can be detected'. It was formed from the H *detektál* (verb) > H *detektálhat* 'can detect' (with the addition of H modal derivational suffix *-hat*) > H *detektálható* 'can be detected' (with adding the H adjectival suffix *-ó*), e.g. *áramlás detektálható* 'flow can be detected/discovered'.

Diszkonnektál (E disconnect) is not given by any of the referred Hungarian dictionaries and MIK does not give any match for it. AHD lists two sememes, and the second one is used in: **2.** (*Electricity) To shut off the current in (an appliance) by removing its connection to a power source*. This verb was always used in USZCCDR in connection with the patient's implanted pacemaker, e.g. *elektródát diszkonnektáltuk* 'the electrode was disconnected'.

Diszlokál (E dislocate) is not given by any of the referred Hungarian dictionaries and MIK does not give any match for it. But BISZ lists the nominal form, *diszlokáció* 'dislocation', which is composed of Latinate elements. Seven sememes are given by BISZ for *diszlokáció*, the 5th of which is related to the medical meaning used in USZCCDR: **5.** *helyzetváltoztatás* 'change in the position'. BOSZ gives only the nominal form: *diszlokáció*. AHD gives three sememes of the word, the first of which is used in USZCCDR: **1.** *to put out of usual or proper place, position, or relationship.* In the studied discharge reports *diszlokál* is rarely used, only in 3 reports, e.g. *a.carotis communisokat diszlokálja* 'the common carotid arteries are dislocated'.

Hospitalizál (E hospitalize) is listed only in BISZ, which describes that it is built up of Latinate elements, and has a medical meaning: *beteget kórházba felvesz, ill. ott kezel* 'admit the patient to hospital or treat him/her there'. EKSZ and TESZ (1803) give only *hospitál* 'to be a guest'. MIK provides 3 matches for the term. AHD defines the verb as *to place in a hospital for treatment, care, or observation.* In the researched reports hospitalizál was infrequently used (only 4 matches were found), e.g. *stroke miatt hospitalizálták* 'he/she was hospitalized with stroke'.

Lokalizál (E locate) is not listed in any of the referenced Hungarian dictionaries. EKSZ and TESZ (1865) list the verb *lokalizál.* EKSZ gives the following meaning of the word: *valami terjedését megakadályozza* 'prevents the spreading of something'. TESZ defines it as *bizonyos helyre szorít* 'restricts it to a certain area'. BISZ and BOSZ give only the nominal form: *lokalizáció* 'localization'. MIK gives 31 matches for the verb. AHD gives three sememes of the verb, and the first meaning is used in USZCCDR: **1.** *to determine or specify the position or limits of.* In the discharge reports, *lokalizál* is always used to describe the position of a certain organ or abnormality, e.g. *a jobb pitvari posterior-posteroseptalis részre lokalizáltuk* 'we localized it to the postero-posteroseptal area of the right atrium'.

Mobilizál (E mobilize) is given by BISZ as a word built up of Latinate elements. Three sememes are listed, the third of which is a medical meaning: *szabaddá tesz* 'making free/mobile'. EKSZ gives *mozgósít, felhasznál* 'mobilize, utilize' as the meaning of *mobilizál.* BOSZ lists only the noun: *mobilizáció* 'mobilization'. AHD gives three sememes of the word, and the first one is close to the Hungarian meaning: **1.** *to make mobile or capable of movement.* MIK gives 21 matches for the word. This verb is relatively frequently used in the studied discharge reports, 8 matches were found for it, e.g. *mobilizáltuk* (*a beteget*) 'we mobilized (the patient)'.

Pozicionál (E position) is not listed in any of the referenced Hungarian dictionaries. BISZ gives a different sememe of the word. TESZ (1604) gives only *positio* 'position'. In AHD two sememes are given, and the first one is used in USZCCDR: **1.** *to put in place or position.* Pozicionál was one of the most frequently used loan verbs in USZCCDR, e.g. *stentet pozicionálunk* 'we position/insert a stent'.

Preparál (E prepare) is listed in BISZ with three sememes: **1.** *előkészít, elkészít* 'to prepare, perform'. The other two meanings are not used in USZCCDR. EKSZ gives *fizikai, vegyi eljárással tartósít* 'conserve by a physical or chemical procedure'. TESZ (1789) gives the meaning of *előkészít, elkészít* 'prepare, make' for *preparál.* BOSZ gives a definition of the nominal form *preparátum* 'preparation'. 28 matches were found in MIK for *preparál.* AHD lists four sememes, and the second one is used in USZCCDR: **2.** *to put together or make by combining various elements or ingredients; manufacture or compound. Preparál* was used only in two of the studied discharge reports, e.g. *zsebet preparáltunk* 'prepared a pocket (for the pacemaker)'.

Provokál (E provoke) is listed in BISZ with 4 sememes, and the fourth meaning is used in USZCCDR: *kivált, előidéz, okoz* 'to trigger, result in, cause'. BISZ highlights that the verb is rarely used with this meaning. EKSZ gives the meaning of *provokál* as *kikényszeríteni igyekszik* 'tries to force', and TESZ (1763) gives two sememes: **1.** *előhív* 'trigger' and **2.** *ingerel* 'stimulate'. BOSZ gives only the noun: *provokáció* 'provocation'. AHD lists four sememes, the third of which is used in USZCCDR: **3.** *to give rise to; evoke. Provokál* is frequently used in the discharge reports (n=11), e.g. *előre dőlés provokálja* 'provoked by leaning forward'. In other cases the adjectival form of *provokál* was used, i.e. *provokálható* 'can be provoked'. It was formed from the H *provokál* (verb) > H *provokálhat* 'can provoke' (with the addition of H modal derivational suffix *-hat*) > H *provokálható* 'can be provoked' (with adding the H adjectival suffix *-ó*), e.g. *slow-fast típusú AVnRT volt provokálható* 'slow-fast AVnRT could be provoked'.

Tesztel (E test) is given in BISZ, EKSZ and TESZ as *teszt segítségével megvizsgál* 'to examine by using a test'. BOSZ lists only the nominal form *teszt* 'test' of the word. MIK gives 22 matches for this verb. Only 4 matches were found in USZCCDR for teszt, e.g. *tesztelni nem sikerült* 'testing was not manageable'

Vizualizál (E visualize) is not listed in any of the refenenced Hungarian dictionaries. BISZ gives only the adjectival form: *vizuális* 'visual', and EKSZ gives *vizuális* 'visual' as *látáson alapuló* 'based on vision'. AHD gives two sememes, the second of which describes the meaning used in USZCCDR: **2.** *to make visible*. Vizualizál was used very rarely in USZCCDR, e.g. *az eltérést vizualizáltuk* 'the abnormality was visualized'. *Vizualizál* was also used as an adjective: *vizualizálható* 'can be visualized'. It was formed from the H *vizualizál* (verb) > H *vizualizálhat* 'can visualize' (with the addition of H modal derivational suffix *-hat*) > H *vizualizálható* 'can be visualized' (with adding the H adjectival suffix *-ó*), e.g. *vizualizálható diagonalis ág* 'a diagonal branch that can be visualized'.

5.1.2.3. Eponyms and trade names

Medical eponyms are terms used in medicine that are based on or derived from the names of persons, and occasionally places or things (Dirckx 2001). New discoveries are often named after the people who made the discovery, which produced a large number of medical eponyms: diseases, fractures, medical signs, devices, therapeutical methods and human anatomical parts named after people. Generally eponyms are frequently used in sciences as an option of term formation, and there are more than 9,000 of them within the field of medicine (Anderson 1996).

Most eponyms in English are formed with the synthetic genitive with *'s* put after a proper name, e.g. *Babinski's sign*, *Hodgkin's disease, Quincke's sign.* This form is the grammatical equivalent of formerly familiar Latin terms such as *morbus Addison* 'Addison's disease' or *tuba Fallopii* 'Fallopian tube'.

The Hungarian language of medicine also uses these eponyms but the structure of eponyms in Hungarian is traditionally different from the English structure: the proper noun is connected to following noun with a hyphen, cf. *Babinski-jel* 'Babinski's sign', *Hodgkin-kór* Hodgkin's disease', *Quincke-jel* 'Quincke's sign'.

Eponyms are frequently used in the language of medicine but in the text type I examined eponyms are rare. In USZCCDR, I found only 4 borrowed eponyms: one English proper eponym: *"Shepherd's crook"*, and 3 assimilated ones: *Holter monitorozás* 'Holter monitoring', *Bruce protokoll* 'Bruce protocol' and *Wood (lámpa)* 'Wood's (lamp)'. The four eponyms show three different features of borrowing: orthographic, lexical and semantic interferences. In *"Shepherd's crook"* the eponym is used in its unassimilated form, the 'foreignness' is indicated by quotation marks (the quotation marks, however, follow the English orthography). *Holter monitorozás* 'Holter monitoring' and *Bruce protokoll* 'Bruce protocol' is orthographically assimilated in not using the hyphen between the proper name and the noun being specified by it (cf. *Holter-monitorozás* or *Holter-féle monitorozás*). In case of *Wood lamp test*, USZCCDR gave data only for *Wood Ø pozitív* 'result of Wood lamp test was positive'. The noun *lámpa* 'lamp' was omitted from the eponym.

A trade name is the trademark name or commercial trade name for a material or product in medicine. Trade names make up a significant part of the terminology of medicine: the majority of trade names that physicians use are patented drug names (e.g. *Aspirin Protect*); others refer to the name of the manufacturer of the medical device.

In English, trade names that refer to the manufacturer of a product, are used as substantival adjuncts, i.e. the proper noun is used as an adjective without change in its form: e.g. *Quinton treadmill.*

In Hungarian trade names are usually used in the same way as eponyms: the proper name is hyphenated with the designated product type: *Wolfram-huzal* 'Wolfram wire', or adding the hyphenated postfix *-féle* 'by' to the proper name: *Voll-féle elektroakupunktúra* 'Voll's acupuncture'.

Several frequently used borrowed trade names were identified in the discharge reports under investigation: *Driver stent*, *JR/JL guiding*, *Maverick ballon* 'Maverick's balloon' and *St. Jude műbillentyű* 'St. Jude's artificial valve'. Each term follows the English orthography for trade names, i.e. they are not hyphenated.

5.1.2.4. Acronyms and abbreviations

There is a universal tendency in medical writing to abridge the utterance when possible, by shortening or omitting words and to abbreviate it (Dirckx 1983, 2006). Initialisms, i.e. acronyms and abbreviations are particularly common in modern medical writing. Initialisms are in some cases better known within the profession than their full name.

An abbreviation made up of the first two or three letters of a word is one common variant: *ab* for *abortion*, *ca* for *cancer* or *syst* for *systolic*. These types of abbreviations are not frequently borrowed from English by Hungarian physicians as acronyms (Bősze 2009).

Initialisms are especially popular for describing names of diseases, and of diagnostic and therapeutic procedures. An acronym is an initialism that can be pronounced like a word, e.g. AIDS.

Though mnemonics (e.g. SOAP for symptoms, observations, assessment, and plan) are very frequently used in the English language of medicine, they do not tend to be borrowed by the Hungarian physicians due to the phenomenon behind the development of these acronyms, i.e. they make it easier for the speaker to remember certain items.

Abbreviations can also be ambiguous, the idea that they stand for can vary according to various fields of medicine, e.g. CAT usually stands for either *computer assisted tomography* or *computed axial tomography*, but it can also initialize cognitive abilities test or *chronic arsenic toxicity* depending on which medical field or what context it is used in.

When an abbreviation has become common and familiar, it may be retained even after the full term has gone out of use. SGOT, which stands for *serum glutamic-oxaloacetic transaminase* is still used in laboratory findings, although the enzyme is now called *aspartate aminotransferase*.

English medical initialisms (especially acronyms) are very frequently transferred into the Hungarian language of cardiology. They can be found mainly in the "Laboratory results" section in the form of a list and the "Medications section" of the report, but less frequently acronyms are also used when the diagnoses or the past medical history of the patient are described.

In analyzing the acronyms and abbreviations that are used in USZCCDR, I relied on data provided by Stedman's *Medical Abbreviations, acronyms and symbols* (2008. Lippincott Williams and Wilkins), the website http://www.medilexicon.com, *Brencsán Orvosi Szótár* [Brencsán Medical Dictionary] and the website www.pirula.net.

Acronyms can sometimes be difficult to identify as borrowings, as the same acronym can stand for the described phenomenon in both English and Hungarian, e.g. *GGT* stands for *gamma-glutamil transferase* in English and *gamma-glutamil transzferáz* in Hungarian. Therefore the below list contains only acronyms in which all the letters stand for English words that have not been borrowed into Hungarian according to the corpus in the discharge reports.

Table 13. Borrowed English acronyms used in the Hungarian discharge reports under investigation.

English abbreviation	**Meaning**	**Hungarian abbreviation if different**	**Meaning**	**Examples form the corpus**
ABPM	ambulatory 24-hour blood pressure monitoring	Ø	24 órás vérnyomás monitorozás	***ABPM felhelyezésre*** **'on pacing the ABPM'**
ACBG	aorto-coronary bypass graft	Ø	koszorúeret áthidaló átültetés	***ACBG műtét*** **'ACBG operation'**
ACE	angiotensine converting enzyme	Ø	angiotenzin konvertáló enzim	***ACE-gátló/inhibitor*** **'ACE inhibitor'**
ALP*	alkaline phosphatase	alk. phos.	alkalikus foszfatáz	**
ASA	acetylsalycilic acid		acetylszalicilsav	***ASA-t szed*** **'(the patient) takes ASA**
AVNRT	atrio-ventricular node reentry	Ø	AV nodalis reentry	**AVNRT *RF ablatioja***

	tachycardia		tachycardiára	***céljából* 'for AVNRT RF ablatio'**
AVR	aortic valve replacement	Ø	az aorta billentyűjének a cseréje	***AVR műtét* 'AVR operation'**
AVRT	atrio-ventricular reentry tachycardia	Ø	AV reentry tachycardia	***AVRT indul* 'AVRT started'**
CABG	coronary artery bypass graft	Ø	koszorúeret áthidaló átültetés	***CABG műtét* 'CABG operation'**
CD CTO	coronary disease chronic total occlusion	Ø	Ø	***proximális RDA és CD CTO* 'proximal LAD and CD CTO'**
CH	carbohydrate	Ø	szénhidrát	***csökkent CH tolerantia* 'decreased CH tolerance'**
*CKMB**	creatine kinase muscle band	Ø	a kreatinin-kináz vázizom és agyi alegységei	**
COPD	chronic obstructive pulmonary disease	(KOLB)	krónikus obstruktív légzőszervi/tüdőbetegség	***COPD-s beteg* ' a patient with COPD'**
DC	direct current	Ø	egyenáram	***DC-shockkal szüntették meg* 'it was ceased with DC shock'**
*eGFR**	estimated glomerulus filtration rate	Ø	becsült glomeruláris filtrációs hányados	**
GERD	gastroesophageal reflux disease	(GORB)	gastrooesophagialis reflux betegség	***távolabbi anamnézisében … GERD… szerepel* '(the patient) has GERD in the past medical history'**
*HDL**	high density lipoprotein	Ø	nagy sűrűségű lipoprotein	**
HUTT	heads-up tilt table	Ø	billenőasztalon történő orthosztatikus terheléses teszt	***HUTT helyzetben* 'in HUTT position'**
IABP	intra-aortic balloon pump	Ø	intraaorta ballon pumpa	***IABP-t vezettek* 'IABP was inserted'**
IBD	inflammatory bowel disease	Ø	gyulladásos bélbetegség	***IBD-szerű* 'IBD- like'**
ICA	internal carotid artery	Ø	arteria carotis interna	**
ICD	implantable cardioverter defibrillator	Ø	beültethető cardioverter defibrillátor	***ICD telepcsere* 'ICD battery exchange'**
*INR **	international normalized ratio	Ø	nemzetközi normalizált hányados	**
IUD	intrauterine device	(IUE)	méhen belüli eszköz/intrauterin eszköz	***uterusban IUD figyelhető meg* 'an IUD can be seen in the uterus'**
JL	Judkins left	Ø	Judkins-bal	***JL guiding***
JR	Judkins right	Ø	Judkins-jobb	***JR guiding***
LAD	left anterior descending/descendent	RDA= ramus descendens anterior	bal elülső leszálló koszorúsér	***LAD, Mid-LAD, dist-LAD***
LAHB	left anterior hemiblock	Ø	bal elülső hemiblokk	**
LBBB	left bundle branch block	BTSZB	bal Tawara-szár blokk	**
*LDL**	low density lipoprotein	Ø	alacsony sűrűségű lipoprotein	**
LIMA	left internal mammary artery	Ø	bal oldali artéria mammaria interna	***LAD-LIMA, LIMA-RDA graft***
LMWH	low molecular weight heparin	Ø	kis molekulasúlyú heparin	**
LVEF	left ventricular ejection fraction	Ø	bal kamra globális szisztolés funkciója	**
LVH	left ventricular hypertrophy	Ø	bal kamra hipertrófia	**
*MCH**	mean cell hemoglobin	Ø	átlagos testecske haemoglobin	**
*MCHC**	mean cell hemoglobin concentration	Ø	átlag vörösvérsejt-test haemoglobin koncentráció	**
*MCV**	mean corpuscular volume	Ø	átlagos sejttérfogat	**
MDRD	modification of diet in renal	Ø	vesediéta	***MDRD formula***

	disease			
MPV	mean platelet volume	Ø	a vérlemezkék átlagos űrtartalma	**
MRI	magnetic resonance imaging	Ø	mágneses rezonancia képalkotás	***szív MRI*** **'cardiac MRI'**
NPDR	non-proliferative diabetic retinopathy	Ø	non-proliferatív diabeteses retinopathia	**
NSTEMI	non st segment myocardial infarction	Ø	nem ST elevációs myocardialis infarctus	**
NSVT	non-sustained ventricular tachycardia	Ø	(non-sustained) pitvari tachycardia	***NSVT-ket regisztráltak*** **NSVTs were recorded'**
NYHA	New York Heart Association	Ø		***NYHA III-IV. stadiumban lévő beteget*** **'a patient in NYHA stage III-IV'**
PCR	polymerase chain reaction	Ø	polimeráz láncreakció	**
PM	pacemaker	Ø		***PM implantáció*** **'PM implantation',** ***PM ritmus*** **'PM rhythm'**
POBA	plain old balloon angioplasty	Ø	hagyományos ballon-angioplastica	***restenosis POBA***
PTCA	percutaneous transvenous coronary angioplasty	Ø	percutan transzvénás koronária angioplasztika	**
PW	posterior wall	Ø	hátsófal(i)	**
RBBB	right bundle branch block	JTSZB	jobb Tawara-szár blokk	**
RCA	right coronary artery	Ø	jobb koszorúsér	***RCA in-stent stenosisa igazolódott*** **'in-stent stenosis of the RCA was revealed'**
RDW-CV*	red cell volume distribution width	Ø	vörösvértest-eloszlási szélesség	**
RIMA	right internal mammary artery	Ø	jobb oldali artéria mammaria interna	**
SAM	septic anterior motion	Ø	septalis anterior mozgás	***SAM jelenség*** **'SAM phenomenon'**
SEC	spontaneous echo contrast	Ø	spontán echo kontraszt	**
SPECT	single photo emission computed tomography	Ø	izotópos szívizom vizsgálat	***szívizom SPECT*** **'myocardiac SPECT'**
STD	ST depression	Ø	ST-depresszió	***horizontális STD*** **'horizontal STD',** ***nem-szignifikáns STD*** **'non-significant STD'**
STEMI	st segment myocardial infarction	Ø	ST elevációs myocardialis infarctus	**
TIA	transient ischemic attack	Ø	átmeneti vérellátási zavar okozta roham, szélütés	**
TIMI	thrombolysis in myocardial infarction	Ø	vérrögoldó kezelés szívinfarktusban	***Merlin-TIMI 36 study gyógyszer*** **'Merlin-TIMI 36 study drug',** ***TIMI III volt a záró flow*** **'the last flow was TIMI III'**
VIDA	viability identification with dobutamine	Ø	dopaminos/dobutaminos viabilitás-vizsgálat	***VIDA vizsgálatot kérünk*** **'a VIDA test is required'**
WPW	Wolff-Parkinson-White syndrome	Ø	Wolff-Parkinson-White szindróma	***WPW sy. /syndroma*** **'WPW syndrome'**

Ø no data available * acronym is used only in the "Laboratory findings" section ** acronym is used/listed only in the "Diagnoses", "Laboratory findings" or "Investigations" sections ( ) the acronym is not used in the researched discharge reports.

Numerically acronyms and abbreviations formed the largest group of borrowings in the cardiology discharge reports. We have to distinguish between initialisms used in the "Laboratory findings" section and in other sections of the discharge report. Certain standardized programs for describing the laboratory findings are used at the department of cardiology (see 5.1.1.2.1), thus, physicians writing the discharge report of a patient rely on these programs[46], which are in English offering English abbreviations for laboratory examinations. Yet the other sections of the report are not ready-made offered to the physicians, and initialisms are also frequently used in these parts of the report.

5.1.2.5. Discussion on lexical changes

Borrowing is the main process that is manifested in the lexical aspects of English–Hungarian language contact. Lexical borrowings form the largest group of all English language contact-induced features identified in the Hungarian cardiology discharge reports under investigation. Borrowed lexical features involve various English morphemes, mainly free morphemes.

In terms of the process of lexical borrowing, loanwords from USZCCDR were subcategorized according to their level of orthographic assimilation into two groups: loanwords proper and assimilated loans. Loanwords proper are words and phrases that are adopted from the English language with no morphemic substitution, i.e. in their original orthographic form, e.g. H *bypass* 'bypass', H *study* 'study'. Loanwords proper involve borrowed English nouns and adjectives. Assimilated loans, however, have already been adapted to conform to the orthographic and/or morphological rules of the Hungarian language, e.g. H *diszkonnektál* '(to) disconnect', H *hospitalizáció* 'hospitalization'. Assimilated loans involve nouns, adjectives and verbs. Borrowed English eponyms and initialisms identified in the discharge reports are also classified as loanwords.

In some contact linguistic studies (cf. Görlach 2001) a distinction is set up between Englishisms and internationalisms based on the assumption that internationalisms are rather words of Latin or Old-Greek origin, and therefore, they should be excluded from the category of English borrowing. Nevertheless, when analyzing the data found in USZCCDR, I did not exclude words that might have a Latin origin, as medical terminology rests on a fundamentally Latin nomenclature with roots, prefixes and suffixes drawn from Greek and Latin. As English words built of Latin word roots and affixes make up for most twentieth century neologisms in the language of medicine (Dirckx 1983), it is almost impossible to say whether a Hungarian medical word containing Latinate elements was directly borrowed from Latin, from the International Scientific

46 Acronysms used in the "Laboratory findings" section are marked (*) in Table 14.

Vocabulary (ISV) or from English. Another feature of the Hungarian language of medicine is that some Latinate words, especially adjectives and verbs, have recently become more widely and frequently used, e.g. *effective* 'effective', *elongál* '(to) elongate', *intenzifikált* 'intensified', *provokál* '(to) provoke'. Their increased frequency in the Hungarian hospital discharge reports can also be attributed to the intensive effect of English language contact.

As an objective criterion to decide whether an English lexical feature has become a fully accepted linguistic phenomenon of the Hungarian language, I checked if the identified loanword was listed in the referenced Hungarian dictionaries. Considering the loanwords proper, most terms were not listed in any of the referenced dictionaries, or the dictionaries contained a lexeme with the same orthography but with a different sememe (see results in Tables 7 and 8). Dictionaries, however, do not contain data on most recently borrowed loanwords, thus, I also checked the presence and frequency of loanwords identified in USZCCDR in the Magyar irodalmi és köznyelv nagyszótárának korpusza/Magyar történeti korpusz [Corpus of the academic dictionary of Hungarian/Hungarian historical corpus]. Approximately half of the borrowed terms from the discharge reports were listed in that corpus, however, it is not a Hungarian medical corpus. Unfortunately no such corpus is available in Hungarian yet.

The process of borrowing is not restricted to the simple transferring of English loanwords into Hungarian; they are subject to phonological, orthographic, morphological and semantic changes. Even some of loanwords proper have undergone these changes considering morphology and/or semantics, e.g. H *flow* 'flow', H *flowt* 'flow (accusative)'.

The assimilation of borrowed words implies their adaptation to the rules of the Hungarian language; the regularly used borrowed items undergo such integration that eventually their foreignness is not noticed by monolinguals. Generally, the borrowed items acquire a 'native status' by the degree of adaptation they undergo. The loanword may be adjusted to the phonetic or spelling norms of the borrowing language (cf. *intenzív* 'intense/intensive', *stressz* 'stress', *tesztel* '(to) test').

Hungarian is a language in which orthography is dominantly based on pronunciation, so the spelling rules of morphemes are mostly determined by the pronunciation used by speakers of standard/everyday Hungarian. Whereas in the case of English, there is a certain lack of correspondence between graphemes and phonemes depending on the context in which they occur.

No phonological examination was undertaken by the present research as Method 1 is based on the analysis of written documents; therefore, no phonological changes of the loanwords are discussed here.

Most English loanwords reveal themselves as foreign because of their orthography. On the orthographical level, loanwords were classified as loanwords proper, i.e. without any orthographic change, and assimilated loans, i.e. there was certain change in the Hungarian orthography of the word compared to the original English one.

The Hungarian language uses the Latin script, thus, it has many items in which the Latin graphemes correlate with phonemes corresponding closely to their English equivalents. Such words are taken over without changes, e.g. E > H *graft, kinking*. However, certain English graphemes and diagraphs are missing or at least are extremely rare in Hungarian so grapheme replacement occurred: *ck, q, sh, th, y* or *w,* e.g. E *levothyroxin* > H *levotiroxin*.

Some English graphemes or combinations are correlated with different phonemes, therefore, the loan may be re-spelt in order to promote a close-to English pronunciation, e.g. H *diffúz* 'diffuse', H *stresszlsztressz* 'stress'. In most cases, however, the English spelling, e.g. *pacemaker, sense, upgrade,* is preserved in the hospital discharge reports. There may be three explanations for this phenomenon. First, these loanwords are still in the initial stage of the borrowing process, and they have not undergone any assimilation yet. They may be used only occasionally in a certain discourse community of bilingual physicians. Nevertheless, it seems to be contradicted by the fact that, on the one hand, I examined a written corpus, i.e. the discharge reports, and on the other hand, these reports are written to members of speech communities who are not necessarily bilinguals (family physicians and patients). The other fact that seems to contradict this explanation is that some of the loanwords proper have undergone morphological assimilation, i.e. they can take up Hungarian suffixes: H *flowt* 'flow (accusative)', H *grafttal* 'with a graft', and H *stentben* 'in a stent'. The second explanation for the unassimilated orthography can be that the spelling of these words correlates closely with their (close-to) English pronunciation and, thus, the original orthography is retained. However, this explanation stands for only a few loanwords proper: e.g. *monitor, penicillin.* But it would not account for the retained orthography of such loanwords proper as *follow up, recovery* or *upgrade*, where the orthography is not close to the pronunciation. The third explanation for unchanged orthography can mostly be derived from social factors: the prestige of the English language is so high that the original orthography is considered to be the standard that should be followed and strictly kept.

On the orthographical level, one of the most frequent changes in spelling is that the English grapheme <c> is usually changed to <k>*:* E *comfort* > H *komfort*, E *(to) disconnect* > H *diszkonnektál*, E *clip* > H *klipp*. The other frequent change is that the English <s> is changed in Hungarian to <sz>*:* E *(to) dislocate* > H *diszlokál*, E *support* > H *szupport.*

Hungarian physicians are not always consistent, however, in the orthography of English loanwords: they use various orthographies for the same source word, e.g. E *flutter* is written with 4 orthographies: H *flutter, flatter, flattern,* and *fluttern*, E *stress* is written either H *stressz* or H *sztressz*, and E *plaque* is written with the English orthography: H *plaque*, with the assimilated orthography: H *plakk* and with a pseudo-English orthography: H *plack*.

Some of the Hungarian endings were written hyphenated (e.g. *flow-val* 'with flow', *spike-ok* 'spikes') and others unhyphenated (e.g. *homografton* 'on the homograft', *stentben* 'in the stent'). Physicians tend to use some of the Hungarian suffixes both hyphenated with the very same loanword and unhyphenated: H *spike-ok* 'spikes' and H *spikeokat* 'spikes (accusative)', *flow-t* 'flow (accusative)' and *flowt* 'flow (accusative)'. Vowel harmony[47] was found in each case of morphological assimilation, but in certain words it harmonized with the orthographic form, e.g. *grafttal* 'with a graft', and in other words with the English phonemic form, e.g., *spikeokat* 'spikes (accusative)', *sprayre* 'due to spray', *scanek* 'scans'.

Hungarian is a Finno-Ugric language that makes extensive use of morphological processes (Fenyvesi 1998). Changes on the morphological level can be described by three processes (Filipović 1996): 'zero transmorphemisation', when there is no morphological assimilation, e.g. H *burst* 'burst', H *defibrillátor* 'defibrillator', H *puff* 'puff', 'partial transmorphemisation', when the English word retains the English suffix of the source word, e.g. H *oversensing* 'oversensing', H *guided* 'guided' or 'complete transmorphemisation', where the original suffix of the English word is completely replaced by a corresponding native suffix, e.g. H *intenzifikált* 'intensified', H *vizualizál* 'visualize'.

Its morphological type is agglutinative, which uses a separate suffix for each morpheme: H *stentelést* 'stenting (accusative)', word root *stent* + verbal thematizing suffix *-el* + nominal derivational suffix *-és* + accusative case ending *-t*. Hungarian nominals inflect for number (H *stentek* 'stents': word root *stent* + plural suffix *-ek*), case (H *graftot* 'graft (accusative)': word root *graft* + accusative case ending *-ot*, H *paceléssel* 'with pacing': word root *pace* + verbal thematizing suffix *-l* + nominal derivational suffix *-és* + instrumental case ending *-sel*) and person – the person of the possessor (H *fluttern-je* 'his/her flutter': word root *fluttern* + possessive ending *-je*). Hungarian verbs inflect through the grammatical dimensions of person, number, tense and mood: H *hospitalizálták* 'he/she was hospitalized', word root *hospitalizál* + third person,

47 Vowel harmony, that is a salient phonological feature that distinguishes it from Indo-European languages (English). The most general Hungarian vowel harmony process restricts the vowels in a word to all back or all front vowels.

singular, past tense, indicative mood, past voice inflectional ending *-ták*'. Both loanwords proper and orthographically assimilated loans can undergo Hungarian nominal, adjectival and verbal inflection.

In loanwords proper morphological assimilation was found in E > H *flow, graft, monitor, pace, pacemaker, scan, spike, spray, stent,* and *study*. Morphological assimilation involved the adding of certain Hungarian endings to the unassimilated orthographic form that is retained: case suffixes – the accusative *-t,* e.g. *flowt* 'flow (accusative)', *stentet* 'stent (accusative)', *studyt* 'study (accusative)', the instrumental *-tal,* e.g. *flow-val* 'with flow', *grafttal* 'with (a) graft', the inessive *-ben,* e.g. *stentben* 'in (the) stent', the plural suffix -*(e)k,* e.g. *pacemakerek* 'pacemakers', *scanek* 'scans', and the verbal thematizing suffix *-l,* e.g. *monitorizál(ás)* 'monitor(ing)', *stentel(ést)* 'stent(ing)'.

None of the loanword proper adjectives have undergone morphological assimilation in the researched cardiological discharge reports. The only exception is *standard,* but this word is used also in other Hungarian discourses in the meaning *szabványos, előírásoknak megfelelő* 'standard, fulfilling the requirements'. Unlike most of the other loanword proper adjectives, *standard* is listed in BISZ and EKSZ. An assimilated orthography is also given in BISZ: *sztenderd.* Other adjectives, e.g. *high* or *low* are also listed in BISZ but only in non-medical compounds: *high-tech, Low Church. Low voltage* and *sick sinus synroma* 'sick sinus syndrome' are listed in BOSZ as compounds borrowed from English, but none of the adjectives are entered in OHSZ (except for *standard*) and TESZ. Thus, *standard* belongs to the group of fully assimilated 'older layer' English borrowings, whereas the other loanword proper adjectives identified in the discharge reports are relatively recent borrowings. It is also supported by the idea that TESZ was published in 1967 and OHSZ was published last in 1992, whereas EKSZ and BOSZ was revised and reedited in 2003 and 2006, respectively.

No loanword proper verb was identified in the discharge reports, though there is indirect evidence for their use in USZCCDR: nominalized verbs such as H *stentelés* 'stenting', word root *stent* + verbal suffix *-el* + nominal derivational suffix *-és, monitorizál/ás* 'monitoring', *pacel/és* 'pacing', and adjectives derived from verbs: H *elongált* 'elongated', word root *elongál* + adjectival suffix *-t, triggerel/t* 'triggered'.

The morphological integration of loans can involve creative processes of adaptation resulting in additional lexical entries. For example English loans are treated as uninflected nouns or stems which can be converted to other classes by the addition of suffixes. Borrowed nouns may be converted into verbs by adding the suffix -z or *-l, e.g. monitoroz* '(to) monitor', *stentel* '(to) stent'. These integrations demonstrate that borrowing involves complex patterns of lexical change that can create new lexical entries or may modify existing ones in response to language contact.

One of the features that make the language of medicine such succinct and economical is its freedom in using nouns as adjectives without any change in form (Dirckx 2006): *bypass operáció* 'bypass operation', *entrainment mapping* 'entrainment mapping', *tamponade jelek* 'tamponade signs'. Another property is that monosyllabic English loanwords are particularly suitable for forming Hungarian compounds, which create even more neologisms to the medical lexicon: H *onkoteam* 'oncology team', H *sludgeképződés* 'sludge formation'.

Besides orthographic and morphological assimilation, loanwords have also been semantically adapted. English loanwords in medicine are usually borrowed in a specific situation and linguistic context (and also with specific intent). This usually means that only one sememe of the polysemic or homonymous lexeme is involved. As the word is borrowed in a specific situation, applied in a specific discourse, cardiology, the meaning may narrow semantically, and become more specific, or referentially it may designate a smaller range of objects stylistically, socially or connotationally (cf. Sankoff 2004).

Most of the borrowed English loanwords in USZCCDR follow a general tendency of narrowing in meaning, a 'restriction of meaning in number' (Filipović 1996), where the English loanword is semantically assimilated into the Hungarian language of cardiology by taking over only one of several meanings, e.g. the English lexeme *pace* has six sememes, and Hungarian has borrowed only one of the technical meanings, the one that is used in cardiology: H *pace* 'regulation of the rate of contraction of the heart muscle by an artificial cardiac pacemaker'.

Borrowing from the English language of medicine can also result in the same lexeme being used by various Hungarian discourse communities, e.g. one sememe of the word E *plaque* is used in cardiology: H *plaque/plakk/plack* 'a deposit of predominantly fatty material in the lining of blood vessels occurring in atherosclerosis', another sememe is used in odontology 'a biofilm noted in the oral cavity', and a third one in dermatology 'a flat, often raised patch on the skin'.

Some of the loanwords, especially compounds are, however, monosemic in both the English and the borrowing Hungarian language, e.g. E *defibrillator* > H *defibrillátor* 'an apparatus for stopping fibrillation of the heart by application of an electric current to the chest wall or directly to the heart', E *hospitalize* and H *hospitalizál* 'to admit or send (a person) into a hospital'. The assimilated loan verbs have all undergone semantic narrowing compared to their English lexeme. The only exception is H *hospitalizál*, which has the same semantic field as E *hospitalize*. It might be due to the fact that the other verbs are used in various fields, but *hospitalize* is used only related to health care. In these cases no change or shift in the semantics of the loanword was found.

USZCCDR provided only one datum for semantic widening/distribution, 'expansion of meaning in a semantic field' (Filipović 1996), where the loanword acquired a new meaning different from its sememes in the English language: *mobilizáció* 'mobilization'. In English *mobilization* means: *to make mobile or capable of movement,* whereas in Hungarian there is a widening in the meaning: *get the patient out of bed.* The scarcity of semantic widening can be explained by the terminological use of these loanwords, i.e. the borrowing was initiated by a terminological gap in the Hungarian language of cardiology.

Considering only the medical meaning of the English words and comparing it with the medical meaning of the borrowed words, as USZCCDR is based on a medical text type, little change could be identified in the semantics of loanwords. None of the adjectives have undergone change in their meaning, which may be due to the fact that most of them are used only with the same noun making a bound phrase, cf. *high rate, sick sinus syndrome* 'sick sinus syndrome'. The borrowed adjectives are usually very short, mostly monosyllabic words (e.g. *fast, high, low, sick, slow, tilt*), and in English they belong to the basic vocabulary. Though in Hungarian, they are used only in compounds resulting in specialized meaning, e.g. E > H (cardiology) *low voltage* 'low R wave in the ECG', E *tilt table test* > H *tilt table vizsgálat* 'orthostatic stress test performed on a tilt table'. Compounds are combinations of two or more free morphemes in English. They are taken over regardless of their compound status if they form a semantic entity. These loanwords become available for use very soon after their adoption since Hungarian has the same pattern for making compounds. The pattern is further strengthened by internationalisms of the *slow-fast* type which are formed on the same principle.

When semantic narrowing of a lexeme was found in USZCCDR, it was, on the one hand, due to the fact that some English nouns can also be used as verbs (cf. *beat, branch, flow, spray, study*) but in Hungarian these loanwords are used only as nouns. However, certain borrowed English lexemes can be used both as nouns and verbs, but in these cases a new lemma is developed: the borrowed lemma can only be used with a nominal sememe, and the Hungarian lemma with the verbal sememe is orthographically different. Verbalization is always marked by the verbal suffix (cf. E n/v *test* > H n *teszt*, H v *tesztel*, E n/v *trigger* > H n *trigger*, H v *triggerel*).

On the other hand, semantic narrowing was due to the fact that some nouns are used with a broader semantic field in English (cf. *puff, sludge*) and only one of these semantic fields is used in the Hungarian cardiology reports. In case of two loanwords the semantic change was not narrowing but rather a shifting in the semantic fields: *burst* and *monitorizál* '(to) monitor' (see details in Section 5.1.2.1.1 and 5.1.2.2.2).

Nouns, adjectives and verbs are open-class content items that can be more easily borrowed (cf. hierarchy of borrowability by Whitney 1881; Haugen 1950; Muysken 1981; Thomason and Kaufman 1988), and closed-class function items like pronouns and conjunctions are less likely to be borrowed. Nouns, adjectives and verbs frequently occur in contexts where they can be isolated and extracted as loans. Verbs tend to be morphologically complex and central to the syntax of a sentence, thus, they tend to be borrowed less than nouns and adjectives. Verbs are facilitated when they can be fitted easily into the Hungarian morphology.

In terms of the parts of speech most English loanwords in USZCCDR were nouns: approximately 80% of all English loanwords. Compounds that contain a noun and a particle are generally considered to be difficult to translate or to translate adequately. This is why they are found in several domains related to medicine (e.g. *bypass*, *oversensing*, *upgrade)*. The economy of expressions given by the *-ing* form also makes the structure frequently be borrowed (*guiding, kinking, mapping*).

Most of the loanwords belong to the nominal category, whereas adjectives comprise a very small rate. Loanword proper adjectives are *fast, high*, *left, low, sick, slow* and assimilated adjectives are *diffúz* 'diffuse', *effektív* 'effective', *elongált* 'elongated', *intenzív* 'intensive', *invazív* 'invasive' and *triggerelt* 'triggered'.

Verbs compared to nouns and adjectives are used relatively rarely in discharge reports due to the generic features of this text type. Verbs are mainly used in the "Presenting symptoms" and the "Past medical history" sections. But the occurrence of verbs is very low even in these sections; mostly copular sentences are used with nominal and adjectival complements. No loan verbs proper were found in the studied corpus, and the assimilated loan verbs are mostly of Latinate origin.

The last three categories discussed in the section of lexical borrowings are: initialisms, eponyms and trade names. A medical eponym is a name for a disease, organ, procedure, or body function that is derived from the name of a person, usually a physician or scientist who first described the condition or devised the object bearing the name. Examples include fallopian tube, Parkinson's disease, or Billing's method. Eponyms are frequently used in medicine as a form of coining new words for recently identified phenomena. Most eponyms in English are formed with the synthetic genitive, with *'s* put after a proper name, e.g. *Babinski's sign*, *Hodgkin's disease, Osler's nodes*, *Quincke's sign.* Though recently, in some cases, it is written as a substantival adjunct, the proper noun is used as an adjective without change of form: *a Colles fracture, the Jones criteria.*

The Hungarian language of medicine also uses these eponyms. The structure of the eponyms in Hungarian, however, is traditionally different from the English structure: the proper noun is either connected to the following noun with a hyphen, cf. *Babinski-jel* 'Babinski's sign', *Hodgkin-kór* 'Hodgkin's disease', *Osler-csomók* 'Osler's node', *Quincke-jel* 'Quincke's sign', or a hyphenated suffix-like element *-féle* is added to the proper noun, cf. *Corrigan-féle pulzus* 'Corrigan's pulse', *Quincke-féle oedema* 'Quincke's edema'.

Eponyms are frequently used in the language of medicine in general but in the text type I examined, eponyms are rare. In USZCCDR, I found only 4 borrowed eponyms: one loanword proper eponym: *"Shepherd's crook"*, and three assimilated eponyms*: Holter monitorozás* 'Holter monitoring', *Bruce protokoll* 'Bruce protocol' and *Wood (lámpa)* 'Wood (lamp)'. The four eponyms show three different features of borrowing: orthographic, lexical and semantic interferences. *"Shepherd's crook"* is orthographically unassimilated, and it is written in quotation marks, which show that it is considered to be in the first phase of the borrowing process when foreign terms are separated by quotation marks. The first quotation mark is at the apostrophe-height, which is an orthographical English language contact-induced feature in itself. In *Holter monitorozás* and, *Bruce protokoll* the more recent form of the English eponyms are borrowed, i.e. Holter monitoring, Bruce protocol. In case of Wood-lámpa the corpus gives matches only for *Wood (poz.)*, which shows that the proper noun in itself substitutes the full eponym (the common noun *lámpa* 'lamp' is not given). The abbreviation in parenthesis after the proper noun, *(poz.)*, refers to the result of the Wood lamp test, i.e. positive result.

A trade name is the trademark name or commercial trade name for a material or product in medicine. Trade names make up a significant part of the terminology of medicine: the majority of trade names that physicians use are patented drug names (*Aspirin Protect*); others refer to the name of the manufacturer of the medical device.

In English, trade names that refer to the manufacturer of a product, are used as substantival adjuncts, i.e. the proper noun is used as an adjective without change in its form: *Quinton treadmill*.

In Hungarian trade names are usually used in the same way as eponyms: the proper name is hyphenated with the designated product type: *Wolfram-huzal* 'Wolfram wire', or adding the hyphenated postfix *-féle* to the proper name: *Voll-féle elektroakupunktúra* 'Voll's acupuncture'.

Several frequently used borrowed trade names were identified in the discharge reports under investigation: E *Driver stent* > H *Driver stent*, E *JR/JL guiding* > H *JR/JL guiding*, E *Maverick balloon* > H *Maverick ballon* or E *St. Jude artificial (heart) valve* > H *St. Jude műbillentyű*. Each term follows the English typology for trade names, i.e. they are not hyphenated.

Initialisms are particularly common in modern medical writing, which consist of first letters of the words that compose a phrase (*ACE, GERD*). Initialisms are in some cases better known within the profession than their full name, e.g. *TIMI* meaning *thrombolysis in myocardial infarction* or *CKMB* meaning *creatinine kinase muscle band.*

An abbreviation made up of the first two or three letters of a word is one common variant in USZCCDR but they are not of English origin, e.g. *k.m.n.* for *külön megnevezés nélkül* 'not otherwise specified', *m.k.o.* for *mindkét oldalon* 'bilaterally' or *sz.e.* for *szükség esetén* 'if needed'. These types of abbreviations are usually not so frequently borrowed as members of the first group (Bősze 2009).

A third type contains a letter for each syllable or morpheme in the base word, e.g. CH for *carbohydrate,* GERD *for gastroesophageal reflux disease*, or it may be a hybrid initialism combining the first or the first two letters of a word, e.g. ALP for *alkaline phosphatase*.

Initialisms are especially popular for describing names of diseases and pathological conditions, e.g. *AVNRT* for *atrioventricular nodal reentrant tachycardia*, *NPDR* for *nonproliferative diabetic retinopathy*, and of diagnostic and therapeutic procedures, e.g. *ABPM* for *ambulatory 24-hour blood pressure monitoring*, *PTCA* for *percutaneous transvenous coronary angioplasty*.

An acronym is an initialism that can be pronounced like a word (ACE, LIMA, POBA, SPECT, and TIMI). Unpronounceable initialisms are turned into acronyms by the insertion of extraneous vowel sounds, e.g. E *NYHA* 'New York Heart Association' is pronounced <njiha> in Hungarian.

Though mnemonics (e.g. SOAP for symptoms, observations, assessment, and plan) are very frequently used in the English language of medicine, they do not tend to be borrowed due to the phenomenon behind the development of these acronyms, i.e. they make it easier for the speaker to remember certain items.

English medical initialisms (especially acronyms) are very frequently transferred into the Hungarian language of cardiology. They behave in the Hungarian discharge reports as morphologically unassimilated loanwords proper. Due to their specific feature, i.e. they stand for English words, no semantic change or assimilation can occur when they are borrowed from English. No assimilation was identified, although there were examples of combining the English loan acronyms with Hungarian/Latinate acronyms, e.g. *LIMA-RDA graft*: E *LIMA-LAD* 'left internal mammary artery – left anterior descending/descendent' > H *LIMA-RDA* 'left internal mammary artery – ramus descendens anterior'.

Acronyms form numerically the largest group of borrowings in the cardiology discharge reports. They can be found mainly in the "Laboratory results" section in the form of a list and in the "Medications" section of the report, but less frequently acronyms are also used in the "Diagnoses" or the "Past medical history" sections.

We have to distinguish between initialisms used in the "Laboratory results" section and in other sections of the discharge reports as certain standardized programs are used at the department of cardiology for describing the laboratory findings (see 5.1.1.2.1), thus, physicians writing the discharge report of a patient rely on these programs[48]. English is the language of these programs and they offer English abbreviations for laboratory examinations. Thus, in this case, the use of the English acronyms is not a real linguistic borrowing, or at least we should consider them as a result of deliberate language planning. Yet, the other sections of the report are not 'ready-made' offered to the physicians, and initialisms are also frequently used in these parts of the report. Acronyms are also used in the "Diagnoses", the "Past medical history" and the "Investigations" sections, where the presence of these acronyms can be considered as instances of unplanned borrowings.

The use of Hungarian proper[49] acronyms and abbreviations was less frequent than that of the borrowed abbreviations, e.g. H *hu.* 'harántujjnyi' 'fingerbreadth', H *ISZB* 'ischemias szívbetegség' 'ischemic heart disease', H *kp.* 'közepesen' 'moderately'. However, not only English borrowed acronyms and abbreviations are used but a significant amount of Latin(ate) ones can also be identified in the studied corpus, e.g. *myoc.* 'myocardial', *RDA* 'ramus descendens anterior'. In some cases it is difficult to say if the acronym stands for the Hungarian/Latin(ate) or the English expression behind it, as it is the same in both languages, e.g. *AMI* H 'akut myocardialis infarktus/acut myocardial infarctus', E 'acute myocardial infarct', *syst.* H 'szisztolés/systoles', E 'sytolic'.

Lexical borrowing is a common form of cross-linguistic influence, which can occur under a variety of conditions ranging from superficial familiarity of the source language, even without real contact with the source language's speakers, to "close interaction between recipient and source language speakers in bilingual communities" (Winford 2003: 29). The English medical terms can often be attributed to the written medium, they are only used occasionally, mainly by the members of the medical discourse community (and very rarely by some patients with checkered medical history), and do not belong to the common word stock of a language. Several parameters have been proposed against which to place a given word technical or non-technical, in the lexicon as a whole (Heller 1970): the extent to which a word is generally understood in the language community as a whole, the extent to which a word is related to a particular technical discipline, or the extent to which a word is normalized or established in its usage (Langslow 2004).

---

48 Acronyms used in the Laboratory results section are marked (*) in Table 14.

49 Hungarian proper means here a non-borrowed item.

Most of the English borrowed lexis is not used by the language community as a whole (e.g. *kinking, sludge, upgrade*), others are understood by certain speakers, usually affected by some related diseases (e.g. *bypass, pacemaker, stroke*) and the rest (mainly terms belonging to the ISV) are understood and used by most members of the Hungarian speech community (e.g. *monitor, penicillin, spray, vitamin*).

An English unassimilated borrowing does not necessarily imply the lack of the native equivalent: E *end stage* – H *end stage*, H *végstádium;* E *spike* – H *spike*, H *tüske;* E *study* – H *study*, H *vizsgálat*. The rules governing borrowing are not yet well defined.

Ardila (2005) hypothesized that several principles are acting simultaneously in borrowing English words:

1. no word corresponds exactly to the borrowed English word in Hungarian, e.g. *oversensing, stent*,

2. the borrowed English word has a very exact referent, like a proper name, e.g. *levothyroxine, penicillin, vitamin*,

3. there are some potentially correct words for the phenomenon in Hungarian, but none has the exact meaning, e.g. the word *study* corresponds in Hungarian to *analízis* 'analysis', *kutatás* 'research', *tanulmányozás* 'investigation', *vizsgálat* 'examination',

4. the borrowed English word is 'compatible' with Hungarian phonology, e.g. *monitor, puff*,

5. the borrowed English word is phonologically simpler (or orthographically shorter) than the corresponding Hungarian word, e.g. E *stroke* > H *stroke/agyérkatasztrófa* 'cerebrovascular catastrophy', E *tilt table test* > H *tilt table test /billenőasztalon történő ortosztatikus terheléses teszt* 'orthostatic stress test performed on a tilt table',

6. highly technical words related to the discourse of cardiological discharge reports are often borrowed from English into Hungarian, e.g.*LIMA-LAD graft, non-sustained VT, Quincke jel* 'Quincke's sign'.

Borrowing English lexical terms may be due to mostly two main motives: the need-filling motive and the prestige motive. However, besides linguistic factors, social factors such as the intensity of the contact, power, professional, economical and political dominance may also play an important role in it. A detailed discussion of motives for borrowing is described in Section 5.3.

5.1.3. Semantic borrowings

Semantic borrowing implies the transference of a semanteme or unit of meaning (Haugen 1950), and words between which this transference takes place show certain formal or semantic analogy.

As Method 1 of the present study involved the research of written documents, the data discussed below are collected from the corpus of 234 Hungarian cardiology discharge reports. Conclusions drawn on the semantic borrowings present in the Hungarian language of cardiology are complemented by the data gained through Method 2, when cardiologists have been asked to reflect on certain phenomena that are present in the reports written by them. Analysis of the data collected through the interviews is discussed in Section 5.2, and overall conclusions are drawn in Section 5.3.

In the present subsection English contact-induced semantic borrowings, i.e. loan substitutions, are discussed. Semantic changes in loanwords, semantic narrowing or shift, have been described above.

According to the categorization of my research data introduced in Section 4.1.4, external borrowing of English lexemes into the Hungarian language of cardiology can be divided into three categories: borrowing of loanwords, loan substitutions and pseudo-loans.

externally borrowed lexemes

loanwords | loan substitutions (hybrid loans) | pseudo-loans

Loan substitutions (hybrid loans) are semantic borrowings; they imply the transference of a semanteme or unit of meaning from English into Hungarian. Loan substitutions[50] involve four types of semantic borrowing: loan translations, loanblends, loan meaning and loan creation.

50 Substitution is not used here to refer to assimilated loanwords (a la Haugen) but as a collective term for semantic borrowings.

loan substitutions
(semantic borrowings)

loan translation | loanblends | loan creation | loan meaning

Loan translations (see Section 5.1.3.1) are calques, showing analogy of meaning between the source and the recipient language, i.e. English and Hungarian in the present case, but the form/orthography is different in the two languages. Loanblends (see Section 5.1.3.2) are hybrid calques which are formed by the borrowing of one or more English morphemes and their combination with one or more Hungarian morphemes. A loan creation (see Section 5.1.3.3) is based on conceptual transmission. It is the creation of a new Hungarian word according to an English conceptual model without any formal relation to this model in terms of lexical structure. A loan meaning is a semantic calque, when only a semanteme but not the form of an English word is transferred to a Hungarian word. Loan meanings are not discussed in this section on semantic borrowings, as I found no data for this borrowing category in USZCCDR. However, with Method 2, I have managed to reveal that there are examples of this phenomenon in the Hungarian language of cardiology, e.g. E *spike* (medicine) 'a sharp peak in an electronic recording' > H *spike,* and H *tüske* (non-technical) 'thorn' > H *tüske* (cardiology) 'a sharp peak in an electronic recording'.

Lexical borrowings discussed in 5.1.2 are usually easy to identify due to the English orthography of these words. Semantic borrowings, however, are more difficult to spot and analyze. Lexical borrowings have been cross-checked in English and Hungarian dictionaries, whereas most of the terms discussed in semantic borrowings are not listed in either English or Hungarian dictionaries. These borrowings are, on the one hand, composed of two or more morphemes not necessarily forming a dictionary entry (lexeme), but, on the other hand, they are highly technical, used only in the language of medicine or even in the language of cardiology only. Thus, their assessment may be less objective than that of the lexical borrowings. Nevertheless, I have had ongoing personal communication about these semantic borrowings with various cardiologists, not only during the interviews but on several further occasions as well.

5.1.3.1. Loan translations

A loan translation is a complete morphemic substitution of lexical complexes or units of the language model, the English language, with morphemes of the recipient language, the Hungarian language. A Hungarian loan translation is therefore the morphemic substitution of a polymorphemic unit of the English language by means of elements, previously existing in the Hungarian language as independent lexemes, but new as a lexical compound with a global sense.

Loan translations are frequently used when new, usually complex phenomena are described, thus, they frequently occur in the language of sciences, and within that in the Hungarian language of cardiology.

Loan translations are particularly common when compounds are involved. Heath (1989) refers to these cases as 'pattern transfer', that is, as instances of structural convergence rather than lexical borrowing per se, e.g. *gócjel* 'focal sign', *magasvérnyomás-betegség* 'hypertensive disease'. Thus loan translations are not discussed within lexical borrowing but under semantic borrowings.

A Hungarian loan translation consists of the reproduction of an English lexical complex by means of the Hungarian material. As the Hungarian reproduction tends to be 'faithful' to the English model, the loan translation may be a borrowing caused by a translation, a 'Lehnübersetzung' (Betz 1939). The new Hungarian lexical complex is an exact 'copy' of the model English lexical unit not only in meaning but usually also in structure.

A loan translation is always a polymorphemic unit, i.e. it is made up of two or more free Hungarian morphemes. By the combination of Hungarian morphemes a word or a lexical complex is resulted that carries the semantic features of that of the English item, but which did not exist in Hungarian earlier, e.g. E *focal sign* > H *gócjel/góctünet*, E *sudden cardiac death* > H *hirtelen szívhalál*. In these cases the English and the Hungarian terms share a primary literal meaning. Loan translations create a new lexical unit not only in the Hungarian language of cardiology but generally in the Hungarian language.

Loan translations may consist of one word only, i.e. a compound or may be formed of a group of words. Compounds found in the discharge reports are mostly nominal, e.g. *alvászavar* 'sleep disorder', *ágynyugalom* 'bedrest', *cukoranyagcsere* 'glucose metabolism, *csúcsáramlás* 'peak flow', *folyadékfelszaporodás* 'fluid accumulation', *góctünet* 'focal sign', *műbillentyű* 'artificial (heart) valve', *szívhalál* 'cardiac death', *várólista* 'waiting list', *zsíranyagcsere* 'fat/lipid metabolism'. The only adjectival compound was *mélyvénás* 'deep vein', but it was used only in the phrase: *mélyvénás thrombosis* 'deep vein thrombosis', therefore, it should be dealt with in the section on loanblends.

Phraseological loan translations are loan translations consisting of several words. These are syntagmatic structures where the relation of the morphemes is more important than the morphemes themselves. They are usually neological means almost exclusive of technical languages: *egy-ér/két-ér/három-ér betegség* 'single/double/triple vessel disease', *folyadékegyensúly zavar* 'fluid balance disorder', *haszon/kockázat arány* 'benefit-risk ratio', *hirtelen szívhalál* 'sudden cardiac death', *képalkotó terheléses vizsgálat* 'stress imaging', *várólista bizottság* 'waiting list committee', *időablakra való tekintettel* 'considering the time window', *szénhidrát-anyagcsere rendelleneség/zavar* 'disorder of carbohydrate metabolism'.

A special semantic subtype can be identified within loan translations: the translated idiomatic expression (Ligeti 1976; Grosjean 1982; Lanstyák 2006): *időablak* 'time window – as the interval between the occurrence of an initial event and the upper limit of the period within which new information can be integrated with the memory representation of that event', *lassú pálya* 'slow path – an anomalous conduction pathway in the heart which has no known functions'.

Besides the above listed loan translations a special tendency of using noun-plus-adjective compounds could be seen in the discharge reports under investigation. Several loan translations have been found to be formed on the pattern of using a noun and an adjective (*mentes* 'free', *szegény* 'low/poor', *dús* 'dense/high/rich') to yield a semantically and morphotactically transparent compound modeling the English phrase.

Mentes 'free' was used in several Hungarian compounds: *eseménymentes* 'event free', *göbmentes* 'nodule free', *kőmentes* 'stone-free', *lobmentes* 'inflammation free', *panaszmentes* 'complaint free', *tejmentes diéta* 'milk/lactose free diet', and *tünetmentes* 'symptom free'. Some of these compounds are loanblends (hybrid calques): *reakciómentes* 'reaction free' *and ritmuszavarmentes* 'arrhythmia free'.

Szegény 'low/poor' and *dús* 'dense/high/rich' were the other two frequently used adjectives with nouns to form compounds: *fűszerszegény* 'low spice', *rostszegény* 'low fibre' *sószegény* 'low salt', *zsírszegény* 'low fat' and r*ostdús* 'high fiber'. Most of these compounds are loanblends: *kalóriaszegény* 'low calorie', *koleszterin/cholesterinszegény étrend* 'low cholesterol diet', *lipidszegény* 'low lipid', *purinszegény diéta* 'low purine diet', and *szénhidrátszegény* 'low carbohydrate diet', and *echoszegény képlet* 'echo-poor structure', *kalóriadús* 'high calorie', and *echodús* 'echo-rich/dense'.

Asymmetric loan translations (a subtype of loan translations) are semantic borrowings in which part of the English model is properly translated and part of it is freely translated. The following asymmetric loan translations were identified in the discharge reports: E *space occupying lesion* > H *térszűkítő folyamat* 'space narrowing process', E *wall motion abnormality* > H *falmozgászavar* 'wall motion disorder'.

5.1.3.2. Loanblends

Loanblends are defined by Haugen (1950) as those instances of lexical borrowing in which both 'importation' and 'substitution' play a role. Weinreich (1953) defined these processes as 'transfer' and 'reproduction'. Loanblends are hybrid calques, they are formed by the borrowing of one or more English/Latinate morphemes and their combination with one or more Hungarian morphemes to form a new sememe, e.g. E *contrast material* > H *kontrasztanyag,* E *peak gradient* > H *csúcsgrádiens*, E *sign of strain* > H *strainjel.*

Loanblends (hybrid compounds) are the most frequent type of loan substitutions in Hungarian cardiology discharge reports. It might be due to the fact that Hungarian uses the Latin script, thus, it has many items in which the Latin graphemes correlate with phonemes corresponding closely to their English equivalents (see 5.1.2 above for details). Thus certain English (and also Latinate) morphemes are taken over without change, and the borrowed morphemes are freely combined with the Hungarian morphemes.

Loanblends may consist of a single word only, i.e. a compound or may be formed of a group of words. Compounds found in the discharge reports are mostly nominal, e.g. *cukorprofil* 'sugar profile' *csúcsgrádiens* 'peak gradient', *kaliberingadozás* 'caliber fluctuation', *pánikbetegség* 'panic disorder', rizikófaktor 'risk factor', *strainjel* 'strain sign', *vérnyomáskontroll* 'blood pressure control', and *volumenpótlás* 'volume substitution'.

Phraseological loanblends consist of a group of words. In these syntagmatic structures the relation of the morphemes is more important than the morphemes themselves: *átmeneti agyi ischaemiás attak* 'transient cerebral ischemic attack', *gyógyszerkibocsátó coronaria stent* 'drug releasing coronary stent', *halmozott rizikófaktorok* 'accumulated risk factors', *intenzifikált inzulinkezelés* 'intensified insulin therapy', *inzulin/nem-inzulin dependens cukorbetegség* 'insulin/non-insulin dependent diabetes', *mellkasi diszkomfort* 'chest discomfort', *mélyvénás thrombosis* 'deep vein thrombosis', *pacemaker tasak/zseb* 'pacemaker pouch/pocket', *pitvarfibrillációs epizód* 'episode of atrial fibrillation', *szoros vérnyomáskontroll* 'tight/close blood pressure control/monitoring', *thrombocyta-aggregáció gátló kezelés* 'thrombocyte aggregation inhibitor therapy', and *24 órás vérnyomás monitorozás* '24-hour blood pressure monitoring'.

Loanblends like loan translations can also form idiomatic expressions, e.g. *kongóvörös* 'Congo red – an azo dye $C_{32}H_{22}N_6Na_2O_6S_2$ that is red in alkaline and blue in acid solution and that is used especially as an indicator and as a biological stain'.

Loanblends are also used to provide the names of certain special hospital units: *Fejfájás Ambulancia* 'Headache Unit', *Invazív Kardiológiai Részleg* 'Invasive Cardiology Unit', *Pacemaker Ambulancia* 'Pacemaker Outpatient Unit', and *Ritmuszavar Ambulancia/ Arrhythmia Ambulancia* 'Arrhythmia Unit'.

Acronyms are also used in loanblends to form a lexical complex: *IUD jelzőszál* 'intra uterine device thread', *PM Ambulancia* 'Pacemaker Outpatient Unit', and *PM beültetés/implantáció* 'pacemaker implantation'.

5.1.3.3. Loan creations

In loan creations the translational equivalence from English into Hungarian is abandoned as it is based on conceptual transmission. It is the creation of a new Hungarian word/term/phrase according to an English conceptual model without any formal relation to this model in terms of lexical structure (Betz 1939). It reflects the English model without being formally related to the English term, e.g. E *temporary collapse in (pulmonary and cardiac) circulation* > H *keringésmegingás* 'a swing in circulation', E *achieving HIS bundle pacing* > (H) *HIS pacelés kötegválaszt igazolt* 'HIS pacing justified bundle reaction/answer'.

5.1.3.4. Loan meaning

A loan meaning is a semantic calque. It refers to the borrowing of a meaning through meaning extension of a word in the recipient language. In this type of semantic borrowing no new lexical item is formed in the Hungarian language but a new semanteme is added to the existing ones of the same Hungarian lexeme (Onysko 2007). Loan meaning presupposes that the English language lexeme and the Hungarian language equivalent have something in common: their phonemic shapes, or their semantic structures or both. A finer classification of loan meanings is given by Haugen (1950, 1972): homophones, homologs and analogs.

Interlingual homophones are words with identical or similar phonemic shape but completely different semantic structure in the two languages, e.g. E *puff* 'vapor'– H *puff* '1. a piece of furniture, 2. special sleeve of a blouse', the newly added meaning is: *(2x3) puff* '(two times a day three) administration(s) of a medicated vapor'.

Interlingual homologs are words with completely different phonemic shapes but identical or similar semantic structures in the two languages, e.g. E *circulation* – H *keringés* 'moving around'. Similarity in meaning usually means at least some overlapping in the meaning of the homologs.

Analogs are words with both similar phonemic shape and similar semantic structure in the two languages. This kind of semantic borrowing arises easily in the process of translation and in the speech of bilinguals: they are known as 'false friends', e.g. E *probe* – H *próba* 'trial', E *visit* – H *vizit* '(ward)round'.

Loan meanings are not discussed in this section on semantic borrowings, as I have found no data for this borrowing category in USZCCDR. However, with Method 2, I have managed to reveal that there are examples of this phenomenon in the Hungarian language of cardiology, e.g. E *spike* (medicine) 'a sharp peak in an electronic recording' > H *spike,* and H *tüske* (non-technical) 'thorn' > H *tüske* (cardiology) 'a sharp peak in an electronic recording'.

5.1.3.5. Discussion on semantic borrowings

Semantic borrowings described in Section 5.1.3 are the transference of a semanteme or a unit of meaning from an English lexeme or lexical complex to a Hungarian word or lexical unit. Loan translations in a narrower sense are created solely by the morphemes belonging to the Hungarian language, whereas loanblends contain at least one morpheme imported from the English language. In loan creations there is only a conceptual transmission, whereas in case of loan meanings there is an extension in the semantic field of the Hungarian term. Instances of the latter two types of borrowing have been found to be relatively infrequent in the studied corpus.

Most of the semantic loans in USZCCDR are polymorphemic units; they are made up of two or more morphemes. Phraseological loan translations and loanblends are the most common type of borrowings within loan substitutions. These are semantic units that are usually used in these forms only in the technical language of cardiology: *thrombocyta-aggregáció gátló kezelés* 'thrombocyte aggregation inhibitor therapy', *24 órás vérnyomás monitorozás* '24-hour blood pressure monitoring'.

Carstensen (1993) points out that, due to the increasingly important role of modern mass communication, neologisms occur ever more as internationalisms rather than neologisms of one language. This tendency can be observed especially in English, and via English and Latin (Latinate elements) they increase the Hungarian word-stock.

5.1.4. Borrowing of grammatical and syntactic features

The problem of grammatical interferences is still debated in general linguistics. Sapir highlighted that "nowhere do we find any but superficial morphological interinfluencings" (1921: 217). An opposite view has been highlighted by Schuchardt that "even closely knit structures like inflectional endings are not secure against invasion by foreign material" (1928: 195).

Several linguists involved in the investigation of language contact-induced features are convinced that grammatical or syntactic borrowing is impossible or close to it (cf. Lefebvre 1985; Prince 1988; King 2000). These authors generally see grammatical change subsequent to contact as a consequence of lexical or pragmatic interinfluence that may then lead to internal syntactic change.

The adoption of bound morphemes has been stated by many authors to be among the most resistant features of language contact-induced change. Only a few cases have come to light, and almost all involve morphemes that are, if not entirely free, not really bound either (Sankoff 2004).

Probably the most popular traditional view is that the grammatical rules of one language can only be transferred to another language through abstraction from borrowed lexical items. That is, the rules themselves are not borrowed at all; instead, lexical items are borrowed, and some or all of their phonological and morphosyntactic structure is adopted as a concomitant feature of the lexical borrowing. No absolute constraint against direct rule transfer can be maintained (Sankoff 2004).

Various definitions of 'rule' can be found in the literature: in this context a rule is "any statement expressing a linguistically significant generalization about the grammatical facts of a particular language, especially when formulated within the formalism of some particular formal description" (Trask 1993: 245).

Even though the mechanisms of rule transfer are not well understood, rules do indeed get transferred as part of contact-induced change. For both phonological and morphosyntactic borrowing, it is quite possible that bilingual speakers simply import a pattern from a second language into their first language for various reasons: adopting a word-order pattern from another language that its speakers use regularly might "lessen the cognitive burden of moving back and forth between languages" (Thomason 2001: 16) or the use of a structure, e.g. passive, might seem prestigious.

Thomason (2003) claims that anything can be subject to borrowing. The change of a grammatical system toward a less explicit form is generally recognized to be quite rare, but some instances have been attested (Vogt 1954).

Although the impact on grammatical structures is less than that of lexical ones in USZCCDR, certain contact-induced grammatical/syntactic features can still be identified. Direct borrowing of structural features is constrained, but it can happen in certain cases: the degree of bilingualism involved and the extent to which bilinguals are dominant in one or the other language. It is well known that situations in which a maintained language has undergone significant contact-induced change invariably involve extensive bilingualism (Winford 2003).

The Hungarian language of medicine may have a mixed grammar, mainly maintaining the original Hungarian grammar but also to a lesser extent changing to become closer to the English one (cf. Poplack 1980). There is evidence that heavy lexical borrowing can introduce new structural features into a language. Nevertheless, direct borrowing of structural elements can occur only when the languages involved are typologically very similar, allowing for the substitution of a Hungarian morpheme by a close counterpart in English (cf. Winford 2003).

In the researched hospital discharge reports, the following changes in grammatical structures and syntax have been identified: changes in the use of the Hungarian articles (indefinite article see Section 5.1.4.1.1 and definite article see Section 5.1.4.1.2), extensive use of impersonalizing and depersonalizing structures (see Section 5.1.4.2), changes in the use of certain tenses (see Section 5.1.4.3), the use of grammatical apposition (see Section 5.1.4.4) and changes in the use of the plural (see Section 5.1.4.5).

5.1.4.1. Articles

There are both indefinite and definite articles in the Hungarian language, which can either precede the noun immediately, or together with their premodifying adjectives holding together the whole noun phrase (Korchmáros 2006). In the Hungarian hospital discharge reports, changes in the use of both types of articles have been found.

5.1.4.1.1. The indefinite article

In Hungarian the indefinite article can stand only with singular nouns or nominals. It usually occurs with countable common nouns, "expressing that the entity referred with the noun is unidentified among the members of its class and has not been mentioned before" (Korchmáros 2006: 175). However, the noun is not preceded by the indefinite article if this noun does not refer to an individual entity from among the members of its class.

The indefinite article was used in the researched discharge reports several instances in the latter mentioned position, where according to descriptive Hungarian grammar it should not be used. The phenomenon was described by Hungarian linguists as early as 1947 by Szamek and then in 1982 by Kontra both identifying the phenomenon in the Hungarian language as used by Hungarians living in the United States. The use of the indefinite article in current colloquial Hungarian is spreading (Kenesei et al. 1998). The use of the indefinite article in this position has also been investigated in Hungarian speakers living in Hungary and being under the effect of the English language (cf. Klaudy 1997; Tótfalusi 1998).

The indefinite article was used in the following examples taken from the discharge reports: *ad hoc angioplasztikáját egy gyógyszerkibocsájtó stent implantációjával elvégeztük* 'we performed his ad hoc angioplasty by the implantation of a drug releasing stent', *Egy 1.5x15 mm Sprinter ballonnal 10 atm. nyomással tágítást végzünk* 'With a 1.5x15 mm Sprinter balloon at the pressure of 10 atmospheres we performed dilatation.', *majd egy 2.5x15 mm Maverick ballonnal* 'and then with a 2.5x15 mm Maverick balloon', *benne egy 22 mm kőreflexió látható* 'a 22 mm stone reflection can be seen in it'.

5.1.4.1.2. Omission of the definite article

The primary purpose of definite noun phrases is to refer to discourse entities that have properties such as identifiability, uniqueness, existential presupposition, and/or totality in the context (Huddleston and Pullum 2002). In Hungarian, the definite article is used even when a demonstrative pronoun precedes the noun and is used as an adjective. The article follows the demonstrative pronoun. Whenever a definite object is referred to, the definite article should be used in Hungarian. The definite article is used before singular and plural nouns that refer to a particular member of a group. When the Hungarian word is without a definite article, it corresponds to a noun in English with an indefinite article.

Several examples of the omission of the definite article have been found in the researched discharge reports. The omission of the article has mostly been demonstrated to occur when it should have preceded a proper noun at the beginning of a sentence. It is a specific feature of the English language of medicine, among them the discharge report and other health documents (Dirckx 2006; Wang and Bai 2007), that the article is omitted. The same phenomenon can be found in the Hungarian discharge reports: e.g. Ø *Belgyógyászat intenzív osztályáról vesszük át a beteget* 'We admit the patient from Ø Internal Medicine Intensive Care Unit', Ø *Haemodinamika küldi Ambulanciánkra* 'Ø Hemodynamics (Hemodynamic Unit) sends him to our Outpatient Department', Ø *SBO-ra érkezéskor* 'On arrival to Ø Intensive Care Unit', Ø Traumatológiai Klinikára szállították 'He was transferred to Ø Traumatology Department'.

The other case when the definite article has been observed to be omitted is when there is a difference in the use of this article between the two languages: the definite article is not used in English before names of materials and abstract nouns. As a result of the English language contact, the definite article is omitted in the Hungarian sentences as well: e.g. *Kb. két hónappal ezelőtt kezdődtek* Ø panaszai 'his complaints started about two months ago', *melynek hátterében Ø ultrahang jobb oldali nephrolithiasist igazolt* 'in the background of which ultrasound has revealed nephrolithiasis'.

However, in structures where the definite article is omitted in front of an improper noun, their omission can be explained by various factors: i. representing a more "archaic" form opposed to the recent spread of definite articles in vernacular Hungarian, ii. they can be the representation of certain individual language variant, or iii. the phenomenon can truly be attributed to English languge contact (Marianne Bakró-Nagy, DSc, DHc, personal communication on 28 April 2010). Further contact linguistic/sociolinguistic research might be carried out in the future to answer the above raised questions. Frequency studies may be performed as well on the discharge reports written by a single cardiologist to study the use or omission of the definite article.

5.1.4.2. Impersonalizing

Medical discourse is characterized by neutrality, impersonality and objectivity. Medical language frequently contains linguistic forms that serve to create a social distance between physicians and patients. This distance develops not only out of poor communication with the patient, but also, and more importantly, arises as the language that a physician uses to modulate his or her experience of the patient. It is suggested that "some of the problem lies in the very nature of language itself as the medical language [i.e. the speakers of it] has adopted special forms and metaphors which further serve to create distance" (Mintz 1992: 223, remark in parentheses by the present author). Impersonalization is a characteristic of medical discourse. Bazerman (1988:14) describes this feature as follows:

"One peculiar aspect of the accomplishment of scientific discourse is that it appears to hide itself. […]. [T]o write science is commonly thought not to write at all, just simply to record natural facts. […] The popular belief of the past century that scientific language is simply a transparent transmitter of natural facts is, of course, wrong."

The use of first person pronouns signifies a personal attitude so that the narration is mediated through the subjective viewpoint of the narrator's consciousness, whereas third person pronouns signify an external point of view (cf. Fowler 1986). An 'empathy hierarchy' ranks discourse elements according to the degree of involvement they create. The first and second person outrank human third persons, which "outrank non-human animates, which again outrank natural forces and inanimates" (De Lancey 1981: 644).

The position of the author of the discharge report, the physician, is neutralized, and the overall textual structure of the report is conventionalized (Taaivitsainen 2000: 67). With the course of the disease in an impersonalized tone with passive constructions and clinical facts, the personal facts of the patient are kept to the minimum. A form of grammaticalization of impersonality that contributes to the creation of the effect of the apparent absence of rhetoric characteristic in the medical discourse is the "removal of explicit agency, resulting in the 'objectification' of the discourse, or the representation of actions, events and qualities as objects" (Halliday and Martin 1993: 52).

In the hospital discharge reports the writer deliberately distances themselves from what is being written. The effect is language that is objective, free of bias or emotion (or at least seems to be objective). The use of formal language is also characteristic of this impersonal style. The literature suggests that beside the passive voice ergative constructions (cf. Lyons 1968; Sinclair 1990), active verbs with inanimate subjects (Master 1991) and deverbalisation and nominalizations (Halliday 1988) can also provide a grammatical context for the creation of this effect.

Some examples from the discharge reports for impersonal style are the following: e.g. *A vizsgálat subcostalis síkból történt* 'the examination was performed from a subcostal plane', *Magasvérnyomás, hyperlipidaemia ismert* 'High blood pressure, hyperlipidemia are known', *ügyelet látta* '(patient) was seen by (the doctor on) duty', *Városi Ügyelet kéri vizsgálatát* 'City Medical Duty Service asks for the patient's examination', *Ügyelet járt kinn nála* 'patient was visited by the medical duty service', *OMSZ hozta az ambulanciára* 'National Ambulance Service has brought (the patient) to the outpatient department', *sürgősséggel Traumatológiai Klinikára szállították* 'was transferred to Traumatology Department as an emergency', *terápiát indítottak* 'therapy was initiated', *ultrahang jobb oldali nephrolithiasist igazolt* 'ultrasound has revealed nephrolithiasis on the right side'. In all these cases the agent of the sentence is hidden, i.e. agentless sentences (Rounds 2009), or referred to as an institution (e.g. Medical Duty Service). These constructions can be considered passive constructions and can be translated into English mainly as passive sentences/structures.

There is no inflectional passive voice in Hungarian; the passive is expressed by means of other constructions with no agency (Rounds 2009). The language has been claimed to have a very restricted passive voice construction (Kenesei et al. 1998). It should rather be considered as a functional equivalent of a passive construction than an inflectional category. Even the existence of the verbal passive is questioned by Horváth and Siloni (2005), who, referring to É.Kiss (2002), deny the existence of the verbal passive as such in Hungarian. In Hungarian, passive voice is used only in a few cases made up with the auxiliary verb *van* 'be' + the suffix *-va/-ve* for the main verb. In complex sentences the use of passive voice sounds strange. However, there is extensive literature on *-T* and *-vA* participles (with the pros and cons of the passive approach) cf. Komlósy (1994), Alberti (1996), Laczkó (1995, 1999), Kenesei (2000), É. Kiss (2002) and Bartos (2009). Passive voice plays an impersonalizing role in scientific discourse (Swales 1985).

The discharge reports contained certain structures that can be considered passive constructions in Hungarian: e.g. *figyelhető meg* 'can be observed', *ábrázolódik* 'is visualized'. In all these examples there is no explicit agency in the sentences leading to the 'objectification' of the discourse.

The transitivity system offers a spectrum of possibilities that allows the writer to move from the assumption of personal responsibility through first person intervention to maximal detachment and impersonality through agency concealment. The use of the passive in the language of medicine is not a 'syntactic innovation' in Hungarian, since this construction is used, however, rarely in Hungarian. It is rather a syntactic borrowing of 'higher frequency', as passive is not so common in non-technical language.

5.1.4.3. Tenses

In English patient notes and hospital discharge reports the present tense is used when the patient's present complaints are described, e.g. *A 32-year old waiter is admitted to our ward. He is complaining of severe chest tightness. He has no dyspnea.* In Hungarian discharge reports, however, the past tense is used to describe the present complaints of the patient, e.g. *A beteget erős mellkasi szorítással vettük fel osztályunkra. Nehézlégzése nem volt* (see English equivalent in the example above).

In some of the studied discharge reports, physicians used the present tense in the *Jelen panasz(ok)* 'presenting complaints' section of the report instead of the past tense, e.g. *A rohamokat mellkasi fájdalom, szédülés, gyengeségérzés kiséri* 'The attacks are accompanied by chest pain, dizziness, and weakness', *Haemodinamika küldi Ambulanciánkra* 'hemodynamic Unit sends [the patient] to our Outpatient Department', *Háziorvos/Városi Ügyelet kéri vizsgálatát* 'Family physician/City Medical Duty service asks for the examination [of the patient]', *Háziorvos utalja be osztályunkra* 'Family physician refers the patient to our department', *Lábai, kezei fájnak* '[the patient] has pain in his/her legs and hands'.

5.1.4.4. Apposition

Grammatical apposition in Hungarian occurs in constructions with verbal predicates and in constructions with possessive restrictors. In this case, the adjective usually precedes the qualified word. In English the adjective can be appositioned.

In Hungarian vitamins are specified by putting the type of the vitamin first and the noun (vitamin) comes after the specifying letter (A, B, C, etc.) with a hyphen: *A-vitamin, K-vitamin.* In most of the studied discharge reports an example of English type apposition was identified: *Vitamin b komplex* 'vitamin B complex', *Vitamin C* 'vitamin C'.

5.1.4.5. Plural

Generally, paired body parts (e.g. ears, kidneys, or lungs) are referred to in the plural in English. In standard Hungarian, however, paired body parts and classes of identical or similar objects are usually used in singular (Tompa 1969; Grétsy and Kovalovszky 1985; Lanstyák and Szabómihály 1996, 1997; Csernicskó and Fenyvesi 2000; Moravcsik 2003). Nevertheless, paired body parts are usually referred to in plural form in Subcarpathian Hungarian dialects (Horváth and Lizanec 1993: 72). Similar result have been found among Hungarian speakers in Romania (Benő and Szilágyi 2005) and former Yugoslavia (Göncz 2001).

When only one of the paired organs is described, an overt singular-marking element, the word *fél* 'half' is used, e.g. *tüdő tiszta* 'lung is clear' but: *jobb/bal/fél tüdejét eltávolították* 'they removed [the patient's] right/left/half lung'. Nevertheless, according to Szepessy (1986), the above rule is only a language myth, and he gives some counterarguments to support that idea.

The analyzed discharge reports contained some examples of the use of the plural in case of referring to paired body parts: *lábai, kezei fájnak* '[the patient] has pain in his/her legs and hands', *bokái nem dagadnak* 'his/her ankles are not swollen', *bokái mérsékelten szoktak dagadni* 'his/her ankles are usually moderately swollen', *Pupillák o=o* 'his/her pupils are round and equal'. In cardiology, there is no need to emphasize that both parts of the paired organ is affected, as opposed to e.g. traumatology or ophthalmology, where the distinction would be relevant (Csaba Lengyel, M.D. PhD[51], personal communication on 28 April 2010).

5.1.4.6. Discussion on grammatical and syntactic borrowing

The Hungarian language of medicine seems to have a 'mixed' grammar, mainly maintaining the features of Hungarian grammar in general, but also, to a lesser extent, changing according to the English one. Heavy lexical borrowing can introduce new structural features into a language as well (cf. Poplack 1980).

Grammatical and syntactic borrowings are debated questions in contact linguistics, though chiefly from the point of view of the extent to which syntactic borrowing is possible (cf. Weinreich 1953; Harris and Campbell 1995). There has accordingly been a concentration on what exactly is to be understood by syntactic borrowing: whether or not it is a function of other kinds of borrowing, especially lexical; whether it is true 'borrowing' or is better construed as 'calquing', 'transfer' or 'interference', and under what conditions it may take place.

In the Hungarian hospital discharge reports, various grammatical and syntactic changes have been identified that might be due to extensive English language contact. Some changes have been found in the use of the Hungarian articles, both the indefinite article and the definite article. The indefinite article has been found to be used frequently preceding a noun that does not refer to an individual entity from among the members of its class. According to descriptive Hungarian grammars, the indefinite article is not used in this position. The definite article was frequently omitted from structures where it should appear: preceding a proper noun at the beginning of a sentence, e.g. Ø *Belgyógyászat intenzív osztályáról vesszük át a beteget* 'We admit the patient from Ø Internal

51 Csaba Lengyel is a leading cardiologist working at the 1st Department of Internal Medicine at the University of Szeged.

Medicine Intensive Care Unit', and also before names of materials and abstract nouns, e.g. *melynek hátterében Ø ultrahang jobb oldali nephrolithiasist igazolt* 'in the background of which Ø ultrasound has revealed nephrolithiasis'.

Impersonalization has been found to be commonly used in each discharge report. In the description of the investigations and the treatment, the passive voice is employed. Its use focuses the action on the patient and reduces the role of the hospital staff; the same impersonal effect may be created by sentences that have a diagnostic method as the subject representing inanimate subjects that are ranked lowest in the empathy scale, e.g. *A szív körül körkörösen kevés pericardiális folyadék ábrázolódik.* 'Small amount of pericardial fluid is visualized concentrically around the heart.', *ultrahang kontroll kóros eltérést nem mutatott* 'ultrasound has not shown any pathologic abnormality'.

These impersonal, passive-like constructions belong to the stock phrases of the discharge reports and serve to list the results of the clinical examinations, laboratory tests, and X-ray findings in a concise, matter-of-fact form. The verbs are limited to a few, such as *ábrázol* 'visualize', *igazol* 'reveal' and *mutat* 'show'. Information is conveyed in extended noun phrases with specialized vocabulary (cf. Halliday 1988).

Halliday and Martin (1993) argue that scientific writing has come to the end of its road, as the impersonalized discourse causes alienation in its readers. According to this view, the language of science is likely to shift toward semiotic explanations and back off from its present rate of nominalization and grammatical metaphor toward more democratic forms of discourse. The new style should also be more tolerant of indeterminacy and flux. On the other hand, well-formalized conventions are learned more easily and serve the function of a *lingua franca* better.

An English language contact-induced change has been identified in the use of the present tense in certain cases, when in Hungarian usually the past tense is used, e.g. describing the patient's presenting complaints: *A rohamokat mellkasi fájdalom, szédülés, gyengeségérzés kiséri* 'The attacks are accompanied by chest pain, dizziness, and weakness', *Háziorvos utalja be osztályunkra* 'Family physician refers [the patient] to our department'.

Grammatical apposition of the restrictive adjective was also found in some reports: e.g. *vitamin B complex* 'vitamin B complex', and changes in the use of the plural in the name of paired organs: e.g. *bokái nem dagadnak* 'his/her ankles are not swollen'.

Considering the above described grammatical and syntactic changes, they should rather be considered as the function of register in the sense that similarly to syntactic calques grammatical transfers take place initially in well-defined circumscribed areas of a language. The above described language changes may not be characteristic of all domains of the Hungarian language but mainly or exclusively for the language of sciences, and especially of medicine.

5.1.5. Other features

The possibility of pragmatic and rhetorical borrowing was first proposed by Clyne (1992), who suggested the study of 'language contact at the discourse level' mentioning several aspects, such as discourse markers, preformulated discourse, and differences concerning speech rules and discourse routines. Starting from the operative concept of communicative competence, he drew the attention to the fact that in different languages differences in discourse routines can lead to a 'communication breakdown' when the intention is not properly understood, and even to a 'communication conflict', when the intention conveyed is just the opposite of the original one.

Pragmatic borrowing seems to occur mostly in bilingual situations, and there are several possible categories of English 'pragmatic interference', which can be identified in various text types of the Hungarian language of medicine.

Discourse markers with phatic function, discourse routines and 'speech rules' were discussed by Clyne as instances of pragmatic borrowing. A Spanish linguist, Zuluaga (1980) identified 'clichés', i.e. phraseological statements which are only allowed to appear in one particular discourse genre. Other possible categories of pragmatic borrowing or interference include modality: interferences in the fields of negation, questions, and statements.

5.1.5.1. Politeness strategies

An individual should follow some communication strategies in defense, which are termed by Brown and Levinson (1987) as politeness strategies. The appropriate use of politeness strategies is important in medical discourse; the most frequently applied strategy is the use of hedging. Hedging is a basic feature in academic discourse (Rounds 1982) that enables academic writers to show their certainty and doubt towards their statements, and to show the amount of confidence they put on their claim. Through hedging, medical writers leave some room for their readers to judge the truth value of their statements. Hedging expressions can also be used in describing methods and results, discussing findings, and drawing conclusions from the evidence. Hedges express vagueness and reflect modesty for achievements and avoidance of personal involvement as well as suggest the impossibility or unwillingness to reach accuracy (cf. Lakoff 1972; Myers 1989; Salager-Meyer 1994; Hyland 1998, 2000). Hedges play an important role in gaining ratification for claims from a powerful peer group by allowing writers to present statements with appropriate accuracy, caution, and humility. They rather express possibility and prudence than certainty and overconfidence (Warta 2005).

Expressions such as *esetlegesen alátámaszt* 'possibly support', *lehet a hátterében* 'may be in its background' and *indokoltnak tűnik* 'seems reasonable' are present in the Hungarian discharge reports, which can contribute to gaining the acceptance of the writing physician's claims by colleagues reading the report.

However, they might have another function as well. They can also be part of the practice of defensive medicine (Csaba Lengyel, M.D. PhD., personal communication on 28 April 2010). Defensive medicine comprises the practice of diagnostic and/or therapeutic measures conducted primarily not to ensure the health of the patient, but as a safeguard against possible malpractice liability (Kevin 2007). Fear of litigation has been cited as the driving force behind defensive medicine (Studdert et al. 2005). Defensive medicine is especially common in the United States of America, with rates as high as 79% to 93% (Manner 2007), particularly in certain high-risk specialties such as obstetrics, emergency medicine or invasive cardiology. Physicians practice defensive medicine to avoid malpractice litigation, as a malpractice lawsuit is the most scarring ordeal that a physician can undergo, both emotionally and financially (Kevin 2007). There is an expectation that doctors have to be 100% accurate with their diagnoses. However, medicine by nature is an imperfect science, and the expectation of perfection is not realistic, nor possible, and almost 40 percent of malpractice cases in the USA were found to be without medical error (Studdert et al. 2005). Due to this uncertainty regarding unfortunate outcomes, physicians err on the side of caution and practice defensive medicine.

5.1.5.2. Depersonalization

Another discursive feature of medical writing is the progressive moderation of the author's own voice; the focus is on facts. The use of first-person pronouns signifies a personal attitude so that the narration is mediated through the subjective viewpoint of the narrator's consciousness, whereas third-person pronouns signify an external point of view (cf. Fowler 1986). An 'empathy hierarchy' ranks discourse elements according to the degree of involvement they create. The first and second person outrank human third persons, which "outrank non-human animates, which again outrank natural forces and inanimates" (De Lancey 1981: 644).

To some extent, the pronoun 'I' is replaced by 'we' in the Hungarian discharge reports, and it is performed neither because of involving the reader, nor because of expressing co-authorship (Gunnarson 2006), e.g. *alakítottunk ki* 'we formed/prepared', *helyezzük vissza* 'we replace', *otthonába bocsátjuk* 'we discharge (the patient) to his/her home', *pozicionáltunk* 'we positioned'.

5.1.5.3. Data organization and conventionalization

Discharge summaries are intended to transfer important clinical information from inpatient to outpatient settings and between hospital admissions. Standards that specify what information should be included in the discharge summary are introduced in many countries and among them in Hungary. These standards are based on mainly recommendations set up by WHO and other international health authorities, and are constructing international discourse markers, which might change the ones used and accepted in certain genres and registers by the national (non-English) discourse communities.

Genre theory suggests that texts fulfilling different functions unfold in different stages or steps (Eggins and Martin 1997). The degree of conventionalization may be seen in the overall textual structure of repeated sequences, in the ways of argumentation and in linguistic realizations. These patterns change over time, when the position of the genre changes in society or when there is intensive cultural and language contact between two languages, especially when attitude and prestige play an important role (Ferguson 1959).

In the studied discharge summaries, subheadings follow the logic used in English (American) hospital discharge reports, they follow the internationally accepted conventions: *Távolabbi/Korábbi kórtörténet/anamnézis* 'past medical history', *jelen panaszok* 'present symptoms', etc. Conventionalization can be seen in various sections in the linguistic formulation of investigation results as well: e.g. *pupillák egyenlőek, kerekek, fényre reagálnak* 'pupils are equal, round, reactive to light', which is an exact translation of the internationally accepted procedure for the examination of the pupils.

5.1.5.4. New occupation with new name

English language contact, English language globalization and internationalization affect not only the language, the discourse and generic characteristics but also the institutional structure of health care. Standardization is achieved through guidelines and recommendations. These guidelines are followed not only in performing certain activities in hospital settings: investigations, operational procedures, therapeutic modalities, but also through the reorganization of health care personnel.

A new post with a new name in Hungarian (*cirkulátor* 'circulator') was set up at the Department of Cardiology following the international recommendations, the OR circulator (operating room circulating nurse). A circulating nurse/circulator is a registered nurse who participates in a surgical procedure coordinating, planning and implementing all the nurse-related activities during an operation (cf. McGraw-Hill Concise Dictionary of Modern Medicine 2002). The circulator monitors the cardiopulmonary pump in operations with extracorporal circulation (Gábor Marton, M.D., personal communication in 2010). The name of the *cirkulátor* is mentioned in several discharge reports.

5.1.6. Conclusions on the results obtained with Method 1

Languages respond to the changing needs of communication, following changes in the world and ways of living. The growing influence of English on the languages of Europe is an example of linguistic change due to contact conditions. It can be traced back to political, economic and technological developments which have been taking place at a growing pace in the past few decades.

English is the international language used in both written and oral communication between health professionals involved in research (Gunnarsson 2001). English may be seen as a neutral lingua franca, or it may be seen as a dominating powerful language (Phillipson 1992; Tardy 2004). The trend to use one lingua franca in medicine, English, leads to the use of technical terms in English even in daily non-English language conversations of Hungarian medical experts.

Englishisms are not only present at the lexico-semantic level, but they also affect Hungarian orthography, grammar and the syntactic level of bilingual physicians (cf. Salager-Meyer et al. 2003; Alcaraz and Navarro 2006; Keresztes 2006b).

English has become the primary source for the creation of new concepts and their corresponding denominations in medicine. New medical nomenclature is built up of English proper roots and affixes or they can be combined with roots and affixes drawn from Greek and Latin (cf. Kontra 1981; Dirckx 1983; Maclean and Maher 2001). In the last 25 centuries, modern languages have borrowed scientific terminology mainly from Greek and Latin, usually through the activity of translators (Montalt and Davies 2007). More than 500 roots, prefixes and suffixes form the basis of fundamental medical terminology. Their multiple combinations expand these initial forms to thousands of terms in most languages. Most neologisms are formed by the help of these Latinate word roots and affixes.

In some contact linguistic studies (cf. Görlach 2001) a distinction is set up between Englishisms and words of Latin or Old-Greek origin concerning the language of sciences. When the corpus of the Hungarian cardiology discharge reports was analyzed, I did not exclude words that might have a Latin(ate) origin in general, as medical terminology rests on a fundamentally Latin nomenclature, and English words built of Latin word roots and affixes make up for most twentieth century neologisms in the language of medicine (Dirckx 1983). Therefore, it is very difficult to decide objectively whether a Hungarian medical word containing Latinate elements was directly borrowed from Latin or from English.

This book deals with contact-induced changes that are due to borrowing, where native speakers of Hungarian adopt vocabulary and structural features from English. The English language-using individuals are thus "the locus of contact" (Weinreich 1953: 1). It is important to note here that not just spoken contact, but also written contact is a contributing factor of language change. In fact, it is the written contact between the English and Hungarian languages (and their speakers) that is investigated through the analysis of English language contact-induced features in the Hungarian cardiology discharge reports. As bilingual Hungarian–English speakers (i.e. Hungarian cardiologists) rarely deactivate their English language totally, even unconsciously and involuntarily they may incorporate almost any type of English language feature into their Hungarian language when they speak and write (cf. Grosjean and Soares 1986).

The influence of medical English on the Hungarian language of medicine affects all linguistic levels: from orthography to lexis through semantics and syntax. Changes in the Hungarian language resulting from the influence of English language contact can be detected primarily in the area of vocabulary due to lexical borrowings.

The discharge summary is the most common method for documenting a patient's diagnostic findings, hospital management, and arrangements for post-discharge follow-up. It is the most common format for communicating information about hospitalization. The hospital discharge summary is a standardized genre: a complex combination of narrative fragments describing what happened to the patient, the steps taken, the outcome of these steps and the follow-up (Iedema 2006). It is a concise summary written for the family physician, who follows the patients after their hospital stay, or for the admitting doctor at next hospitalization. Therefore, the discharge summary is a vital tool for communication and information transfer between members of the medical society. Writing these documents is part of the daily routine of Hungarian cardiologists, as each discharged patient in Hungary receives their own discharge report before leaving the health institute. It is essential that the cardiologists and family physicians share a great deal of special knowledge, use the same specialized vocabulary, thus the family physician can decode the message written by the cardiologist in an adequate way.

Internationalization is an increasingly important factor in medical writing, including the hospital discharge summary, and the position of English as the lingua franca in medicine has an influence on the writing conventions of these medical texts as well (Taavitsainen and Pahta 2000).

Cardiology is one of the most technologically sophisticated, professionalized, institutionalized, and highly invasive medical disciplines. There have been great innovations and scientific progress in this medical field since the last decade of the 20th century. To name all the new diseases, structures, surgical and other therapeutic options an extensive neological process is needed in the language of medicine, which has become the English language since the middle of the last century. National languages mainly turn to the process of borrowing to enrich their scientific lexicon (Haugen 1950; Hope 1971), thus, solving the problem of neologisms. The speakers of the Hungarian language of medicine are also involved in this borrowing process in response to internal lexical needs in Hungarian (Kurtan 2003). Medical neologisms are the new terms composed to represent and transmit the new concepts in the specific field. These neologisms are the result of the process of terminologizing new medical knowledge either by newly formed words or by existing words to which new meanings are attached.

In the Hungarian language of cardiology, term formation is mainly produced by lexical borrowing and semantic borrowing from English. Standardization and unification is very important in the language of sciences, and among them in the language of medicine. At the beginning of the 21st century English seems to be the lingua franca of medicine, therefore, English origin neologisms are very common in most native languages of medicine.

Besides extensive borrowing from English, another feature of the Hungarian language of medicine is that some Latinate words, especially adjectives and verbs, have recently become more widely and frequently used, e.g. *ineffectív* 'ineffective', *intenzifikált* 'intensified', *lokalizál* 'localize'. As these words are frequently used in the English language of medicine, their increased frequency in the Hungarian hospital discharge reports can also be attributed to the intensive effect of the English language.

Lexical borrowing is a common form of cross-linguistic influence, as it is one aspect of a creative process of lexical change under contact, which builds on both native and foreign resources. Lexical changes due to contact involve not just direct importation of words but a variety of other processes leading to innovations in the lexicon of the Hungarian language: borrowed English loanwords are combined with Hungarian suffixes, become assimilated morphologically to the Hungarian language, and expand vocabulary in other word classes as well, e.g. E n/v *stent* > H n *stentelés* 'stenting', word root *stent* + verbal thematizing suffix *-el* + nominal derivational suffix *-és*, L/E v *elongate* > H adj *elongált* 'elongated', word root *elongál* + adjectival suffix *-t*, E n/v *trigger* > H v *triggerel* 'to trigger', word root *trigger* + verbal thematizing suffix *-l*. Morphological adaptation may seem difficult as Hungarian has complex rules involving case and number, but, in many cases, the borrowed words are treated like Hungarian word roots of equivalent categorical status, and they take the bound morphology and other properties appropriate to the class they are assigned to.

English lexical borrowings are integrated to varying degrees into the orthography, morphology, and syntax of the Hungarian language. They are also subject to different kinds of semantic change. Many of the borrowings are not strict lexical borrowings but innovations that have no counterparts in the source language: loan substitutions. They build on both Hungarian and English resources.

Few borrowed words have shown no semantic change. In most cases semantic narrowing can be seen, the borrowed word (lexeme) has retained only one or two of its original (English) sememes, when used in the Hungarian language of medicine, e.g. E *support* has 3 sememes, whereas H *szupport* has only one sememe in medical Hungarian: *a mechanism or arrangement that helps keep something else functioning*. After the borrowing process has taken place, the borrowed item (the English word) may lose (semantic narrowing), change it/them (semantic shift) or develop new meanings (semantic widening) in the Hungarian language of medicine, e.g. E v/n *burst* 'to break suddenly/a sudden break while under tension or expansion' > H n *burst* 'sorozatos külső ingerület' 'serial external stimuli'. Borrowings are generally eligible for the same type of semantic changes as native words, i.e. metonymic extension, metaphorical shift, polysemous extension, or loss of a polysemous meaning.

Unassimilated loanwords (e.g. *guided, spike, upgrade*) and semantic borrowings such as loan translations (e.g. *mélyvénás* 'deep vein', *sószegény* 'low salt', *várólista* 'waiting list') and loan blends (e.g. *echodús* 'echo rich/dense', *pacemakertasak/-zseb* 'pacemaker pouch/pocket', *vérnyomáskontroll* 'blood pressure control') make up the largest portion of English contact-induced changes in the cardiology discharge reports.

Considering the word class of these lexical and semantic borrowings, the majority of these terms are nouns (n=62): nouns proper, e.g. *branch, graft, stent,* or nominalized verbs, e.g. *kinking, mapping, stentelés* 'stenting'. Noun compounds are also very common, in which a noun is used to modify the head noun, both in loanwords proper, e.g. *end stage, entrainment mapping*, and in loan substitutions, e.g. *ágynyugalom* 'bedrest', *szívhalál* 'cardiac/heart death', *tamponade jelek* 'tamponade signs'. The 4 most frequently used nouns – considering their derived forms as well – are: 1. *stent* with altogether 282 occurrences, 2. *block/blokk* with altogether 240 occurrences, 3. *pacemaker* with altogether 211 occurrences, and 4. *pace* with altogether 194 occurrences.

Adjectives are the second most frequently borrowed terms forming only a fragment of all lexical and semantic borrowings, e.g. *gyógyszerkibocsátó* 'drug releasing', *intenzív* 'intense', *sick, slow-fast, tilt, tünetmentes* 'symptom free/asymptomatic'. The 4 most frequently used adjectives were: 1. *panaszmentes* 'symptom free/asymptomatic' n=74, 2. *diffuse/diffúz* and *lobmentes* 'inflammation free' n=50, 3. *koleszterinszegény* 'low cholesterol' n=31 and 4. *invazív/invasive* 'invasive' n=22.

From the borrowed word groups verbs were the least frequently borrowed items. Only 11 borrowed verbs have been identified altogether in the discharge reports, all of them are assimilated loanwords. The 4 most frequently used borrowed verbs are 1. *pozicionál* '(to) position' n=16, 2. *detektál* '(to) detect' n=14, 3. *diszkonnektál* '(to) disconnect' and *provokál* '(to) provoke' n=9 and 4. *lokalizál* '(to) localize' n=5.

English medical initialisms (especially acronyms) are very frequently transferred into the Hungarian language of cardiology. They can be found mainly in the "Laboratory results" and the "Medications" sections of the discharge reports, e.g. *LIMA, NYHA, TIMI*. Initialisms form the largest group of borrowed items in the cardiology discharge reports. The 4 most frequently used borrowed acronyms are 1. *SEC* 'spontaneous echo contrast' n=375, 2. *LAD* 'left anterior descending' n=355, 3. *INR* 'international normalized ratio' n=260, and 4. *MCH* 'mean cell hemoglobin' n=248.

Borrowed orthographic, grammatical and syntactic features are not as varied as the above described lexical and semantic borrowings, but the number of their appearance is very high. Each cardiological discharge report contained the English-type decimal separator and the capitalized L for liter. Capitalized L for liter has altogether 1,246 occurrences in the 234 discharge reports.

Although the impact of English language contact on grammatical structures in the discharge reports is less than that on lexical ones, certain contact-induced grammatical/syntactic features can be identified in the former as well. The frequency of impersonal structures is unusually high in the discharge reports. The point of view of the discharge report is distanced and objective focusing on the clinical facts. The language of the discharge reports is characterized by the "progressive phasing out of authorial identity" (Gunnarson 2006: 714), e.g.

ultrahang jobb oldali nephrolithiasist igazolt 'ultrasound has revealed nephrolithiasis on the right side', i.e. the physician performing an ultrasound examination found that the patient has nephrolithiasis. On the other hand, the passive and other impersonal structures are employed as a strategy for avoiding the use of personal object pronouns, i.e. avoiding having the patient as the direct object, e.g. *magasvérnyomás, hyperlipidaemia* *ismert* 'high blood pressure, hyperlipidaemia are known', i.e. the patient suffers from high blood pressure and hyperlipidaemia. In most discharge reports the agent of the sentence (the physician or the patient) is hidden, i.e. agentless sentences are used, or the agent is referred to as an institution, e.g. *Ügyelet járt kinn nála* '[patient] was visited by the medical duty service', i.e. a physician who works for the medical duty service visited the patient, or *OMSZ hozta az ambulanciára* 'National Ambulance Service has brought [the patient] to the outpatient department', i.e. health workers from the National Ambulance Service transferred the patient to the outpatient department.

Internationalization is an increasingly important factor in scientific writing, and the position of English as the lingua franca in medicine has an influence on the writing conventions of medical texts today. Medical writing is a general label with a great deal of variation across several genres, including the hospital discharge reports. Corpus-based studies have shown that genres of writing may be very heterogeneous in their linguistic features and that there is variation even within a narrowly defined genre. Due to intensive language contact, changes in society, in the discourse community, or in scientific methods, the name of a genre may remain constant although its internal linguistic features change. It has been claimed that scientific discourse evolves and emerges in relation to the scientific practices and that texts within professions give us insight into how the professions constitute themselves and carry out their work through texts (cf. Bazerman and Paradis 1991; Bazerman 1998; Taaivitsainen and Pahta 2000). Changes in modulation and data organization of the discharge reports were identified pointing toward efforts to internationalize the rhetorical and generic features of this text type: hedging and defocusing of agents appear in the Hungarian reports, and new subheadings are introduced (e.g. *távolabbi kórtörténet* 'past medical history') to follow the structure of the English/American hospital discharge reports more closely. Even a new post in hospital care was introduced at the Department of Cardiology, the post of the *cirkulátor* 'circulator', a nurse who monitors the patient's circulation during the surgical intervention.

Discharge reports are neutral, fact-recording documents with a high degree of conventionalization and internationalization. Conventions help physicians to record details in an economical form, and internationalization makes contact with physicians from other countries available. The target group (physicians) shares a great deal of special knowledge, uses the same specialized vocabulary and can decode the message in the appropriate way. Due to the intense English language contact, new lexical fields may be created in Hungarian in the field of medicine. The spread of English 'medicalese' can be detected in the Hungarian language of medicine as well as in other languages of the world (Fielding 1995; Ogden 2007).

English lexical morphemes may be introduced into Hungarian directly via code-switching from English as bilingual physicians often use code-switching in their speech. These code-switched items can change from code-switches to borrowings through increasingly frequent usage by the code-switching speakers (in our case Hungarian cardiologists), they are also used in writing, e.g. in the hospital discharge reports. And then as not all members of the medical discourse community engage in code-switching (cf. family physicians are not necessarily bilingual speakers of English beside Hungarian) by adoption by these non-bilingual speakers (cf. Thomason 2003). The accommodation continues after the word is borrowed. Unless the Englishism remains a synonym to a Hungarian word it may develop distinctive semantic features (usually restricting the meaning, i.e. semantic narrowing) and it may develop new meanings by contextual restrictions, metaphorical and metonymic applications, or even euphemistic uses. The terminological use of the loanwords in which the borrowing is indicated by a terminological gap is slightly different and some type of a language planning is employed to ensure that the meaning remains constant in order to provide a stable equivalent for the phenomenon behind the term.

Another criterion mentioned by scholars involved in research on contact linguistics is what has been termed as the 'frequency hypothesis'. Code-switching forms are considered ephemeral and non-recurrent; however, frequently repeated forms gradually become more or less stable loans. This is the view maintained by those who contend that code-switches and borrow-ings occur at the beginning and end of a continuum (Gardner-Chloros 1995; Myers-Scotton 1993; Backus 1996). According to Scotton's (1993) classi-fication, the borrowings identified in USZCCDR can be divided into cultural and core borrowings: the former are widely used by Hungarian speakers, e.g. *hormon* 'hormone', *teszt* 'test', *standard* 'standard', *vitamin* 'vitamin', the latter are commonly restricted to the medical discourse community, e.g. *komplience* 'compliance', *pace* 'pace', *triggerelt* 'triggered'.

Loanwords proper, regardless of unassimilation, may be embedded into the Hungarian morphological system, i.e. may act as word roots in accor-dance with the Hungarian syntax rules or as roots taking over Hungarian suffixes. Speakers may handle them as foreign words putting a hyphen in writing between the unassimilated root and the Hungarian suffix (e.g. *flow-t* 'flow (accusative)', *flow-val* 'with flow') or considering them loanwords and writing them without a hyphen (e.g. *grafttal* 'with graft/grafting', *pacelés* 'pacing'). Thus, morphological assimilation can precede orthographic and probably semantic assimilation.

Variation in the amount of integration may also depend on the 'degrees of bilingualism'; a loanword can be subject to continuous interference from the source language to the other language, so that different writers use diffe-rent forms of the same loanwords (cf. Haugen 1950). As a result, various orthographic and morphological realizations of the same word can coexist in the same discourse community.

Factors influencing the degree of integration of loanwords into the Hungarian language of medicine can be linguistic or extra-linguistic relating to the speakers' attitudes and frequency of use of the loanwords. One of the factors influencing integration is the linguistic nature of the loanword itself, whether it conforms to the orthographic and morphological patterns of the Hungarian language.

Specificity is an indicator of modern scientific writing (Taavitsainen et al. 2002), in this sense, the lexicon plays a crucial role. We have seen that lexical and semantic borrowings represent most of the English contact-induced features in the Hungarian language of medicine, and international scientific words with Latin and Latinate elements also have a great impor-tance. The increasing international influence of English has been welcomed by many, but criticized by many others. While some appreciate its political, economic and cultural advantages, others are sensitive to a possible threat to other languages and cultures. Language theoretically belongs to all, but is often changed by only a few, many of them anonymous. Resentment at interference or sudden changes in the language has a long history.

Goethe, the German poet elucidated that "the strength of a language does not lie in rejecting what is foreign but in assimilating it". The Hungarian language is extremely flexible and able to accept and integrate new terms. However, a balance should be found between the puristic approach to use only Hungarian terms and the acceptance/integration/adoption of all English language items. Pál Bugát, reformer of the Hungarian medical terminology, composed more than 40,000 medical terms in Hungarian but in current Hungarian medical language only approximately 100 of them are used, e.g. *gyógyszer* 'medication', *láz* 'fever', *visszér* 'varicose vein'. Grétsy (2004) admits that in the language of medicine the semantic identity is difficult as the frequently used and accepted borrowed medical terms are usually very accurately demarked/circumscribed and difficult to translate into Hungarian as they have various meanings, therefore, English borrowing sometimes cannot be avoided.

Every professional group is formed by the establishment of an internal role structure, group identity, group attitudes, and group norms. The need for professional identity for a professional 'us-ness', for separation from the out-group, has played an important role in the construction of professional group language and constantly motivates people to adapt and be socialized into professional group behavior. It also means establishing distance from people outside the group (Gunnarson 2006).

When and for what the English language is used by physicians has been asked during semi-structured interviews. Attitudes of the members of the Hungarian medical discourse community and of their patients toward the English language, the English language contact-induced change and the motives for the borrowing have been analyzed with Method 2.

5.2. Results and discussion of data obtained by Method 2

The aim of the interviews is to measure, on the one hand, how dominant a role English plays in the professional life of physicians and how their patients are affected by it, and, on the other hand, what the attitudes of the interviewees are to this dominance.

The interviews are not aimed at getting quantitative data, therefore, in discussing the results of these interviews, emphasis is laid on the quality of responses rather than on the exact numbers of interviewees giving a specific response.

5.2.1. Demographic data of the interviewees

Method 2 involves the conducting and analysis of interviews with cardiologists working in secondary and tertiary care, primary care physicians, and patients having received cardiology care. Originally, I intended to examine secondary and tertiary care cardiologists separately, but at the beginning of 2008 all secondary care health institutions were integrated into the university (as part of the Albert Szent-Györgyi Clinical Center), therefore, the same regulations and requirements now apply to physicians working at both levels of care. The other fact that made me consider them as a homogenous group is that each secondary care cardiologist (involved in the study) began his/her career and spent at least 5-10 years at the Department of Cardiology. According to my findings, there is relatively flexible mobility between the two levels.

Participants in the study were selected on the basis of their willingness to participate in it. More than 40 physicians work as cardiologists (or cardiology residents/candidates for specialty examination) in secondary and tertiary care in Szeged. Some of them refused the participation on the basis of lack of time, and others were not available for various other reasons. Therefore, 11 cardiologists were interviewed during the period of September 2008 and January 2009. Most interviews were recorded in the office of the physicians, and some of the cardiologists came for the interview to my department.

The age distribution of tertiary and secondary physicians is presented in Table 14. Students usually finish their graduate medical studies at the age of 24 or 25; therefore, no younger subjects were interviewed. The number of cardiologists working at the department over the age of 60 is very low (only two), therefore, I excluded them from this survey to keep up confidentiality, as they would have been easy to identify for the readers. The youngest participant works as a resident at the department. Two other interviewees are studying for their subspecialty examination in cardiology. The rest of the participants, 8 physicians, are consultants in cardiology working either in invasive or in non-invasive cardiology. 6 of the interviewed physicians are males and 5 females (see Table 15).

Table 14. Distribution of the interviewed persons according to their age.

	Age groups (in years)				
Number of participants	**25-29**	**30-39**	**40-49**	**50-59**	**60-**
Cardiologists (n=11)	2	4	3	2	–
Family physicians (n=6)	–	1	2	1	2
Patients (n=8)	–	2	1	–	5

Primary care physicians were very difficult to convince to participate in the study. In the first cycle, when I contacted 5 family physicians by telephone, each one refused the interview reasoning the negative answer by lack of time, interest or willingness to participate in an interview. Therefore, I asked my colleagues and acquaintances to approach their own family physician and help me get an appointment with them. This way, I managed to arrange interviews with 6 family physicians working at various sites of Szeged during the period of January 2009 and March 2009. Each interview was performed in the office of the physicians.

Their age distribution is summarized in Table 14. I could find no interviewee from the first age group and 2 family physicians belonged to the age group over 60. Each interviewed family physician was female (see Table 15).

Patients in the study were selected by the help of the nursing officer at the Department of Cardiology. All the 8 patients were interviewed on the day of their discharge while waiting for their discharge report to be prepared. Interviews with the patients were prepared at the Department of Cardiology in April 2009.

Table 15. Distribution of the interviewed persons according to their sex.

	Male	**Female**
Cardiologists (n=11)	6	5
Family physicians (n=6)	–	6
Patients (n=8)	2	6

The age distribution of the interviewed patients is shown in Table 15. Most patients were over 60 years of age representing the most typical age group of the patients being hospitalized at the Department of Cardiology. 2 of the interviewed patients were males and 6 of them females (see Table 15).

5.2.2. Background information on the role of the English language at the Faculty of Medicine

Every doctor working at a clinical department of the University of Szeged is expected to be involved in patient care, research, pharmaceutical trials and teaching. Patient care at the Department of Cardiology involves the emergency care provided by anyone in need, therefore, care is provided not only for local Hungarian patients but for tourists, transit workers, i.e. truck drivers from various countries, and foreign students studying in Szeged. The department also provides elective care for patients from neighboring countries, mostly Romania and Serbia, whose care is not financed by the Hungarian Health Insurance System.

Research involves participation in certain national and international surveys and presenting results of these surveys at national and international forums, as well as publishing the results in Hungarian and international medical journals. PhD dissertations are expected to be handed in in English, and the impact factor that is required from the candidate can be achieved only by publishing in international medical journals in English.

Pharmaceutical trials are financed by large international pharmaceutical companies. University departments are involved in these trials not only to benefit from the knowledge gained through these investigations but the various types of financial support provided by the companies can also be attractive for them.

Teaching involves graduate training of Hungarian medical students as well as of non-Hungarian students in the English language program. The Faculty of Medicine, University of Szeged has been running an English program for medical students arriving from all over the world since 1986. Each medical subject is taught in English, all the lectures and practicals are in English as well as exams and patient presentations.[52] Postgraduate training of physicians in primary health care, i.e. of family physicians, is also provided by the Department of Cardiology.

5.2.3. Results of the interviews with secondary and tertiary care cardiologists

At the beginning of the interview, cardiologists have been asked about the languages they have learnt. 5 physicians have learnt German and 5 have learnt Russian. Three other languages have been mentioned (Dutch, French and Italian) by 1 interviewee each. All the 11 physicians have learnt Latin (medical Latin) at university. English has also been learnt by all of them: 3 of them started learning English in primary school, 4 in secondary school and 4 at the university over age 18 (see Figure 9).

52 As Hungarian patients usually do not speak English, the tutor of the presentation has to mediate between the students and the patients. Students in their 3rd and 4th years at the university study Hungarian for medical purposes, which they can also rely on during these presentations.

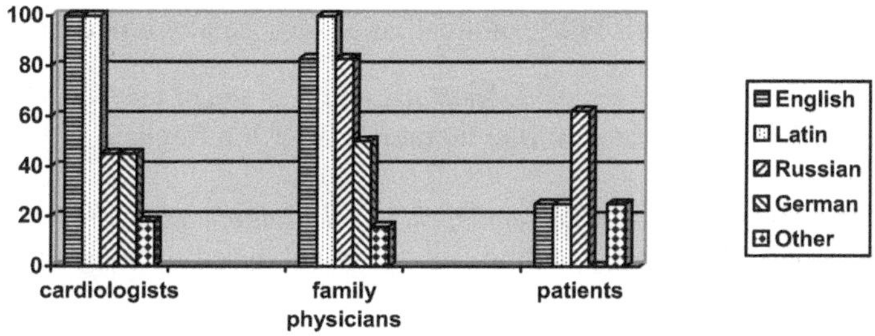

Figure 9. Languages spoken by the interviewees (results are given in percentage).

Interviewees have been also asked about the time spent in English-speaking countries. Most of them have been to countries where the working language was English for them (Spain, Italy, the Netherlands) and some of them to Britain, Canada, Ireland or the USA. They worked in these countries for some time, or participated in workshops, congresses or short visits.

After the introductory questions, physicians have been asked about the role of the English language in their professional life: what they use the English language for. Answers can be grouped around four major areas: accessing professional information and acquiring medical knowledge (see Section 5.2.3.1), publication (see Section 5.2.3.2), conference presentation (see Section 5.2.3.3), and daily professional life (see Section 5.2.3.4).

In the next section of the interview, cardiologists have been asked if they consider their English language competence important, and if it is a drawback for a cardiologist if he/she does not speak English (see Section 5.2.3.5).

In the last phase of the interview, they have been shown a discharge report that has been written at the Department of Cardiology and questions have been asked about its language (see Section 5.2.3.6).

5.2.3.1. Accessing professional information and acquiring medical knowledge

Each interviewee has mentioned accessing professional information and acquiring medical knowledge at the first place when asked about what they use the English language for in their professional life. Physicians read English language publications on a regular basis for gaining the most recent information or when preparing for their PhD examination or subspecialty board examination:

(1) C4[53]: ... *folyamatosan irodalmazunk, ami [...] angol nyelven folyik* '...we always read the literature, and it [the literature] is [...] in English'

(2) C7: *A mértékadó közlemények, azok angol nyelvű folyóiratokban jelennek meg.* 'The quality publications are published in English language journals'.

(3) C9: *ugye a szakirodalom [...] nyelvezete az angol* 'well, the language of medical literature is English'.

(4) C10: *Hát rendszeresen kell cikkeket olvasni, a cikkek nagy része angolul van* 'well, you need to read articles regularly, and the majority of the articles are in English'.

(5) C3: ... *nem tudja letenni a kardiológusi szakvizsgát, ugyanis nincs magyar könyv, én ... angol könyvekből próbáltam, meg angol nyelvű internetről összeszedni az adatokat ... angol nélkül nagyon nehéz* '...you cannot pass the subspecialty exam in cardiology, as there is no Hungarian textbook. I ... tried to collect data from English-language books and from the Internet ... without the English language it's very difficult'.

(6) C2: *Ugye én a PhD képzésem kapcsán kénytelen vagyok angol irodalmat forgatni, illetve gyakorlatilag én az internetet másra nem is használom, ... legfőképpen a szakmámon belüli fejlődésre, illetve cikkek olvasására, irodalomra, illetve hát a PhD-m ... nyilvánvalóan angolul fog elkészülni, úgyhogy ahhoz mindenképpen kell* 'I have to read the literature in English because of my PhD studies, and practically, I use the Internet for nothing else ... but mostly for developing myself professionally, to read articles, literature, and my PhD ... will obviously be written in English, thus I need it [English] for that'.

Books and journal articles on cardiology are available at the library of the department mostly in English, and the Internet provides an unrestricted access to scientific/cardiological knowledge. Literature is mainly used for research, teaching and self-training. The pressure for reading texts in English starts during the university years of students, and then it continues and even increases when physicians start their career at university departments. Cardiologists have to be up to date on the most recent guidelines and recommendations issued by

53 'C' refers to cardiologists, and the number after it refers to the number of the interviewee.

international health organizations (cf. website http://www.cardiologyonline.com). They have to start reading about medicine in English already during their graduate studies at the university:

(7) C2: *az egyetemen is rászorultunk arra, hogy angolul olvassunk* 'we were forced to read in English during the university studies'.

(8) C3: *ott [az egyetemi tanulmányok alatt] a tudományos dolgokhoz a cikkeket angolul kellett olvasgatni* 'there [during the university studies] we had to read the articles for the scientific things in English'.

Reading in English is essential not only for physicians but also for medical students, therefore, the leadership of the faculty is planning to introduce the requirement of having an intermediate level English language examination certificate on entrance to the medical studies. 81% of the students accepted to begin their studies at this faculty in 2009 have an intermediate (52%) or an advanced level (29%) English language examination certificate (information provided by the Dean's Office in November 2009). It is a requirement for PhD students at the Faculty of Medicine to have an intermediate level English language examination certificate.

Cardiologists read not only the medical literature in English but the newest guidelines and recommendations are also available in this language:

(9) C1: *az új irányelvek, ezek a legeslegújabbak, azok csak angolul vannak* 'the guidelines, the most recent ones are available only in English'.

(10) C8: *És akkor jöttek ezek a guideline-ok, amerikai ajánlás, európai ajánlás, ezek angolul jöttek, mentek* 'and then these guidelines appeared, the American recommendations, the European recommendations, and these were all in English'.

The most recent publications in the field of medicine are usually available via the Internet; therefore, cardiologists often research the Internet for medical websites, the language of which is mainly English:

(11) C1: *... ha interneten valamit keresek, akkor is angol oldalakra keresek rá* 'if I search the Internet, I always go to English language websites'.

(12) C9: *az interneten bármit nézek, angolul van* 'whatever I search for in the Internet is in English'

(13) C11: ... *ha az ember a Google-n rákeres bizonyos emberekre, akiknek mondjuk keresne esetleg cikkeit, természetes, hogy talál egyébként mindenféle nyelven cikket, de az elfogadott nyelv az angol, és a jobb lapok, azok is mind angolul vannak és az teljesen mindegy, hogy norvég, dán, francia vagy japán [a szerző] mindenképpen angolul található meg [a cikke]* 'if you search the Internet for certain people, whose articles you are interested in, naturally you can find articles in several languages, but the accepted language is English, and all the high level journals are in English, and it does not matter if [author is] Norwegian, Danish, French or Japanese, [the article] can be found exclusively in English'.

Appropriate literature is not available in Hungarian, books, reference materials and journal articles are rarely translated from English into Hungarian or only with considerable delay:

(14) C10: ... *hogyha a legfrissebb szakmát akarja az ember olvasni, akkor csak angolul lehet* '... if you want to read about the most recent advances in your profession, they are available only in English'

(15) C3: *Bármire kíváncsi vagyok, nincsen meg magyarul ... már régóta nincs se könyv, se adat, se cikk, semmi sincs meg magyarul. Nem is keresem úgy, mert nincsen. Nincsenek tisztességes magyar nyelvű könyvek* 'if I'm interested in anything, it is not available in Hungarian ... there have been no books, data, articles, nothing in Hungarian for a long time. I don't even look for them, because they aren't there. There are no proper books written in Hungarian'.

(16) I[54]: *Kardiológiából van magyar nyelvű folyóirat?* 'Is there a cardiology journal in Hungarian?'
C3: *Igen, van, de általában nem azok a referenciák, tudományos munkák, ami magyar nyelvű folyóiratban leírnak, fel lehet használni egyértelmű, de hogyha valaki minimum egy PhD szintű dolgot, vagy ilyesmit készít, ahhoz komoly cikkekről van szó, azok mind angolul jelennek meg, vagy legalább is németül vagy franciául, de az kevésbé* 'Yes, there is, but the scientific papers published in it are not considered as references, if they are published in a journal that is in Hungarian. You can obviously use them, but if you want to write at least a PhD or something like that, then you need more 'serious' articles, and they are all published in English, or in German or French, but the latter ones are less frequent' .

---

54 'I' stands for the interviewer.

Translation of scientific texts or textbooks into Hungarian is commercially mostly unprofitable, only a fragment of the published research articles written in English are translated into Hungarian, sometimes with a delay of 6 to 12 months after their first publication in English. Textbooks are very rarely translated, and the translated books are mostly appropriate for graduate and not for postgraduate training. These books are published in Hungarian usually years after the original publication in English. Therefore, if a physician wants to have up-to-date knowledge in his/her own field of special interest, information is accessible only in English.

5.2.3.2. Publications

Researcher cardiologists must be able to express themselves in English if they want to be fully accepted members of the international medical community. Publishing in English has become more and more important over recent years as the pressure to produce work and publish internationally has increased. Within academia researchers have to "publish or perish" (Bakewell 1992; Viereck 1996), and everything that is not in English is simply disregarded (Weinreich 1988; Treanor 1999). Publications in major international medical journals are considered more valuable,[55] and these medical journals are almost all in English; in addition, most medical journals publishing in English refuse to accept contributions in other languages (Treanor 1999).

Publication in English is very important in the professional life of cardiologists:

(1) C4: Az irodalomból angol nyelven idézzük be a különböző cikkeket, hivatkozásokat, ezek alapján elkészítjük a [kutatási] tervet, magát a kutatási részt, az experimentális részt elvégezzük, folyamatosan irodalmazunk, ami szintén angol nyelven folyik, és utána ebből később először absztraktokat írunk szintén angol nyelven kongresszusokra, vagy hát előadunk, ismertetünk, és utána maga a cikk is angol nyelven íródik 'we cite the articles, citations from the literature are in English, and prepare the [research] design and the study itself, we perform the experimental phase, and continuously search the literature, which is also in English, and then we first write the abstract for the congresses in English, of course, present the paper, and finally the article itself is written in English'.

55 No Hungarian medical journal has an impact factor. The impact factor of a journal measures the frequency with which the journal has been cited in a given period.

(2) C2: Egy cikkben voltam társszerző. Gyakorlatilag most egy-két cikk van folyamatban 'I have already been a co-author of an article. Practically, one or two articles are being written at the moment'

5 of the interviewed cardiologists (n=11) report that they have already written articles in English. English language scientific texts produced by non-native speakers represent the highest level of their specialized language skills (Kloss 1929), the highest density of accumulated knowledge and the highest grade of "readiness for global intercommunication" (Haarmann and Holman 2001: 238).

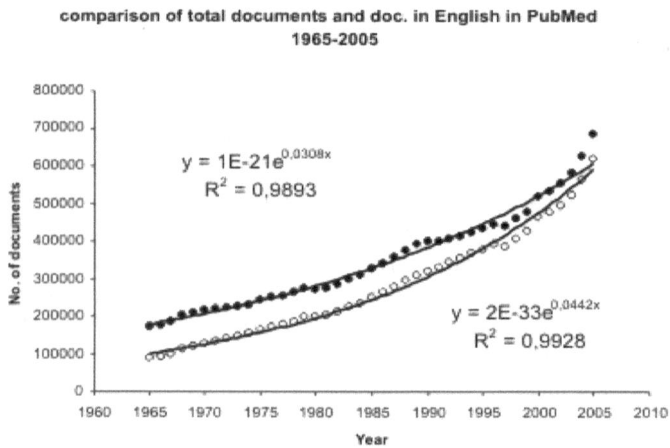

◦ English language publications; • total number of publications

Figure 10. Comparison of total number of publications and number of English language publications in PubMed 1965-2005 (Biglu and Umstätter 2007 at website http://bvs.sld.cu/revistas/aci/vol *16_3_07/ac06907.html).*

Figure 10 shows how the number of English language publications increased between 1965 and 2005. The percentage of papers in English has increased steadily, and going from 52% in 1965 to 90% in 2005. The International Federation on Documentation says that approximately 85% of all the scientific and technological information in the world today is written and/or abstracted in English (cf. website http://www.informaworld.com), thus, it has become necessary for the members of the medical community to be able to publish their research articles in English.

All the 11 cardiologists are involved in writing abstracts in English. Abstracts are written for two purposes: they are sent to conference committees for consideration to indicate what the researcher intends to speak about, or they can be an integral part of a journal paper. Even if the paper is published in Hungarian, the abstract has to be written in English beside the Hungarian version:

(3) C4: … először absztraktokat írunk szintén angol nyelven kongresszusokra 'first, we write abstracts for congresses in English'

(4) C5: Próbálkoztam absztrakttal. … magyarul is kell, meg angolul is kell, mert szerintem magyar lapokban is úgy van, hogy kell angol verzió, meg magyar verzió is 'I tried to write abstracts … both in Hungarian and in English, because in Hungarian journals both the English and the Hungarian versions are needed'.

(5) I: És olyan volt-e már, hogy cikkhez absztraktot kellett angolul írni? 'And did you have to write an abstract in English for your article?'

C7: Volt. 'Yes.'

I: És azt egyedül oldja meg ilyenkor? 'And do you prepare it yourself?'

C7: Hát igen. 'Well, yes.'

(6) I: Absztraktokat, hogyha kell leadni, azokat általában angolul kell megírni. 'If you have to send in an abstract [for the conference committee], does it usually have to be in English?'

C9: Igen, azt mindig angolul. 'Yes, always in English'

I: És ezt Te meg szoktad írni, vagy hogy csinálod? 'And can you write it or how do you prepare it?'

C9: Hát azt is úgy, hogy én lehet, hogy megírom, és akkor valakivel átnézetem. 'Well, I write it myself and then have somebody check it for me'.

Depending on the English language competence of the interviewed subjects, they write the abstracts themselves, some of them write the abstract themselves and then have somebody to check it, and one cardiologist mentioned that she always has somebody else to translate it for her.

5.2.3.3. Conference presentations

Each interviewed cardiologist participates in conferences regularly. Conferences or as they refer to these gatherings, congresses are very important forums of exchange of up-to-date scientific knowledge. Participation is a must, on the one hand, if a scientist wants to keep up with the most recent advances in their scientific field, on the other hand, this is the very forum where they can publicize their own scientific achievements:

(1) C9: de hát ugye nálunk a kardiológiából azért a nemzetközi konferenciák nyelve az angol. … Barcelonában is a nemzetközi kongresszuson angolul történt, Bécsben, de említhetném Horvátországot is, de mindenütt angol az előadói nyelv 'but in cardiology, you see, the language of international conferences is English … There was an international congress in Barcelona and it was in English, and in Vienna or I can mention Croatia, but everywhere the language of presentations is English'

(2) C5: Most, ahol legutóbb voltam ősszel, az Nagyszebenben volt a Közép-Európai Vándorkongresszus, ott az angol volt a hivatalos nyelv … a résztvevők 95%-a helyi országban dolgozók, és csak mutatóba van egy-egy külföldi …bementünk az egyikbe [szekcióba] és románul ment az egész. … és akkor észrevette az egyik szervező, hogy ott vagyunk, odaszaladt az ülés elnökhöz, szólt, az szólt az előadónak, és azonnal váltott angolra, és onnan angolul mondta 'most recently I was in Sibiu [Romania] in autumn at the Central European Annual Congress and the official language was English … 95% of the participants were working in the host country, and only one or two foreigners were present … we entered one of the sections and it was all in Romanian … and then one of the organizers noticed that we were there, and went to the chairman and told him that we were foreigners, he warned the presenter and he immediately changed the language and from there he continued in English'

(3) C5: Volt Magyarországon is nemzetközi konferencia, ahol angolul kellett előadni. 'There was an international conference in Hungary, and we had to present our papers in English'

(4) C3: … most volt egy kardiológus, kimondottan katéteres kongresszusunk itt Szegeden, magyaroknak, de sok külföldi volt, ezért a hivatalos nyelv angol volt. '… recently we have had a cardiological conference on catheterization here, in Szeged, for us Hungarians, but there were many foreigners present, therefore, the official language was English.'

I: Tehát annak ellenére, hogy Magyarországon volt? 'So, despite the fact that it was in Hungary?'

C3: Igen, sőt 90%-unk magyar volt, de a 10% külföldi vendég miatt a 3 napból másfél napig angol volt a hivatalos nyelve a dolognak. 'Yes, and 90% of the participants were Hungarians but because of the 10% whi were from abroad, in a day and a half out of the 3 day program English was the official language'

(5) C8: ... most pl. Szegeden az ECHO kongresszus is angol nyelven ment. Ez Európai akkreditált kongresszus volt, és angol nyelven ment. '... well, we had the ECHO congress here in Szeged and it was in English. It is an accredited European congress, and it was all in English.'

English is the main language of international conferences beside the local, national language of the organizing country, or in some cases the only language used even at national meetings, as Gunnarsson (2000) outlines and as the cardiologists in the interviews attest.

Except for the youngest participant in my research, each cardiologist has participated in national and international conferences and presented their papers in English. Two of the interviewees mentioned that they prefer presenting posters as they think that, because of their lower English language competence, this can be done with less stress.

5.2.3.4. Professional daily life

Beside the above described three academic domains where cardiologists use the English language, they also mentioned several further occasions when they speak English. All of them, except for the youngest participant, are (or used to be[56]) involved in teaching students in the English program: members of the senior staff deliver lectures to the students and junior cardiologists are involved in giving practicals[57] on a weekly basis. But even the youngest participant has mentioned that she works together with foreign students in their final-year when examining and diagnosing patients at the department:

(1) C5: Volt olyan, mikor tantermi előadást is kellett tartani. 'On some occasions I had to give a lecture'

I: Devizásoknak? 'To the foreign students?'

C5: Igen. Ötödéveseknek. Valahogy megoldottam, egyszer 90 perc volt, egyszer 45 perc, és ráadásul ilyen, hogy a szívultrahangnak a fizikai alapjai.

56 All three cardiologists, who are now working in secondary health care used to be involved in teaching foreign students when they worked at the Department of Cardiology.

57 A practical is a class similar to a seminar, it is less formal than a lecture, and in clinical subjects patients are also presented in these classes.

Senkinek nem volt ideje, és akkor be kellett ugrani. … Sőt, már most nyolcadik éve, vagy hogy is, hogy dolgozom, gyakorlatilag minden évben van angol csoportom, mármint devizás csoportom. 'Yes, to the fifth year students. I managed somehow, once it was 90 minutes and on another occasion it was a 45-minute lecture, and it was the physical basics of cardiac ultrasound. Nobody was available so I had to fill in … And now for 8 years, I have had my own English group every year, I mean of foreign students'

(2) C11: Persze gyakorlatot mindenkinek kell tartani. 'Of course, everybody has to give a practical.'

(3) C6: A másik nagyon sarkalatos pont, ez az angol oktatás. Tehát egyre kevésbé tud az ember kibújni alóla. … Elmondom, hogy mit kell hallgatni, vagy szívet vizsgálnak vagy valami, és akkor utána meg megbeszéljük, hogy mit találtunk, és akkor borzasztó sokat kérdeznek. 'Another important thing is teaching in the English program. You can hardly avoid it any more … I tell them what they should listen for, or they examine the heart or something, and then we discuss what we have found, and then they ask a lot of questions, an awful lot.'

Each participant has mentioned that they have to take history in English more or less regularly and the language of the examination instructions is also English in this case:

(4) C11: általában a külföldi betegek közül vannak kelet-európaiak, norvég, dán, amerikai, de van egyébként török, angol, aki itt lesznek rosszul. 'usually there are patients from Eastern Europe, Norway, Denmark, US but there are patients arriving from Turkey, and England, and they get sick here.'

(5) C9: Mindig [van] valami, például ma volt egy indiai fiú, akit vizsgálni kellett. 'There is always something happening, for instance today I have had an Indian boy to examine.'

(6) C8: például tegnap volt egy angol évfolyamos orvostanhallgató. 'for instance yesterday there was a medical student here from the English program'

I: Mint beteg? 'As a patient?'

C8: Mint beteg, mint páciens inkább. De egyre több külföldi jön, és azért angolul nagyjából mindenki meg tud szólalni. Tegnap pl. egy norvég gyerek volt, nyilván norvégul én nem fogok soha megtanulni, viszont tud jól angolul, mert az angol nyelvű évfolyamra jár 'Yes, as a patient, or rather a client. But more and more foreigners come to us, and almost everybody can speak a little English. Yesterday, for example, a Norwegian guy came to me, naturally I would never learn Norwegian, but he spoke English as he attends the English program.'

(7) C1: ... a devizások jönnek le az ambulanciára, és velük tényleg csak angolul [lehet beszélni]. '...the foreign students come to us to the Outpatient Department, and you can speak to them only in English'

(8) C3: ez [az angol] volt a közös nyelv, gyakran ez a közös nyelv, tehát több ilyen beteg volt ... Általában Szerbiából, Romániából érkező nem magyar ajkú betegekről van szó. De egy-két itt ragadt kamionos, vagy ilyesmi is van. 'and it [English] was the common language, frequently it is the common language with several patients... They usually come from Serbia, Romania, and are non-Hungarian speakers. But sometimes there are truck drivers or similar people who get stuck here'

Most of the cases, when English is used in history taking, comprise students from the English program, but, less frequently, tourists and truck drivers also visit the Emergency Outpatient Unit. Patients also arrive from Serbia and Romania for elective cardiological care.

Further domains where English language performance is required are participation in 'studies' sponsored by pharmaceutical companies, visits to departments in other countries, writing CVs and study plans, talking to colleagues from other countries on the phone, writing e-mails to colleagues involved in the same scientific project, and talking to and teaching colleagues from abroad, who are here on postgraduate training, since the Department of Cardiology is a European Postgraduate Training Center as well.

5.2.3.5. The importance of English language competence

Participants have been asked in the third section of the interview about the importance of their English language competence in their professional life, and if it is a disadvantage for a physicians to not speak English.

As described in Section 5.2.2, each cardiologist has studied English and can speak it at an upper-intermediate or advanced level, and they use the English language in their profession on a daily basis in various situations: doing research, giving lectures and practicals as well, examining English-speaking patients, etc.

The interviewed cardiologists all agreed on the importance of the English language, and have used strong, emphatic adjectival and adverbial phrases to describe its importance: the English language is *elfogadott* 'accepted', *nagyon fontos* 'very important', *mindenképpen fontos* 'important by all means', *rendkívül fontos* 'extremely important', *egyértelműen* [fontos] 'obviously [importantg', *minden nap kell* 'necessary every day', *lényeges, napi szinten használatos* 'essential, it is used on a daily basis', *elengedhetetlen, nem lehet lépni sem* [angol nyelvtudás nélkül] 'indispensable, you can't do without it [without English language competence]'.

Cardiologists have all agreed that those colleagues who do not speak English or not at the appropriate level are at a disadvantage:

(1) C2: *... mindenképpen hátrány [ha nem beszél angolul] ... Minden szakterületen az angol dominál.* 'It is definitely a disadvantage [if they cannot speak English] ... English dominates in each specialty.'

(2) C9: *Egyértelműen hátrány. Hát igyekezzen felzárkózni, én azt csinálom.* 'Obviously it is a disdavantage. Well, they should try and catch up, that's what I'm doing, too'

(3) C1: *Egyrészt azért, mert a legeslegújabb irányelvek, ... azt ő nem tudja, illetve le kell neki fordítani. ... A másik az, hogy annak, aki feljebb akar lépni a ranglétrán, annak kell különféle előadásokat, ilyen publikációkat készítenie, ... [a] jó értékűek azok angolul vannak, úgyhogy mindenféleképpen kell.* '[they are at a disadvantage] On the one hand, because the most recent guidelines ... they are not familiar with them or the guidelines need to be translated for them ... And on the other hand, if they want to be promoted, they have to give various presentations and prepare publications ... but the high quality [medical journals] are in English, thus, it is essential [to speak English].

(4) C3: Az baj. Az most ebben a mai világban, az baj. ... Biztos vagyok benne, hogy – ez nem pejoratív – bizonyos szint alatt meg lehet angol nélkül lenni. ... de ha valaki bővebben utána akar nézni csomó dolognak, ha nem is búvárkodik, az angol nyelvvel, az angol nyelvű tankönyvvel fog szembe kerülni, ami adatokat fog szolgáltatni. 'That is a problem [if you can't speak English]. In this world now it is a problem ... I'm sure, I Don't mean to be pejorative, that under a certain level you can do without English ... but if you want to read about various things, even if you don't want to research something, you will meet the English language, you will be faced with an English textbook which can provide you the data.'

(5) C3: ... így, nem tudja letenni a kardiológusi szakvizsgát, ugyanis nincs magyar könyv, ... angol nélkül nagyon nehéz. '[without English] they cannot

pass the cardiologist subspecialty exam, as there is no Hungarian book ... without English it is very difficult.'

(6) C4: Ezt [hátrány] teljes mértéken így gondolom, ... az az orvos, aki nem beszél valamilyen szinten angolul, ő nem tud a mindennapos/tudományos élettel lépést tartani. ... iszonyatosan fejlődik az orvostudomány, számtalan technikai dolog van, fejlődik nap mint nap, s ezeket leginkább angolul tudja követni az ember. ... egy orvosnak, aki most végez, mindenképpen kell beszélnie valamilyen szinten angolul. 'it is [a disadvantage] I think ... a doctor who does not speak English at some level cannot keep up with the daily/scientific life ... medicine is developing at a terrible speed, there are many technical innovations, they are being developed and you can get informed about them only in English ... a doctor who graduates these days need to speak English at a certain level'

(7) C5: Biztosan [hátrány], mert nem tudja a legfrissebb dolgokat. Nálunk ... probléma lenne. 'It is [a disadvantage] surely, as they are not informed about the most recent advances. Here [at the clinic] ... it would be a problem.

(8) C6: Szerintem ez [hátrány] teljesen így van. Hát eleve minden irodalom angolul [van]. ... Minden nap kell az angol. 'I think it is [a disadvantage], absolutely it is. Well all the literature is in English ... You need your English every day.'

(9) C11: Mindenképpen hátrány, minden szempontból. ... az angol nyelvtudás pedig szinte elengedhetetlennek tűnik az orvostudomány szakmai területén. 'It is a disadvantage, in every respect. ... English competence seems indispensible in the field of medicine.'

And what happens to a cardiologist if they do not speak English:

(10) C7: Hát itt, aki kardiológus, az beszél. 'Well, if you are a cardiologist working here, you must speak English.'

(11) C8: Pechjük van. Tényleg. ... Megtanul. Muszáj megtanulnia 'They are out of luck. Really. ... You must study, then. You must learn English.'

(12) C6: Az itt hagyja a klinikát. Tehát az angol az annyira fontos a klinikai életben, munkában, hogy gyakorlatilag itt nyelvtudás nélkül nem lehet itt maradni. 'They will leave the department. English is so important in the clinical

life, in our work that practically you cannot stay here without having English knowledge.'

5.2.3.6. The language of Hungarian discharge reports

In the last part of the interview, cardiologists have been asked to read through a discharge report that was written at the Department of Cardiology, and to tell me if they would have written anything differently. They have made several remarks on the professional content of it and that they would have written certain things, from a medical aspect, differently. But they have made very few remarks on the language, expressing that it is the way they themselves would have written it:

(1) C5: *hát szerintem ez így jó. Nyilván, hát miután én is hasonlóan szoktam, nem tűnik idegennek.* 'Well, I think it is fine this way. Certainly, as I do it in a similar way, it does not seem strange at all.'

(2) C8: *Teljesen korrekt* 'Perfectly fine'

(3) C9: *Ez egy kórlefolyás, és ez jól le van írva … Hát ugye rengeteg a latin kifejezés benne, most ezen belül nem veszek észre [angolos dolgokat]* 'This is the course of the disease described here, and it is described well… Well, there are a lot of Latin expressions in it, aren't there. And I can't recognize any [Englishisms] within this part'.

(4) C11: Szerintem *jó. Orvosok megértik, és a betegek is általában megértik egyébként.* 'I think it is fine. Doctors can understand it, and by the way, the patients can usually also understand it'.

On direct questioning, the cardiologists have mentioned that in some cases the conjunction is missing and probably the word order used is not standard Hungarian.

(5) C4: *Tehát én úgy gondolom, hogy aki foglalkozik ezzel napi szinten, tehát olyan szinten, hogy az irodalommal, illetve el kell neki mennie kongresszusokra, prezentálnia kell, ő már azért többé-kevésbé angolul gondolkodik.* 'So I think that those who deal with it on a daily basis, so at a level that [he/she reads] the literature, or has to attend conferences or present at conferences, [those doctors] are thinking more or less in English.

(6) C9: *Igen, vannak itt nekem idegennek tűnő rövidítések ...mondjuk a 'study' kifejezést, most ezt vesszük példának, ... hogy ezt azért mindenki érti, még aki nem tud angolul, az is.* 'Yes, there are some abbreviations that seem to be foreign ... well, let's take the word *study* as an example, ... but everybody understands it, even those who do not speak English.'

(7) C6: *Nem tudok. Ezt így hívjuk. A sztent, az sztent. ... Ja, hogy ponttal [írta a tizedestörtet]? Nem vesszővel. Igen [én is így szoktam].* 'I don't know. This is what it's called. A stent is a stent. ... Oh, have they written it with a [decimal] point? Not with the comma. Yes [I also write it this way].'

(8) C8: *Igen, ez egy másik érdekes, hogy ugye vagy eredeti latin, vagy magyarított. Ez is egy általában mixelt dolog szokott lenni a zárójelentésekben. Hát nehéz egy ilyet megírni magyarul, mert ugye ez rögzül az emberben, ezt tanulja hat évig, így látja a könyvekben, használja, tehát nehéz átmagyarosítani. Ez külön odafigyelést igényel, hogy átmagyarítsa.* 'Yes, that's another interesting thing, the issue whether it is original Latin or Hungarianized. There is usually a mixture in the discharge reports. Well, it is difficult to write this in Hungarian, this is what you get used to, you study this for six years, you see in the textbooks, you use them this way, therefore, it is difficult to translate them into Hungarian. It would require special attention to make it Hungarian."

(9) C10: *Nem is nagyon lehet lefordítani, mert nagyon hülyén nézne ki, és akkor inkább úgy döntött a szakma ebben, hogy azokat a kifejezéseket megtartjuk az eredeti formátumban.* ''You cannot really translate it, it would look very silly, and therefore, the professional community has decided to keep these expressions in their original form.'

The interviewed cardiologists have identified very few English contact-induced features in the sample report, only some of the words (e.g. *study*) and abbreviations (e.g. *LIMA-LAD*), but no other features (e.g. orthographic, syntactic features) seem 'foreign'[58] to them. They claim that this is the way how they write the reports themselves and they think this is the way they should be written.

58 The term 'foreign' is used here to refer to any English language contact induced feature.

5.2.3.7. Attitudes to the use of English

English is the dominant language in several medical domains: postgraduate studies, research publications, presentations and the daily work of cardiologists. The interviews demonstrate that the cardiologists' knowledge of English (or a lack of it) can affect their careers. Physicians claim that English is their working language most of the time when they are doing research, and English also appears in teaching, when instructing the medical students in the English program. English is present in doctor–patient interactions as well, however, not on a daily basis, and also in collegial talk, when talking to colleagues from other countries working at the university as part of their postgraduate training program.

Responses given by the cardiologists for the questions if they like the fact that English has become the lingua franca of medicine, and if they can benefit from it indicate that few of them consider the dominance of English to be a handicap in any way for them. Only one physician has said that she is embarrassed by it, as her English is not good enough, though she works hard to improve her English. Other two physicians have also mentioned that they have to have private classes in English to improve their English, which is essential for their work:

(1) C7: *egy szakmai zsargont meg kell, hogy tanuljon valamilyen szinten.* 'you have to learn the professional jargon at a certain level.'

(2) C8: *egyre több külföldi jön, és azért angolul nagyjából mindenki meg tud szólalni* 'more and more foreigners are coming [to Hungary], and because of this almost everybody can speak some English'

(3) C9: *Úgy gondolom, hogy a magyar után angolul kéne legjobban beszéljünk.* 'I think English should be the next best language spoken for us after Hungarian.'

(4) I: *Van még valami, amit el szeretnél mondani így az angollal kapcsolatosan?* 'Is there anything else you'd like to tell me in connection with the English language?'

C6: *Azt, hogy nagyon szeretnék jobban megtanulni angolul.* 'I would love to have a better command of it.'

Cardiologists' explanations for considering the dominance of the English language in medical sciences as an advantage fall into the following three categories (i-iii):

(i) it is an advantage to have a single agreed language in scientific communication:

(5) C8: ... *mindenki az integrációra törekszik ugye, Unió, meg na mindegy. El kell fogadni.* 'everybody aims for the integration, don't they, the Union and that's it. We have to accept it.'

(6) C9: *Én azt gondolom, hogy globálisan jó, mert hiszen ablakot nyit a világra, mert bárkivel tudunk kommunikálni, nem ijedünk meg, ha valaki felhív Angliából és érdeklődik a rokona felől,*'I think that globally it is beneficial, as it opens a window to the world, as we can communicate with everybody, we are not scared off if somebody calls us from England to make an inquiry about their relative,'

(7) C10: *én azt gondolom, hogy nekünk, mint külső használóknak, nekünk jó, mert így bárhol tudunk beszélni.* 'I think it is good for us, external users, it is beneficial for us as we can speak to other people anywhere.'

(8) C11: *Én azt gondolom, hogy mindenképpen kell egy univerzális nyelv, vagy legalábbis az, amit egyébként mindenki a világon bárhol, fórumokon, konferenciákon szakmai szempontból elő lehet venni. Erre nyilván nemzeti nyelvek nem alkalmasak, az eszperantó nem alkalmas erre, ezért úgy gondolnám, hogy miután azért univerzális nyelvvé vált, és az univerzális nyelvek közül lehet, hogy a spanyolt többen beszélik világszerte, mégsem vált elfogadottá és nyilván a nyugati kultúra miatt valami nyugatibb nyelvet kellett választani, történelmi okok miatt ez az angol maradt, ami egyébként azt gondolom, hogy orvosi szempontból támogatható.* 'I think a universal language is needed, anyhow, or at least a language that anybody can use in all parts of the world at forums, conferences for professional purposes. National languages are obviously not suitable for this purpose, Esperanto is not suitable for this purpose, thus, I would think, as [English] has become a universal language, and from universal languages Spanish might be spoken by more speakers in the world, it has still not become accepted, and obviously because of Western culture a more western language should be chosen, so because of historical reasons, English has become this language, which I think, from a medical aspect, can be supported.'

(ii) physicians study English since their childhood or adolescence, therefore, they acquire sufficient language competence:

(9) C1: *könnyebb, ha úgy tanuljuk meg, hogy már angolul, és akkor nem kell fordítgatni.* 'it is easier if we learn this way [in English] and then we don't need to translate it.'

(10) C4: *hogy most per pillanat én már inkább angolul gondolkodom, mikor írok egy absztraktot,* 'and nowadays, I am thinking rather in English when I'm writing an abstract'

(11) I: *melyik nyelven olvasol szívesen?* 'Which language do you prefer reading in?'
C11: *Csak angolul.* 'Only in English.'

(iii) for certain reasons the English language is inherently more suitable than other languges to be the language of medicine (English-intrinsic argument):

(12) C2: ezért nevezünk el eszközöket vagy beavatkozásokat angolul, mert sokkal egyszerűbb és könnyebben érthető a szakma számára. 'Therefore, we give the devices and interventions English names, as it is much simpler and easier to understand for the members of the professional community.'

(13) C3: inkább angolul jegyzetelek … , mert néha angolul tömörebben lehet leírni egy-egy dolgot, magyarul sokkal szebben, sokkal kifejezőbben … , de angolul tömörebben lehet leírni. 'I prefer taking notes in English … as sometimes it's more concise to put a thing down in English, it is much nicer and more expressive in Hungarian …, but you can write more concisely in English.'

(14) C3: valahogy funkcionális, gyakorlati értéke [van] ennek. 'somehow [the English language] has a functional, practical value'

I: … könnyebben jön angolul? 'Is it easier to say it in English?'

C9: Könnyebben, vagy jobban fedi azt a dolgot. 'Easier, it describes that thing more adequately.'

5.2.4. Results of the interviews with primary care physicians

At the beginning of the interview, family physicians (n=6) have been asked about the languages they studied. All the 6 physicians studied (medical) Latin as part of their university studies, 5 physicians have studied English, 5 have studied Russian and 1 interviewee has studied French (see Figure 9). 3 of them started learning English in secondary school and 2 of them at the university over age 18.

Interviewees have also been asked about the time spent in English-speaking countries. Only one family physician spent some weeks in England at a hospital during her university studies. The others have not been abroad for professional purposes.

After the introductory questions, physicians have been asked about the role of the English language in their professional life: what they use the English language for. Answers can be grouped around two main areas:

(i) 5 out of 6 physicians have mentioned that they need it rarely in their daily practice: some patients (Chinese or Serbs, students of various nationality, or truck drivers) visit them in their office, but it happens only 4–5 times a year:

(1) F3: Tehát azért hozzám befutnak, a [szállodához]-hoz közel vagyok, és azért ott vannak külföldiek, tehát volt már rá precedens, hogy mondjuk kellett használnom az angolt. 'So they do visit me, as my office is close to [hotel], and there are a lot of foreigners there, so there were some occasions when I had to speak English.'

(2) F4: a múltkor volt egy kínai gyakorlaton, hát azzal angolul kellett [beszélnem], ... azért úgy hellyel-közzel megértettük egymást. Ritkán előfordul, hogy kamionosok jönnek. 'The other day, there was a Chinese student here on practice, and I had to [talk to] this student in English, ... and more or less we were able to understand each other. And rarely, some truck drivers come to see me [for medical advice].'

(3) F5: meg itt vannak ezek a külföldi tanulók, tehát függ attól, hogy milyen betegkört lát el az ember. 'and there are the foreign students here [in Szeged], so it depends on what clientele you have.'

(4) F6: mert kínaiak vannak most már, egyre több, ő velük is [angolul beszélek], nyilván kínaiul nem, ... aztán egyszer-egyszer egyetemisták befutnak, ... akkor volt jugoszláv területről, nem magyar területről, azok is inkább angolul

[tudnak] 'as there are the Chinese [patients], there are more and more of them, and I speak English with them, obviously not Chinese, ... and once in a while university students come in, ... and patients from the former Yugoslavia, from non-Hungarian speaking areas, they rather speak English...'

(ii) the other area where they use the English language is in searching the medical literature; however, only 2 of them have mentioned that they regularly do it in English.

(5) F3: Nyilván, hogyha bármit elolvasok [angolul], akkor azért azt megértem. 'If I read anything [in English], no doubt, I understand it.'

(6) F4: Hát cikkek vannak angol nyelven, azt szoktam ritkán. Tehát nem vagyunk rákényszerítve. 'Well, there are articles in English, I read them rarely. We are not compelled to do it.'

The other 4 physicians read about medical achievements and recent advances in Hungarian:

(7) F5: Van néhány [magyar nyelvű anyag], kapunk ilyen lapot. Azokat azért úgy el szoktam olvasni. 'There are some [materials in Hungarian], we receive these journals. I usually read them.'

(8) F2: Igen [olvasok]. Inkább szaklapokból. Orvostovábbképző szemle, Praxis, akkor a Diabetológiai Társaságnak vannak, annak vagyok a tagja és az szokott küldeni, ... jó le van a másik oldalon angolul is írva, de itt meg magyarul. 'Yes I do [read]. Mostly medical papers. The Medical Postgraduate Review, Praxis, and the Society of Diabetology also has a journal, and as I am a member of this society, they send me the journal ... and it is translated into English, so on the one page it is in Hungarian and on the other page it is in English.'

(9) F4: hozzáférhető [a szakirodalom magyarul]. Nagyon széles a paletta. Tehát, ha ... akarjuk magunkat tovább képezni, azt meg tudjuk magyarul is csinálni. 'it [the medical literature] is available [in Hungarin]. There is a wide spectrum. Therefore, if we want to develop ourselves, we can do it in Hungarian.'

(10) F6: Nem [olvasok angolul]. Szakirodalom van lefordított is, mert a British Medical-t is, mindent kiadnak magyarul. 'I do not [read in English]. The

medical literature is also available in Hungarian, as everything, the British Medical Journal and everything is also published in Hungarian.'

All of them attend postgraduate trainings regularly but the language of these trainings is always Hungarian. Sometimes presenters come from abroad but in these cases an interpreter helps in understanding the presentations:

(11) F2: Igen magyarul mondja, de ha például azt mondja, hogy mit tudom én milyen vizsgálatnak a formációja, akkor azt nyilván angolul mondja, ... de azokat megértjük. 'Yes, they [the presenters] speak Hungarian, but if they mention, for instance some form of examination, they give the English word for it, ... but we can understand them.'

(12) I: Értem. És akkor gyakorlatilag ugyanazok fordulnak elő rendszeresen, azért érti meg, mert azok többször előjönnek? 'I see. Then practically they are used regularly, and do you understand them because they are used frequently?'
F2: Igen rendszeresen, ugyanaz fordul elő, és ezt magyarul is így tudjuk, hogy relatív, vagy reverzibilis, vagy irreverzibilis, ugyanezek vannak az angolban is, amikor következtetünk valaminek a végkonklúziójára vagy a végpontokra. Meg mortaltás, morbiditás, ez mondjuk nem tudom, hogy a latin, meg az angol vagy a magyar, de annyira már a betegek is megértik, hogy mi az. 'Yes, they are used frequently, the same expressions are mentioned, and we use them in Hungarian the same way: relatív 'relative', reverzibilis 'reversible' or irreverzibilis 'irreversible', the same can be found in English, when we come to the conclusion or deduce the endpoints. And then the words mortalitás 'mortality', or morbiditás 'morbidity', but I don't know if these are Latin, English or Hungarian [words], but even the patients can understand them, what they mean.'

(13) F4: angol nyelven van [a dia], az mondjuk nagyon jó, mert az ember látja, hogy úristen, tényleg ezt értem, 'it [the slide] is in English, well, it is really good, because you can see that, my god, you can really understand this.'

(14) F5: Hát előfordul az, hogy véletlenül bennefelejtik és akkor belekerül... elmagyarázzák, de hát azért elég érthető, nincs, amivel különösebb gond lenne. Ezt így érti mindenki. 'Well, it can happen that they accidentally leave them [the English language slide] in, and if it is so ... they explain, but they are quite comprehensible, we have no real problem understanding them.'

(15) F6: az elkészült diákat nem írják át magyarra ... Elég sok meghonosodott, ami angol nyelvű már a gyakorlatban is, vagy eleve úgy

mondják, tehát már a magyar szövegekben is úgy jelenik meg. … ezért is jó, ezekre el kell járni. 'the prepared slides are not translated into Hungarian … There are a lot of assimilated [loanswords], which come from the English langauge and which are used in medical practice, or we simply say it that way, and they appear [in English] in the Hungarian texts. … thus, it is beneficial to attend these [postgraduate courses].'

English words are regularly projected in these trainings as the slides, the presenters' (even the Hungarian presenters') shows, are frequently in English. Physicians say that it is not embarrassing for them because, on the on hand, they studied some English so they can understand these texts; on the other hand, the presenter always explains them in Hungarian. Thus, they get familiarized with the most recently used medical terms in both Hungarian and English. Therefore, it is no problem for them to understand these terms when they see them again in the discharge reports. However, it can happen that they meet an English term in the discharge report, which has been written by a tertiary or secondary care physician, which they are not familiar with, but even in these cases they can make out the meaning from the context:

(16) F6: a szakszövegeket könnyű kikövetkeztetni is. 'medical texts are easy to figure out.'

(17) I: Volt-e már olyan esetleg, hogy valami olyan szót használtak, amit Ön nem értett, esetleg olyan rövidítés? 'Has it ever happened that they [those who write the hosptial discharge reports] used a word or an abbreviation that you could not understand?'

F2: Volt, nagyon sok ilyen volt. Most például volt egy EKG-ban volt egy ilyen couplet, így írja, hát arra nem tudtam rájönni, hogy micsoda. … tudtam, hogy mik voltak az előzmények meg a következmények és akkor hát valahogy úgy silabizáltam ki. 'Yes, there have been many cases, for instance in an ECG report the word couplet was used, and I wasn't able to figure out what it means. … I knew about the past history and the consequences and then I somehow managed to figure it out.'

(18) F3: van, aki annyira túlspanolja magát, hogy ő milyen profi, … ott is bőségesen angol eredetű szavakat használ magyar toldalékolással, ahol már nem kellene. … ez nem feltétlen az angol tudás eredete, ez szerintem inkább az, hogy milyen alkatú, 'There are some physicians who overdo their job, how professional they are, … there you can find plenty of English words used by them with Hungarian suffixes, which they would not necessarily have to use. …

it does not necessarily originate in their English knowledge, I think it depends on your attitude,’

Several English abbreviations are used in the hospital discharge reports, and family physicians know what the most important ones stand for, e.g. WBC ‘white blood count’, as they have seen them several times during the postgraduate trainings:

(19) F3: Abban [a zárójelentésben] úgy van rövidítve, hogy WBC, fehérvérsejt. Akkor ezek [a többi rövidítés], például a laborban. ’In the discharge report it is abbreviated as WBC, white blood cell. And then these [other abbreviations] for instance in the “Laboratory findings” section.’

(20) F4: Kardiológiában van nagyon sok rövidítés, amit csak akkor tudunk követni, ha továbbképzéseken halljuk ’There are many abbreviations in cardiology, which we can understand only if we hear them at the postgraduate training courses.’

(21) F6: Valószínű, hogy úgy van beletáplálva, és akkor úgy kapjuk azt. Mindig úgy kapjuk. ... Bár leírni [mi] is így szoktuk. ’Probably, they are programmed like that, and we receive them [the abbreviations] like that. We always get them like that. ... Although we also write them [the decimal with point] like this.’

None of the physicians think that the lack of English knowledge can be a disadvantage for a primary care physician, at least not at the moment:

(22) F2: itthon elboldogul, de innentől kezdve, ha szeretne külföldi kapcsolatot tartani, vagy kutatómunkában részt venni, vagy kongresszuson részt venni, vagy egy kicsikét mondjuk egy több szabadidővel vagy pénzzel rendelkezik, magyar nyelven nem boldogul. ’you can do without [English competence] in Hungary, but later on, if you want to have some contacts abroad, or you want to participate in congresses, or let’s say, you have a little bit more free time and money, you can’t make it if you speak only Hungarian.’

(23) F4: Magánszorgalomból lehet ezt [angol tanulás] csinálni. És én azt gondolom, hogy alapellátásban nem [hátrány] ... egy klinikai orvos az jobban rá van a tudományos munkája alapján erre kényszerítve, mi nem sajnos. ’You can learn English as an individual initiative. I think that in primary care it is not [a disadvantage if you don’t speak English] ... a clinical physician is forced to speak English, as it is necessary for their scientific research, but, unfortunately, we are not.’

(24) F5: Hát olyan nagyon még nem hátrány, De ez annyira nem mérvadó, mert mi nem is a szakrendelésen vagyunk, nem is az egyetemen vagyunk, tehát a betegeknek a környezetében vagyunk inkább. Tehát igazándiból egy klinikán azért más, mert azért ott sokan vannak kollegák is, ugyanúgy szakrendelőkben is, tehát itt azért mások az arányok. Én úgy gondolom, hogy mi inkább a betegeknek vagyunk, ezért nincs annyira szükségünk rá. 'Well it is not a huge disadvantage at the moment. But it is not relevant, as we don't work either in secondary outpatient care or at the university, well, we are rather in contact with the patients. It is rather different if you work at the clinic, as there are several other physicians working there, and the situation is the same in secondary care, thus the [doctor–patient] ratio is different. I think, we are here for the patients, therefore, we do not need [the English language] so much.'

(25) F6: Hát egyelőre nem. Nekem eddig még nincs hátrányom, hogy nem igazán tudom aktívan a nyelvet, de azért csak rá kell szorítanom magam, mert hát ugye egyre több a külföldi, vagy lesz itt Magyarországon, vagy ha csak átutazóban és valami történik, akkor azért nyilván jobb, ha az ember tud kommunikálni, úgyhogy hátránynak semmiképp nem hátrány, de egyelőre előny se származna belőle most a jelenlegi helyzetemben. 'Well, at the moment, it is not a disadvantage for me that I cannot speak English actively, but I think I must make myself learn it, as more and more people arrive from abroad to Hungary, or they just travel through Hungary, and if anything happens to them, it is better if I can talk to them. So it is not a disadvantage at all [if you can speak English], but it is not an advantage either, at least not in my present situation.'

And they also add that English competence does not mean a real advantage for them in their daily work. However, 5 out of 6 physicians agreed that it is very useful to have a common language in medicine, and 4 out of 6 agreed that it should be the English language:

(26) F1: … jó dolog, hogy van egy közös nyelv… az angol a latinnal együtt, így jó. '… it is a good thing that there is a common language … English together with Latin, it is fine this way.'

(27) F3: … szerencsés vagyok, hogy pont angolul tanultam, …Szerintem jó, mert azért nagyon sokan ezt a nyelvet beszélik a világon, tehát ez olyan elég elterjedt, meg Amerika, a vezető gazdasági potenciállal rendelkező országokban az angol az anyanyelv, így tehát automatikusan ez adódott. ' … I am lucky that I studied English, … I think this is good since many people speak this language in the world, so it is very widespread, and in the USA, in countries which have an

economical potential, English is the first language, so it is natural that English became [the common language].'

(28) F4: már fiatal korom óta maga a nyelv nagyon tetszik, tehát amikor egy angol ember beszél, akkor az egy nagyon szép dolog, ... Szerintem nagyon jó, mert ugye hát nemzetközi. Mert mindenki tud angolul, aki tud angolul, az meg tudja a szakirodalmat magasabb szinten nézni. De az orvostudomány nyelve az angol. Ezt mindannyian tudjuk. Szerte a világon, és ez így jól is van. Nem? 'Since my younger age, I have loved the English language, it is beautiful when an English person speaks, ... I think [the English language] is very good, as it is international. Since everybody speaks English, and those who speak English can read medical literature at a higher level. But the language of medicine is English. We are all aware of it. All over the world, and that's just fine, isn't it?'

(29) F5: Szerintem ez egy nagyon jó dolog. Anno még mondták, hogy az eszperantó, én azt nem ismertem, de azt mondják, hogy a legkönnyebben tanulható, de szerintem ez sem annyira nehezen tanulható. És hogyha azt nézzük, hogy inkább németet kellene vagy oroszt, vagy nem tudom, akkor szerintem ez sokkal jobb így. Nem beszélve arról, hogy hát azért angolul nagy többsége a világ lakosságának valamilyen szinten beszélget. ... nagyon sok angol szó van a mi nyelvünkben, vagy a szavak közt is, vagy lehet, hogy már annyira nemzetköziek ezek a szavak, hogy már itt is, meg ott is azt jelentik. Szerintem ez így jó. 'I think it is a very good thing. In the past, some people talked about the Esperanto language, but I am not familiar with it, but it is said to be easier to learn, but I think [the English language] is also not so difficult to learn either. And if we consider that we would have to study German or Russian instead or something like that, then I think it is much better this way. Not to mention that the majority of the population of the world can speak English at some level ... we have lots of English words in Hungarian, a lot of words, or these words might be international words meaning the same here and there. And I think this is just fine.'

One physician highlights that it is harmful that English has become the language of medicine internationally, she would prefer using the Hungarian language with the Latin language and would exclude English from her professional life:

(30) F2: Szerintem rossz. Most nem azért, mert hogy politika, vagy Amerika, vagy angol nyelv a világnyelvek egyike, de épp úgy mondhatnánk akkor az oroszt is, vagy a kínait, hogy akkor miért nem az. Sokat romlott a magyar nyelvhelyesség, a stílus az utóbbi 10 évben...'I think it is bad. Not

because of politics, or the USA, or because English is one of the world languages, but then we could mention the Russian or the Chinese languages, why not those instead? The correct Hungarian usage and the style have been corrupted considerably in the past 10 years …'

According to 5 family physicians, English used together with Latin can make international communication possible between doctors, and English can also help doctors communicate with foreign patients. 5 physicians have mentioned that they think that more and more patients come from various countries to Hungary, to Szeged, and they turn not only to secondary and tertiary care physicians but also to primary care physicians. Therefore, family physicians should develop or review their English knowledge:

(31) F3: Hát nem hátrány semmiképpen sem. Nyilván azért, a szakmai cikkek, ha az embernek van rá ideje, vagy azért tényleg, ha szerintem bármilyen területen van Magyarországon, már jó lenne, ha valamilyen szinten beszélnének angolul, mert bárki szembejöhet az utcán és úgy sem értik meg a mi magyar nyelvünket. Szerintem az a minimum, hogy azért egy nyelvet ebben az országban tudni kell. 'It is not a disadvantage at all [if you can speak English]. Obviously, the medical articles, if you have time for reading them [are in English], or if you work in any specialty in Hungary, it is beneficial if you can speak English at some level, as you can meet somebody in the street and foreigners don't understand our language, the Hungarian language. So I think, in Hungary you should speak at least one [foreign] language.'

(32) F5: Hát ez mindenféleképpen fontos, nyilván ott [a klinikákon] azért ez nagyon fontos, tehát nem egy háziorvosi gyakorlatban, … vannak nekik [a klinikusoknak] ezek a nemzetközi kapcsolataik, és sokkal jobban [szükségük van az angol nyelvre], mint mondjuk a periférián [háziorvosi gyakorlatban]. …de ha majd jönnek itt az Unióból jobbra-balra, tehát sokkal több külföldi illetőségű lehet, … mindenféleképpen egy városi intézménynél ott rá kell készülni, hogy ott azért lesznek olyanok, akikkel azért kommunikálni kell. 'Well, it is important by all means, of course, it is very important there [at the university clinics], but not in the family practice, … they [tertiary care physicians] have international relations, and [they need the English language] much more than let's say on the periphery [in family practice]. … but when people start coming from the EU, there might be much more foreign citizens here, … in a municipal institution we have to be prepared for the task that we will have to communicate with some of them somehow.'

5.2.5. Results of the interviews with patients

At the beginning of the interview, patients (n=8) have been asked about the languages they studied. 5 patients studied Russian at school, 2 patients studied English, 2 patients studied Latin and 2 patients studied another language (see Figure 9). None of the interviewed patients have been to English speaking countries.

It is not the first time for 7 out of 8 patients to have been hospitalized at the Department of Cardiology. So they are relatively familiar with the hospital surroundings, they know much about their own condition, and about the investigations performed at the department.

After the introductory phase of the interview, they have been asked about the language used by their doctors at the Department of Cardiology. Two patients have mentioned that everything, all the examinations and interventions, are performed in Hungarian:

(1) I: Volt olyan esetleg, hogy olyasmit beszéltek, amit nem értett? Vagy nem teljesen volt világos? 'Can you remember a situation when they [the physicians] were speaking about something that you could not understand?'

P4[59]: Nem teljesen volt világos, volt olyan, persze, amit nem teljesen értettem, de mindig magyarul ment [a beszéd]. 'No, everthing was completely clear, of course, there were things I could not fully get, but they were always [speaking] in Hungarian.'

(2) P7: [katéterezés során] mindig magyarul beszélgettek. '[during the catheterization] they were always talking to each other in Hungarian.'

But the other patients have explained to me that they could hear doctors speaking English in various clinical situations:

(3) P1: Tegnap a folyósón figyeltem fel arra, hogy angolul beszéltek, valószínű, hogy orvostanhallgatók lehettek, és angolul tette fel a doktor úr a kérdéseket. Angolul beszélt hozzájuk. 'Yesterday, I heard in the hallway that they were speaking in English, probably, they were medical students, and the doctor asked his questions in English. He talked to them in English.'

(4) P4: Jaj igen. Sokat vizsgáltak engem angol orvosok. 'Oh, yes. I was examined by a lot of English doctors.'

---

59 'P' stands for patient, and the number refers to the number of the interview.

I: A hallgatók? 'Medical students?'

P4: Igen, nagyon sokat vizsgáltak januárban is, mert egy ritka betegségem volt, 'Yes, they examined me a lot in January as I had a rare disease,'

(5) P3: … angolul beszéltek. Mert egy magyar orvos volt, meg egy angol, aki nem tudott egy szót sem magyarul és akkor mondták is, hogy nem azért beszélnek angolul, hogy én ne értsem, hanem azért, mert az orvos nem tudott magyarul. '… they were speaking in English. As there was a Hungarian doctor and English one, who could not speak a word of Hungarian, and they mentioned that they were talking to each other in English not because they did not want me to understand them, but because one of the doctors could not speak Hungarian.'

(6) P4: volt olyan, mikor az angolok vizsgáltak, és volt, aki beszélt magyarul egy kicsit, és akkor, ahogy ultrahangozott a doktornő, akkor nevettek valamin, valamit meséltek, és akkor mondom megkérdezhetem, hogy min nevettek? És akkor mondják, hogy semmi, csak ahogy kivágták nekem, ami itt volt, olyan banán alakú volt, és azt nevették. 'there was one time, when I was examined by some English doctors and there were some of them who could speak a little Hungarian, and then, as my doctor was performing an ultrasound scan on me, they laughed at something, they were telling something to each other, and then I asked, may I ask what you were laughing at? And they answered that it was not important, they said that my incision was shaped like a banana, and they were laughing at that.'

(7) P6: Igen, a műtétem fele is angolul zajlott, mert egy nagyon aranyos spanyol orvos volt bent a műtétemnél. … Ő is műtött, ő volt, aki feltárt és utána közösen csinálták a … doktorral. Igen, ők angolul beszéltek. Volt, amit megértettem, ugye mert azért sok minden ragad a tévéből, ebből-abból az emberre, és elég jól ment a dolog, úgyhogy nem volt probléma. 'Yes, half of my surgical intervention went on in English as there was a very cute Spanish doctor present at my operation. … He was also operating on me, he performed the exploration and then they did it together with doctor … . Yes, they were talking to each other in English. There were certain things I could understand, as from TV or from other sources you learn certain things, and everything went on well, so it was no problem for me.'

(8) P8: Csak angolul beszéltek most, amikor sütöttek ki, csak angolul beszélt a doktor úr. 'They were speaking only in English during the intervention, the doctor was speaking only English.'

I: Mert angol volt a kollégája? 'You mean that his colleague was an English person?'

P8: Szerintem nem, hanem a ... doktor volt belülről a pultnál, és ő meg csinálta magát a műtétet, és akkor ő az, aki azt hiszem, hogy bolgár, ha jól tudom, és így a közös nyelvük az angol volt, és így beszéltek.... attól [hallottam], aki csinálta a gépelést. És elmesélte nekem előre, hogy nyugodjak meg, nem azért beszélnek angolul,hogy én ne értsem, meg ne halljam, hanem azért, mert hogy ő így tud beszélni, és úgy látszik, hogy a magyarok inkább megtanulják az angolt, mintsem, hogy a bolgár a magyart. 'I don't think so, but ... doctor was sitting at the desk, and the other doctor was performing the operation, and I think he is the Bulgarian doctor, and English is their common language as far as I know, and thus, they were talking to each other in English. ... I heard it from the person who did the typing. And she explained to me before the intervention that I had no reason to worry about it, as they were speaking in English not in order that I not understand them, or hear them, but because he can only speak this way, and I think the Hungarian doctors learn English rather than the Bulgarian doctor learning Hungarian.'

I have asked the patients what they think about this situation that doctors speak English at a Hungarian hospital, how they would evaluate this situation. The answers were various, some patients think that the English language is very useful to connect those working within one profession, and it can be a drawback if a physician cannot speak this language:

(9) I: *Hátrányban lenne az az orvos, aki nem beszélne angolul?* 'Do you think a doctor would be disadvantaged if they can't speak English?'

P8: *Igen, a mai világban igen.* 'Yes, in today's world they would.'

(10) P1: *Mindenképpen jó, mert nagyon sok ember beszéli az angol nyelvet. Meg ugye az Unióban elfogadott nyelv az angol nyelv.* 'It certainly is good, as a lot of people can speak English. And in the European Union English is an accepted language.'

(11) P5: *Hát én jónak találom, hiszen egy nyelvtudás az nyilván mindig jó. Tehát teljesen mindegy, hogy a munkánkból vagy, civil emberként. Én jónak tartom,... hát ez természetes mindenképpen. Semmiképpen, én nem látom ennek hátrányát.* 'Well, I think it is good as competence in a foreign language is always good. So it doesn't matter if you learn it for professional or non-professional purposes. I think it is good, ... yes, naturally. I can't see that it has any disadvantages.'

(12) P8: *Jobban tudnak kommunikálni, főleg az ő területükön* 'they can communicate much better, especially in their specialty'

(13) I: *Mit gondol, ha valaki ma az orvosok közül nem beszél angolul az hátrányt jelent neki?* 'Do you think it is a disadvantage for a doctor nowadays if they can't speak English?'

P6: *Nagyon nagyot. A mai világban, pillanatnyilag nagyon nagyot. Igencsak talpalni kell neki, vagy bizonyítani, hogyha valamit el akar érni. Egy az. A másik, hogy nem tud elmenni tanulmányi utakra, meg nem tud ösztöndíjat szerezni, szóval nagyon nagy hátrány neki. ...nem is ajánlom egyetlenegy orvosnak sem, hogy kihagyja az angolórát.* 'Yes, a huge disadvantage. In the present world, these days a huge disadvantage. On the one hand, the doctor has to work hard or give evidence of hard work if they want to achieve something. On the other hand, they can't go for study trips or cannot apply for scholarships [if they can't speak English], therefore it is a huge disadvantage for them. ... I would not recommend to any doctor to skip their English classes.'

Other patients, however, see the situation differently, they are concerned about the future of the Hungarian language:

(14) P6: *Na most állatorvosok, építőiparba, a középvezetőtől felfelé, de hát szerintem a melósnak is jobb, ha érti, hogy mit mondanak neki, akkor vendéglátósok például, mint a falat kenyér. Mint például a tanárok, ezeknek nagyon kell, de nem kell egész Magyarországot elangolosítani.* 'You see, [it is important to speak English] for veterinary surgeons, in the construction industry, from the post of a middle manager, but I think also for the worker it is better if they understand what is told to them, and, for instance for people in catering, it is essential. For example for the teachers, it is very important, but we should not 'Anglicise' the whole of Hungary.'

(15) P2: *Szerintem nem jó [hogy az angol a szakma nyelvévé vált]. ... mert az átlagember a mai Magyarországon nem tájékozott annyira angol nyelvben, hogy külön az angol orvosi szakkifejezéseket elsajátíthatná, tudhatná, tehát nem fogja megérteni.* 'I think it is not good [that English has become the language of medicine]. ... as nowadays, an average person in Hungary is not so competent in the English language to be able to learn the English medical terms, therefore, they will not understand them.'

(16) P6: *én kicsit féltem emiatt a magyart, meg a magyar betegeket, hogy valahogy nem szabadna ennyire elangolosodnunk. Ez a véleményem. Amúgy meg hát ahány nyelvet beszél egy ember, annyi ember, szóval annyi személy. Azt nem mondom, hogy ne tanuljunk, de valahogy azért magyarok vagyunk. Úgyhogy én így vagyok vele, hogy a beteghez azért magyarul szóljanak, ... és,*

aki idejön, tanuljon meg magyarul. 'I'm worried a bit about the Hungarian language, and the Hungarian patients, we should not be so much 'Anglicised'. This is my opinion. Otherwise, the more languages you speak, the more valuable it is, I mean you are. I don't suggest that we should not study [English], but somehow we should stay Hungarian. Therefore, I think that patients should be talked to in Hungarian, … and, if somebody comes here, they should learn our language.'

Patients see the importance of a common language, but they think that it should not necessarily be the English language:

(17) P7: *biztos, hogy kell a magyar nyelven kívül más nyelv is. Hogy ennek angolnak kell-e lenni, azt nem tudom. ... angolul tanulni kell-e, ... szerintem igen. Mert ugye világnyelv. De az sem baj, hogyha németül, mert lehet, hogy ott is kap egy olyan tudományos munkát, vagy éppen olaszul, vagy francia, vagy bármelyik nyelv. De még akkor is hozzáteszem, hogy akár oroszul is.* 'I'm sure that you need another language beside Hungarian. Whether this other language should be English, I don't know. .. Should you study English? … Yes, I think so. As it is a world language. But it's not a problem if you learn German, as it is possible that you get scientific work there, or Italian or French or any other languages. But then I must mention Russian as well.'

Obviously, patients want to understand what is going on around them at the clinic, and they need explanations in simple Hungarian:

(18) P2: *Hallottam idegen szavakat, de nem tudtam különválasztani, nyilvánvalóan a latin kifejezéseket, de azért voltak angol kifejezések, szavak is, amik ismertek voltak számomra. És nem volt kellemes hallgatni, mert rejtjeles beszéddel beszéltek az orvosok – nem úgy mondom, az ember sorsa fölött – de viszont az egészségi állapota fölött, amit viszont mindenféleképpen jó volna tudni, de nem idegen nyelven, ami számára érthetetlen* 'I heard foreign words, and I could not differentiate them, obviously they were Latin expressions, but there were also English ones, words which were unknown to me. And it was not convenient for me to listen to it, as the doctors were using this coded language – I don't mean about your fate – but at least about your state of health, and by all means, it would be nice to know [about it], but not in a foreign language that is incomprehensible to you'.

(19) P5: *Tehát előfordult, hogy ők szaknyelven megbeszélték, és akkor csak néztem, hogy húha. Most akkor mi van?* 'So, it happened that they talked about it

in a technical language and then I just looked and thought well-well. So what's going on?'.

(20) P7: *A viziteken is olyat lehet csak hallani, hogy az orvosi kifejezéseket. Szoktam mondani, hogy idegen nyelven mondják, merthogy viccesen határozzák meg, nem a mi nyelvünkön, ugye az orvosi szakszavakat mondták, amiből sok mindent nem értünk.* 'At the ward rounds you can hear only such things, the medical terms. I usually say that they speak in a foreign language, as they define it in a funny way, not in our language, you see, they used the medical technical terms, which we could not understand too much of'.

But patients have admitted that when they asked their physician about something they did not understand, they received a detailed answer:

(21) P2: *a beavatkozás előtt, és 100%-os választ kaptam magyar, érthető nyelven* 'before the intervention, and I received 100% answer in Hungarian, in a comprehensible language'.

(22) I: *meg szokta kérdezni, hogy most miről van szó?* 'Do you ask the doctors what is going on?'
P4: *Igen és akkor jól elmondják, hogy mindent értsek.* 'Yes, and then they tell me properly, in a way to make me understand everything'.

Finally, I asked the patients about the discharge report, how much they can understand of it, what the things are that they do not understand in it:

(23) P4: *Ezekből itt semmit nem értek ... Nem tudom a magyar megfelelőt, biztos latinul van vagy ilyesmi* 'I don't understand any of this here. ... I don't know the Hungarian equivalent of it, it must be in Latin or something like that'.

(24) P6:*... amúgy, ha kórházba megyek, nekem mindig segít [a latin nyelvtudás] a mai napig. ... amiben nem voltam biztos, azt meg hazamentem, elővettem az orvosi szótárt és megkerestem, hogy mi van benne* '... anyway, if I go to hospital, I'm always helped by [my Latin knowledge] even nowadays ... if I was not sure in something, I went home and took the medical dictionary and looked it up in it'.

(25) P6: *jobb lenne, ha egy kicsit „magyarabbul" írnák [a zárójelentést], ha az az érdekük, hogy a beteg tájékoztatva legyen* 'it would be better, if it [the discharge report] were written a bit 'more Hungarian' if their interest is to make the patient be informed'.

(26) P6: CABG ezt abszolút nem értem...Na most, ha ez [a zárójelentés] az enyém lenne, akkor hazamennék, és akkor a szótárba nincs benne, akkor gyerünk az internetre, mert akkor ott keresném meg. Ezek a mozaikszavak nem mondanak semmit. Szóval nagyon ritkán mondanak valamit 'CABG: I don't understand it at all ... Well, if it [the discharge report] were mine, I would go home, and if I can't find it in the dictionary, I would search the Internet, then I would look for it there. These abbreviations very rarely mean anything to me'.

5.2.6. Discussion and conclusions on the results obtained with Method 2

Professional groups are formed through the establishment of an internal role structure, group identity, group attitudes, and group norms. There is a need for professional identity and for separation from the other groups in health care, and this need plays an important role in the construction of the language of cardiologists, and it constantly motivates doctors who want to belong to that group to adapt and be socialized to the group behavior. At the same time, it also means establishing distance from people outside the group, i.e. other physicians or patients (cf. Gunnarson 2006).

English is the international language of medicine, the language used in both written and oral communication between those involved in sciences. In medical discourse, communication takes place in "cooperative networks formed among invisible colleges of scholars" (Baldauf and Jernudd 1987: 98), who normally speak among themselves in the same language – these days overwhelmingly in English. Unless a scholar is able to use English, he or she will not be admitted to these 'exclusive clubs' by the gatekeepers of the medical profession. Gatekeeping refers in its metaphorical sense to the control exerted by a group over access to something (Bates and Jenkins 2007), which, in case of medicine, is most up-to-date knowledge and promotion.

The domains in which English has attained the status of a dominant language for medical discourse in Hungary at the beginning of the 21st century have been examined in this paper with Method 2. Hungarian scientists have always had to master themselves in some foreign languages: in the Latin language in each period of Hungarian medical history, the French and German languages between the 18th and 20th centuries, in Russian from the 1950s, and finally, in English since the mid-1980s, however, only Latin, German and

English can be considered as lingua francas of certain periods in the history of medicine.

The Hungarian medical discourse community has experienced the trend toward an increasing influence of English in the field of research especially since the 1990s. The same trend can be found elsewhere in Europe as well (cf. Haarmann and Holman 2001; Truchot 2001; Fischer 2008).

The presence of the English language in Hungary is, however, not restricted to scientific domains as English is the first language of choice in most Hungarian primary and secondary schools (Dörnyei et al. 2006), and then almost exclusively the language of choice in non-linguistic tertiary education. Figure 11 shows how language choice changed in Hungary between 1993 and 2004.

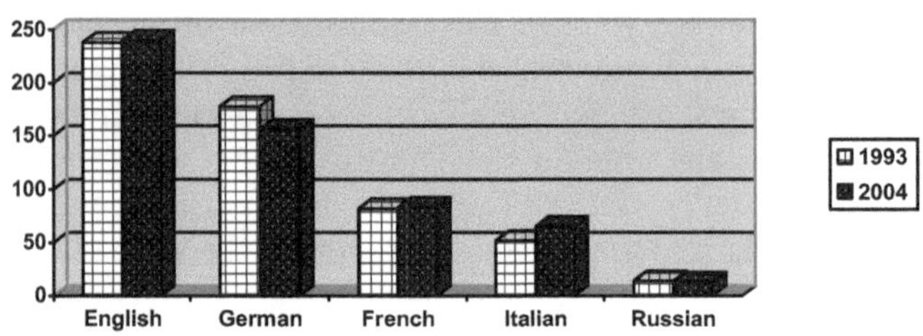

Figure 11. Changes in language choice between 1993 and 2004 (Dörnyei et al. 2006: 53) – data show the popularity index calculated by the means based on answers to language attitude questionnaires.

Results of the present study show that each cardiologist (or 11 in total) and most of the family physicians (5 out of 6) who have been interviewed have studied English, just like one-third of the patients. Results on language learning, i.e. practicable language competence, has also been asked about, and it has been found that each physician who studied English also uses it, if not on a daily basis but quite regularly, whereas patients do not use their English knowledge regularly.

Comparing my results with the ones published in 2005 and 2006 on the total population of Hungary (CEF results; Brux), we can conclude that English is considered very important in certain professions: 62% of all Hungarians consider English very important in their professional career, though the great majority of the population is monolingual, and only 16% claim that they have a working knowledge in English (cf. the European average is 47.6%). The English language and English competence seem to be more important and also a requirement in certain domains, especially in the field of medicine.

Physicians use the English language for various purposes: both family physicians and cardiologists read scientific publications in English, but family physicians read mainly in Hungarian and rarely in English, whereas clinicians read almost exclusively in English. Research efforts concentrate and become dependent on English literature to such an extent that information in other foreign languages (and to some extent even in Hungarian) is practically ignored or discarded (cf. Ammon 1998, 2001; Benfield 2006; Haarman and Holman 2001; Kiss 2009).

Cardiologists not only read publications in English, but they also prepare their own publications, abstracts, conference papers in English. English also dominates exclusively as the language of PhD dissertations at the Faculty of Medicine in Szeged.

Both groups of physicians have mentioned that they speak English in their daily work when examining non-Hungarian speaking patients, but, again, this is done frequently by clinicians and very rarely by family physicians. Cardiologists are also involved in teaching the students in the English program of the medical faculty, giving both lectures and practicals, they are involved in postgraduate trainings, and colleagues from abroad are trained here by them. When teaching students or colleagues, cardiologists have to mobilize their high-level proficiency in English.

Cardiologists also participate in international conferences, where the official language is usually English even if the conference is held in a non-English speaking country. They participate in international studies mostly organized by pharmaceutical companies, and they write the reports in English, talk to colleagues from abroad in English, and present the results at various forums in English.

Patients hospitalized at the Department of Cardiology have also remarked that their doctors spoke in English in various situations: teaching or instructing the foreign students, and talking to colleagues from abroad. Patients seem to be used to doctors speaking in English, and they can understand the situation, however, they tend to be slightly disturbed by the fact that they cannot understand what the cardiologists are talking about at such occasions. Although, they claim that whenever they needed information on their condition or management, they received the explanation in Hungarian.

Both family physicians and cardiologists consider English knowledge very important, however, English is not present in the professional daily life of the former. Cardiologists have a very supportive attitude towards the use of the English language in sciences, since it is considered indispensable in the life of clinicians, and only one physician has expressed embarrassement by the fact that her English was not good enough. For cardiologists English competence is essential, whereas a lack of English knowledge is considered a drawback by each interviewed tertiary and secondary care physician.

Cardiologists have agreed that a common language is needed in scientific communication, and that this common language should be English, as the medical terminology in English is more concise than, for example, the Hungarian terminology, and somehow functionally more appropriate for them to describe complex investigations and interventions. In addition to using this English-intrinsic argument, cardiologists have explained their positive attitude toward the English language by its utilitarian or instrumental function, i.e. English helps them in gaining rewards both professionally and financially, and, thus, English competence is obviously an advantage in their career. There is another practical reason for favoring the English language: physicians who are younger than 45 studied mostly English as their first foreign language at school, and even at the medical university English was offered to them as the main option of foreign languages.

The knowledge function of the English language is also emphasized: English is the medium of scientific texts, thus, it can help physicians keep up with the most recent advances. The dominant role of English is a fact for them which can no longer be questioned, but it has to be acknowledged as such (cf. Ammon 1998). None of the cardiologists refer to any negative effects of the English language in any respect.

Family physicians are also aware of the importance of the English language in medicine (they are learning the language or wish to learn it in the future), but they think that at the moment they are not very much affected by it, as all the needed information is available to them in Hungarian. English has made its way into primary scientific/medical information, in the medical journals disclosing the results of most recent international research. The Hungarian language is present mostly in secondary information. Primary physicians say that there are journals devoted mostly to secondary information (reviews, studies, or reports) written entirely in Hungarian.

It is not a disadvantage for a Hungarian family physician if they cannot speak English, but they consider the existence of a common language important for communication between members of the international medical community. Most of the family physicians interviewed have agreed that this common language should be English (together with Latin). As a vehicle of scientific communication, English enjoys high acceptance among them. Although one of them has mentioned that the international use of English can be harmful as it has a negative impact on the Hungarian language of medicine, with the Hungarian language deteriorating and being corrupted by the English influence.

Half of the interviewed patients have had positive feelings about the English language and argued that a common language is very important within certain professions, and in medicine this common language can be English. Others have expressed concern about the future of the Hungarian language of medicine as well as negative feelings about the domination of the English language as, according to them, it can lead to miscommunication between doctors and patients and, thus, the country should put a halt to Englishization.

In conclusion, we can safely say that for Hungarian cardiologists working in tertiary and secondary care English is not only the language of research (cf. Ammon 1998), but it is the language of medicine in general, used in various domains of their profession for various purposes. However, it is unquestionable for them that the Hungarian language of medicine should be used in other professional domains such as graduate and postgraduate training of Hungarian doctors, and Hungarian is also the language used with the Hungarian patients who make up most of their daily turnover. The global spread of the English language in the field of medicine may be construed as a move toward diglossia (Ferguson 2009). Phillipson and Skutnabb-Kangas (1996: 446) claim that "evidence in western and Eastern Europe shows that diglossia, with English as the intrusive dominant language, may be imminent". This diglossia may give rise to fears that the spheres of use of the Hungarian language will be diminished and the language marginalized (cf. Bősze 2009; Kiss 2009). English may be the high language (the language used in research and advanced academic teaching), and Hungarian may be the low language used only for teaching at lower levels and for popularizing medicine. The spread of English in academic circles is likely to widen the communicative gap between scientific and non-scientific communities and, thus, lead to further social stratifications (Gunnarson 2000; Murray and Dingwall 2001). The medical terminology might in the future lack Hungarian terms and the English ones will predominate, and Hungarian researchers might lose the ability to talk about their research in Hungarian. Therefore, linguistic effort may be required to ensure communication between various Hungarian discourse communities and the Hungarian language will continue to need some form of scientific register, and this function should not be entitled to the English language (cf. Grétsy 2002a; Zimányi 2004; Bősze 2010).

5.3. Complex evaluation of data collected with Methods 1 and 2

Data gained through the semi-structured interviews with cardiologists, family physicians and patients (Method 2) contribute to the interpretation of the results achieved with Method 1, as the results of Method 2 highlight the human factors behind the written data collected by Method 1.

Subjective viewpoints of all three parties have promoted a better understanding of the object of this research. Complex relations from the distinct data are attempted to identify the complexity of the examined issue by including context. The results of the two analyses have been compared, and to the extent possible, integrated: results gained with Method 1 provide the opportunity for generalizability, whereas results collected with Method 2 provide a better understanding of the context and meaning.

Two cases can be distinguished in interpreting and discussing the results collected with the two methods:

when the English language is used by physicians for various purposes in various situations, domains of professional life, and

when the Hungarian language is used (especially in writing) exhibiting certain English language contact-induced features.

The two cases, however, are correlated and cannot be examined separately, as the second one, i.e. the use and presence of the contact-induced features, is a consequence of the first one, i.e. the extensive use of the English language.

In the hospital discharge reports under investigation, native speaker (L1) cardiologists of Hungarian adopt vocabulary and structural features from their second language, English (L2). The Hungarian cardiologists rarely deactivate their L2 totally (cf. Grosjean 1992), they may incorporate almost any type of L2 feature into their L1, when they speak and write in Hungarian.

English lexical morphemes may be introduced into Hungarian directly via code-switching from English, as bilingual speakers often use code-switching in their speech. Code-switching forms are considered ephemeral and non-recurrent; however, frequently repeated forms gradually become more or less stable loans. Due to what is called the 'frequency hypothesis' (cf. Myers-Scotton 1993), the code-switched items can change to borrowings through increasingly frequent usage, and finally, they are also used in writing, e.g. in the hospital discharge reports.

And then, as not all members of the medical discourse community engage in code-switching (cf. family physicians, who are not necessarily fluent speakers of English), these borrowed items are adopted by the non-bilingual speakers of the Hungarian medical community (cf. Thomason 2003). Variation in the amount of assimilation of these borrowings may depend on the 'degrees of bilingualism', as a borrowing may be subject to continual interference from the model in the L2 (cf. Haugen 1950). Therefore, different writers may use different forms of the same item, and as a result, various orthographic and morphological realizations of the same word can coexist in the same medical discourse community.

The position of the English language as the *lingua franca* in medicine does not only have an influence on the lexis of the medical professionals' L1 but it also has an impact on the structural features (syntax and grammar) and affects even the writing conventions of medical texts today, including texts written in L1 for L1 monolinguals (patients and family physicians).

Cardiologists (see Table 16) and family physicians (see Table 17) use the English language for various professional purposes. Both family physicians and cardiologists read scientific publications in English, but family physicians read mainly in Hungarian and rarely in English, whereas cardiologists read almost exclusively in English. Both groups have mentioned that they speak English in their daily work when examining non-Hungarian speaking patients, but this is done frequently by cardiologists and only very rarely by family physicians.

For cardiologists being involved in research, publishing and attending conferences is very important as these are the arenas of presenting their achievements. Publishing in English has a positive effect on citations, thus, the English language medical journals have high impact factors. No Hungarian medical journal has any impact factor, which can also deter cardiologist from publishing in their L1.

Cardiologists use the English language extensively, both in international professional collaborations and in several domains of their daily work, whereas family physicians do not use it or only rarely do so.

The extensive use of the English language results in contact-induced changes in the L1 of Hungarian cardiologists, and these changes can be seen in the documents examined with Method 1. Most changes have been identified at the lexico-sematic level, but changes are also present at orthographic, syntactic/grammatical and rhetorico-pragmatical levels.

Table 16. Domains of professional L1 and L2 use of cardiologists.

	L1 (Hungarian language)	**L2** (English language)
Gaining information (reading textbooks, medical journals, guidelines, searching the Internet)	rarely	almost always
Publishing (research articles, case reports, abstracts)	rarely (writing for L1 readers)	frequently (writing both for international readership and L1 readers)
Attending conferences (presenting papers, posters)	rarely (at national forums)	frequently (both at international and national forums)
Daily work (teaching, patient examination, doing research)	regularly (when in contact with Hungarian speakers)	regularly (when in contact with non-Hungarian speakers)

Lexical and semantic borrowings form the largest group of English language contact-induced features in the Hungarian cardiology discharge reports. English loanwords have been categorized according to their orthographic and/or morphological assimilation to the Hungarian language: loanwords proper and assimilated loans. Loanwords proper are words and phrases that were adopted from the English language in their original orthographic form, e.g. H *non-sustained* 'non-sustained', H *postbranch* 'postbranch'. Assimilated loans had already been adapted to conform to the orthographic and/or morphological rules of the Hungarian language, e.g. H *elongált* 'elongated', H *sheat* 'sheath'. Loanwords proper identified in the hospital discharge reports are nouns and adjectives, and assimilated loans involve nouns, adjectives and verbs. Altogether 89 loanwords have been found in the discharge reports. The total number of all loanwords is 1,705, which means that English loanwords make up approximately 0.8 % of all the words used in the discharge reports.

Table 17. Domains of professional L1 and L2 use of family physicians.

	L1 (Hungarian language)	**L2** (English language)
Gaining information (reading textbooks, medical journals, guidelines, searching the Internet)	almost always	rarely
Postgraduate training (as trainees)	always	never
Daily work (patient examination)	almost always	rarely

But this number is significantly higher if we consider the English eponyms and initialisms (abbreviations and acronyms) used in the studied documents. Initialisms borrowed from English are used altogether 3,079 times, and eponyms (e.g. *Holter monitor*) and trade names (e.g. *Maverick ballon* 'Maverick balloon') 102 times. Thus, all English loanwords comprise 2.25 % of the words in the studied Hungarian cardiology discharge reports.

Two main categories of semantic borrowings (loan substitutions) have been identified in this study: loan translations and loanblends. Loan translations are created solely from Hungarian morphemes (e.g. *két-ér betegség* 'two-vessel disease'), whereas loanblends contain at least one morpheme adopted from the English language (e.g. *cukorprofil* 'sugar/glucose profile'). Most of the semantic loans are polymorphemic units, they are made up of three or more morphemes (e.g. *nem-inzulin dependens cukorbetegség* 'non-insulin dependent diabetes'). Semantic borrowings, especially loan translations, are very commonly used in the discharge reports, e.g. *falmozgászavar* 'wall motion abnormality' is used 88 times in the 234 reports and *gócjel/góctünet* 'focal sign' is used 86 times altogether.

English language contact-induced features are also present at the orthographic level. Some examples of re-Englishization, e.g. E *shunt* > H *sönt* >

(re-Englishized) H *shunt*, have been found in the discharge reports, as well as changes in punctuation and spelling.

In the investigation of the Hungarian hospital discharge reports some grammatical and syntactic changes have also been identified that might be due to English language contact. Changes are seen in the omission or addition of the Hungarian definite and indefinite articles, in the use of the present tense instead of the past tense in certain cases, in using the plural in the name of paired organs, and in grammatical apposition of certain restrictive adjectives. Impersonalization and passive-like constructions are commonly used in the discharge reports.

Changes have also been recognized at the rhetorico-pragmatic level in the presence of certain attenuating rhetorical patterns (cf. Hyland 1998; Salager-Meyer et al. 2003; Warta 2006) in the epistemic use of words expressing possibility, e.g. *lehet* 'may' or *esetlegesen* 'possibly'. Data organization in the discharge reports also attests to efforts toward internationalization in the generic features of this text type.

The changes made by individuals may become institutionalized at the societal level in discourse communities where bilingualism is widespread, or changes may also be due to certain language planning performed by the institutions, as it will be described lbelow.

Although language choice (i.e. the use of L1 versus L2) and the use of contact-induced features are not arbitrary, through the selection of one language over another and by the exhibition of certain contact-induced features, speakers may display what is called 'acts of identity' (cf. Le Page and Tabouret-Keller 1985). Speakers may have various motivations behind their language choice and use, and the two main motivations identified by scholars are *need* and *prestige* (cf. Weinreich 1953; Hockett 1958). Nevertheless, these two main motives, on the one hand, cannot always be sharply distinguished, and, on the other hand, numerous culture and profession specific motivations showing relation to these two main ones can also be involved.

Filling a gap in L1 vocabulary is one of the motives that seem to play an important role in borrowing in the field of sciences. It can involve the importation of a concept and introduction of new phenomena that are not available in L1. In certain cases, especially in the language of medicine, using ready-made designations is in some cases more economical than describing phenomena afresh.

Generally, there might also be a need for synonyms or euphemisms in L1. The borrowed term may help speakers make more specific differentiations in semantic or conceptual fields, or introduce finer distinctions of meaning. Stylistic effects can also play a role: the text might appear more technical, professional, authoritative, precise and objective due to contact-induced change.

Scientific dominance of the English language is accompanied by its high prestige and value of L2 knowledge. Speaking in L2 or the use of L2 contact-induced features can raise in-group identity and social solidarity. It refers to the speaker's accommodation to the conventions of the discourse community and acceptance of its norms. Being a member of the discourse community may result in high social status that can be concomitant with economic advantages. High level L2 competence means advantage in education, employment, research and, generally, in the professional career. As L2 has high value of knowledge and there might be pride in its use, it can lead to the 'show-off' of its speakers as well.

Using L2 or L2 features does not only express in-group identity or solidarity, it can also be the means of authority or exclusion of those (e.g. patients or non-bilingual health workers) who are not members of the bilingual medical discourse community.

Weinreich (1953: 57) explains that the main extralinguistic reason for lexical borrowing is "the designative inadequacy of vocabulary in naming new things", that is, a denotative deficit in the lexicon. Communicative needs are added to denotative needs (English loanwords as specific denotata lacking Hungarian equivalents), and connotative needs (emotional implications entailed in the use of Englishisms). The latter can be termed "the aura of English" (Onysko 2007: 321) in Hungarian, which radiates a variety of connotations such as education or modernity, invention, wealth and power. The denotative and connotative reasons interact and can vary for the same English loanword according to the communicative intention of the speaker. The incidence of an English loanword in Hungarian is tied to the psycholinguistic state of the speaker's mental lexicon and the speaker's motivation for lexical selection.

Heavy lexical borrowing may be due to the need for vocabulary reflecting different levels of style, when both the Hungarian and the borrowed English words are retained. There is sometimes a distinction between the more formal, borrowed English vocabulary and the more informal Hungarian lexicon (E/H *kinking* and H *megtörés/megtöretés,* E/H *recovery* and H *lábadozás*).

Motivation for borrowing can be various, involving prestige (individual or collective), and need (objective need to express new ideas, or name scientific and technological discoveries). Both reasons for borrowing can be identified in the Hungarian language of medicine and cardiology. Apart from the very general distinction between 'necessity borrowing' and 'luxury borrowing' and the two frequently named motives 'the need to designate new, imported things', e.g. *defibrillátor* 'defibrillator', *stent* and 'prestige', e.g. *branch* (H *ág/branch*), *potassium* (H *kálium/potassium*), *study* (H *tanulmány/vizsgálat/study*), the following aspects, among others, can be mentioned as causes for lexical borrowing in medicine: the need to differentiate special nuances of expression (e.g. H *tüske* same as E *spike* but in H *spike* 'a sharp peak in an electronic recording'), a feeling of insufficiently differentiated conceptual fields or rise of a specific conceptual field (e.g. *bridging, graft*), the need for a euphemistic expression (e.g. *diszkomfort* 'discomfort' for expressing pain), and the bilingual character of the medical discourse community (cf. cardiologists typically speak English at an upper-intermediate or advanced level and use it everyday).

Most of the semantic loans in the field of cardiology seem to be introduced first into written Hungarian, mostly through the translation of research and review articles, instruction manuals, guidelines and recommendations from English into Hungarian (Keresztes 2007). Many of such loans appear as a result of the translation process: since neologisms without an existing Hungarian equivalent frequently appear in the original English texts, translators have to solve the problem of term formation.

Changes are mostly introduced by the members of the bilingual medical discourse community as a result of the motivations described above, but in some cases, changes might be due to certain language planning as well. International recommendations and guidelines are very important in medicine, influencing not only health care itself, but the language used during the performance of health care as well. The Department of Health of the Hungarian government, the university/faculty leadership, and the head of the department may also have a role in language planning by establishing certain standardization, e.g. standardized format for discharge reports, programs for reporting the laboratory results or describing the dosage of medication.

Scholars approach the phenomenon of borrowing, especially lexical borrowing in different ways. Lexical borrowing may be considered, on the one hand, as a natural process of language contact, as borrowing from other languages facilitates and enriches communication, loanwords and other borrowed structures may be integrated into the existing language structures. On the other hand, there might be extensive resistance against borrowing as such.

But the critique of the Englishisms is not so much about the fact that language is a means of communication, but rather about language being a symbol of the national and cultural identity of a speech community. Englishisms, according to some scholars, embody British or American social and cultural structures and values, which can be perceived as a threat to one's own values (cf. Phillipson 1992; Kontra 1997a; Skutnabb-Kangas 2000). Attitudes toward some kinds of code-switching, mixing and borrowing may also be negative based on the fear that borrowing would lead to the corruption of the native language (cf. Wexler 1974; Shapiro and Schiffmann 1981; Jernudd 1989, or the Hungarian language purists Deme 1965; Fábián 1993; Grétsy 2002b; Balázs 2005).

In order to avoid the negative connotations of English borrowings, *languages of communication* and *languages of identification* can be distinguished (cf. House 2005). The advantage of this distinction is that English and one's own national language are not perceived as competitors but rather as complementary possibilities of communication. Accordingly, Englishisms should function as means of communication and not of identification. Moore and Varantola (2005: 150) highlight the following:

"As long as a language can assimilate the linguistic loan, play with it and mould it to fit its own patterns, there is no danger. On the contrary, the changes are normal developments in language contact. What would be worrying, however, is if ... speakers began to underestimate the status of the language spoken in their own country and instead began to overestimate their skills in English."

Gardner-Chloros (1995) argues that there can be a 'native synonym displacement' in the language of sciences. Native (Hungarian) words may be replaced by English loanwords, e.g. E *flow* > H *flow* parallel to or instead of H *áramlás* 'flow'. There is little doubt that most Europeans, and among them Hungarians, do not want their national language be replaced by English, and in the domain of scientific discourse both a lingua franca and a national language are considered desirable. While English is seen as a foreign language, serving as a useful means of communication with members of the international (and Hungarian) medical discourse community, the Hungarian language is used in communication with members of the Hungarian speech community in general.

Acquisition of a foreign language is usually associated with high prestige by most speakers. To demonstrate their knowledge of a foreign language, some bilinguals refrain from producing the standard, phonologically-integrated loanwords and insist on making their utterances sound foreign. Speakers with a positive attitude to foreign languages, in this case to the English language, usually regard the English language as prestigious and want to identify with the lingua franca of medicine, and project themselves as competent in it.

On the one hand, some other speakers may be apprehensive to the use of loanwords, considering them as a form of cultural and/or linguistic 'invasion', English language globalization, and resisting the English borrowings. As a result, they either choose to treat loanwords as Hungarian words through maximal phonological and morphological integration into Hungarian to preserve the language from 'alien elements', or they may avoid using them altogether if there is a Hungarian alternative, thus minimizing the feeling of the intrusion of the English language and showing loyalty to the Hungarian language (cf. medical language purists, e.g. Bősze, Buvari, Grétsy, and Keszler).

Sometimes interference features are introduced by speakers whose competence in the source language is strictly passive – that is, a speaker may borrow a feature from a language that he or she does not speak actively at all. At the beginning of this book it was highlighted that not all members of the

Hungarian medical discourse community are fluent speakers English, but this refers mostly only to those physicians who are involved in research, basically working in tertiary/secondary health care. Physicians working in primary care are bilingual speakers of Latin and Hungarian but not necessarily of English. As they also attend workshops and postgraduate training events organized and held by research physicians, they are also 'exposed to' some of these borrowings. For them the language used by the research physicians is similar to an interlanguage. They share this common interlanguage with the research physicians, but they are not necessarily speakers of the English language. They have acquired only certain features of the English language that they incorporate into their medical Hungarian. Most of the features transferred this way are lexical. The adoption of loanwords is usually a deliberate decision. A reason for it, besides need and prestige, may be the fact that the discourse community deliberately tries to withhold their 'real' language from outsiders, emphasizing in-group status, or differentness from other groups/communities. The newly developed bilingual language may serve as a symbol of the medical discourse community.

It is likely that passive familiarity is the mechanism by which English features contribute to the emergence of medical Hungarian, an interlanguage that is used by these speakers only in one domain of their language use. The discourse community of medical Hungarian comprises both bilingual speakers of English and Hungarian and members of a group who speak Hungarian and understand the interlanguage that is used by the bilingual members. Those belonging to the latter group may never speak English itself, but their passive familiarity with the English language, or at least the interlanguage that they use, makes them introduce some English features into their medical Hungarian.

As a consequence of the above described changes, we may come to the conclusion that changes have lead to the development of a specific language, which might be considered a special jargon, the medical jargon or in a narrower sense the cardiological jargon. Though the changes do not affect only the lexis but each linguistic level, therefore, we might consider it a type of 'interlanguage'. This medical interlanguage contains mostly Hungarian elements with Latin medical vocabulary, and it also comprises several English language contact-induced features. It is not an interlanguage in the classical meaning of the word (cf. Selinker 1972; Corder 1975, Barron 2003), but it is rather a reversed interlanguage. In interlanguage proper learners of L2 transfer certain features from their L1 into L2, whereas in the case of the Hungarian medical language, bilingual speakers transfer elements from L2 into their L1. Hungarian–English bilingual cardiologists use their L1, L2 and the medical/cardiological interlanguage (CI) in different domains of their professional life, e.g. L1 is used when they take patients' history, L2 when they teach medical students in the

English language program, and CI when a cardiologist speaks to another cardiologist.

Selinker (1972) defines interlanguage as an autonomous or independent language system. CI is a system that is in constant change, just like other language systems, except for the dead languages, e.g. Latin, but the end point, the aim of its speaker is not to achieve complete mastery in L2. It should be noted, however, that the distinction between interlanguage and language change effects is mostly very hard or even sometimes impossible to draw.

Interlanguages are described by many scholars as permeable, dynamic, changing and yet systematic (cf. Selinker 1972; Corder 1975). An interlanguage may undergo relative fossilization and relative change, but it always reveals an underlying cognitive process (Andersen 1984). There are certain features which are fossilized in IC, and these features make it possible for multiple speakers to speak and understand it. IC is understood not only by bilingual cardiologists but also by family physicians who are not necessarily fluent speakers of English, and also by other health workers at the Department of Cardiology such as nurses and assistants. Members of the latter two discourse communities may acquire this IC during their work or at postgraduate trainings.

IC can be considered a bridge between tertiary/secondary care physicians and primary care physicians, as well as other health workers, who are involved in tertiary care. But at the same time, IC also has a gate-keeping function: those who cannot acquire it and do not have at least a passive knowledge of it will have restricted access to certain medical information, knowledge and other benefits, e.g. patients who are excluded from it have restricted access to information on their health status, management and prognosis of their disease.

Pidgins and creole languages are considered interlanguages (cf. Hymes 1971; Selinker 1972, 1992; Bickerton 1977; Muysken et al. 1995). It has also been argued that 'English as an international language' may be looked at as an interlanguage (cf. Davies 1989). We might consider a technical/scientific language an interlanguage as well, but in a different aspect, as IC is not understood by either English monolinguals (e.g. British cardiologists) or Hungarian monolinguals (e.g. Hungarian patients).

Physicians use "different languages for different activities in different circumstances: perhaps a regional language [or a dialect of Hungarian] at home, the official language of the medicine [Hungarian and Latin] or English at work, English on the Internet" (Carmichael 2000: 289). This use of different languages expresses an unwillingness to commit to one particular identity and a preference for keeping open several means of expression. Here it is clear that a new sense of identity is forming. This identity is not only connected to nationality.

Physicians have layers of identity at local, national, European and global levels. As Pennycook (2003: 517) suggests, English is part of these users' "identity repertoire", and these identities are partially connected to the use of English as an additional means of expression.

Popular attitudes towards some kinds of code-switching and interference features are often negative even among community members themselves who engage in this kind of multilingual behavior frequently (cf. Romaine 2003). However, there is no evidence to indicate that multilingualism is an inherently problematic mode of organization, either for the society or for the individual. As languages are often symbols of class, gender, ethnic, and other kinds of differentiation, it is easy to think that language underlies conflict in multilingual societies (cf. Nelde 1997). Yet disputes involving language are really not about language, but instead about "fundamental inequalities between groups who happen to speak different languages" (Romaine 2003: 532). Each language or variety of language in a multilingual community may serve a specialized function and is used for particular purposes. The degree to which the outside world is engaged is justified only to the extent that it contributes to the maintenance of the discourse community.

Attitude to a language can be measured by looking at the internal state of the examined person caused by certain previous influential factors that make them behave in a specific way in a given situation. In the behaviorist view, attitude is the way in which a person responds to a given situation. We could see it in the language choice of physicians, how much they use the English language in certain academic activities or when writing the hospital discharge reports (Method 1). The mentalist view on language attitudes, however, claims that the speakers' (in our case, the physicians') self-report should also be taken into consideration in order to have access to their internal state and their attitudes (Method 2).

There is a definite connection between attitudes and language behavior (Ammon 2004) during social interaction. Similarly to the status of the language, language attitudes and their social functions are closely interrelated. Attitudes can serve one or a combination of four attitude functions (cf. Katz 1960): the utilitarian or instrumental function where physicians' language attitudes depend on the rewards received due to the attitudes. For example, publishing in English is accompanied by certain benefits, i.e. reputation at the department, or even international reputation; teaching in the English program results in financial reward and reputation from students; and attending international conferences and presenting posters or papers are also rewarded by colleagues. Therefore, Hungarian cardiologists prefer publishing, attending conferences and teaching in English.

Another function is the ego-defensive function, which means that physicians tend to take up attitudes that ensure their inner security and defend them from internal conflict. Baker (1992) highlights that being a peripheral member of a group may result in changes in one's attitude that can help achieve a higher status in the given group. Physicians all consider English very important, and those who do not have a high command of English try to attend courses to better their knowledge of the language, and, therefore, be more suitable for the professional tasks that should be performed in English. One of the cardiologists interwieved for this study has claimed that she was very much afraid of giving lectures and practicals in English as the students ask a lot of questions, but she has convinced herself that she must cope with this task and wants to study more English. Her attitudes to language choice have changed as she now wants to accommodate herself to the requirements of the discourse community she belongs to.

The third function of language attitude is the value-expressive function, which means here that physicians' attitudes are in accordance with their personal values. It also expresses central values and a concept of self.

The fourth function, the knowledge function, has a role in all attitudes, as they all help to simplify interaction with the environment by classifying objects according to their positive and negative implications. We should consider that attitudes held by the individual physicians are not isolated entities, as physicians are members of groups: members of the department, members of the teaching staff, and members of a research community in the narrower sense, and also, in a much broader sense, members of the internal medical community.

Baker (1992) claimed that membership in a given language community has an impact on the member's language attitudes. Peer groups (both the closest colleagues and the international scientific community) may have considerable effects on the individual's language attitudes. As the use of English is considered a norm in the international medical community, individual cardiologists would also consider it a norm. Institutions may have an effect on language attitudes as well. Baker (1992: 110) claims that "through the status given to a language [...] and through the teaching of a language [...], attitudes to a language may change".

Nevertheless, the attitudes of individuals may also have an effect on institutions: they can influence decisions on language policies (Zámbori 2004). The presence or lack of measures against the dominance of English in a given country may be indicative of the attitudes of the community toward the dominance of English in that given community. Graddol (2006) describes one of the main challenges that many countries face, namely, how to maintain their identity in view of globalization and growing multilingualism. In response to the spread of English and increased multilingualism arising from immigration, many countries have introduced language laws in the last decades. In some, the use of languages other than the national language is banned in public spaces such as advertising. One of the first such legal provisions was the 1994 'Toubon law' in

France, but the idea has been copied in many countries since. Such attempts to govern language use are often dismissed as futile by linguists, who are aware of the difficulty of controlling fashions in speech and know from research that code-switching and borrowing among bilingual speakers is a natural process.

In Hungary, there are no governmental measures taken against the dominance of English. The only exception is Act XCVI of 2001 on the Publication of Business Advertisements, Shop Signs and Certain Announcements of Public Interest in the Hungarian language, which stipulates that the Hungarian language must be used in all public service announcements, in all signs purporting economic advertisement, and in all signs indicating shops and businesses (cf. website www.ec.europa.eu). But even eight years after the Act was put into force, no real measures have been taken to have it enforced.

The need to protect national languages is, for most western Europeans, a recent phenomenon – especially the need to ensure that English does not unnecessarily take over too many domains. Public communication, pedagogic and formal genres and new modes of communication facilitated by technology may be the key domains to be defended.

Public reactions to the presence of English in Hungary show that this trend has not come about without debate. As mentioned in Section 2.2, there have been frequent discussions about the increasing presence of English in Europe at the beginning of the 21st century as a result of increased globalization and European unification. While many Hungarians accept the practical necessity of English, there is a fear that it may 'damage' or 'deteriorate' the Hungarian language or that monolingual Hungarian speakers might lose power in the face of English. There is some insecurity expressed about the future of the Hungarian language, especially in the field of sciences and medicine. Standard Hungarian is more prestigious among Hungarians outside Hungary, and contact-induced features from other languages have low prestige: loan words proper are stigmatized whereas "hidden" types of borrowing, such as semantic loans are not even noticed (cf. Péntek 1997; Lanstyák 2000; Keresztes 2006a).

In international communication, when international functions are performed, national (i.e. non-English) languages are always in a disadvantageous position (cf. Phillipson 2000; Fergusson 2006). In a globalized world this trend has to be changed, otherwise it may imply too many risks for the less powerful languages (cf. Skutnabb-Kangas 2000; Ammon 2004).

Arguments are raised, however, not only against English as the global language of sciences and medicine, but there are various arguments for English language dominated medicine. The English intrinsic argument was raised, among others, by Crystal (1997: 212), who argues that there may be "something inherently beautiful or logical about the structure of English". English intrinsic arguments describe the language as God-given, rich, noble and interesting, these arguments usually assert what English is and other languages are not (cf. Jespersen 1955). This idea was advanced by one of the interviewed family physicians as well: due to the simplicity of its grammar, English is suitable for being a lingua franca of medicine.. English extrinsic arguments point out that English is well established, there are trained teachers and a multitude of teaching material, and there are also immaterial resources like knowledge of the language (cf. Graddol 2006).. English functional arguments emphasize the usefulness of English as a gateway to the world (cf. Galtung 1980; Nelde 1993). Other arguments for English are its economic-reproductive function enabling people to operate technology, and its ideological function according to which it stands for modernity and is a symbol for material advance and efficiency (Phillipson 1992).

Arguments for an international use of English in the field of sciences are also approached from a personal side. Siguan (2001: 59) argues that a common language is needed "to serve as a vehicle for scientific communication and production". English as a common language of science makes international communication possible and more efficient. De Swan (2001) claims that English allows to reach everybody who counts, although it is possible only if you speak the language. Therefore, we can conclude that "those who count" inevitably speak English. This statement has two implications: namely, first, that those who are in the inner and probably the outer circles (cf. Kachru 1986) are at an advantage which others in the expanding circle cannot make up for, and, second, that those who lack an appropriate competence in English are severely handicapped in medical sciences.

Arguments advanced from a linguistic aspect support the idea that the dominance of English as the lingua franca of medicine is beneficial to the careers of non-native, English speaking physicians; however, it can have negative effects on the native tongue of these physicians. Disadvantageous effects of the dominance of English on the position of other languages have also been described in the literature (cf. Kontra et al. 1999; Skutnabb-Kangas 2000).

More publication in English leads to less publication in Hungarian (cf. Péntek 2004; Bősze 2009). Kaplan (2001: 19) highlights the risk that English might "still the voice of science in languages other than English". It may have several serious consequences: domain loss in the field of sciences (cf. Gunnarson 2001), and a general neglect of the Hungarian language (Grétsy 2002b; Bősze 2002).

Ammon (2001) expresses his fear that modernization may be slowing down in languages other than English. The scientific terminology of Hungarian will preserve gaps, leading to the condition when the Hungarian language will fail to provide an effective means of academic communication in medicine (cf. Grétsy 2002b; Zimányi 2004). It can also widen the gap between physicians and the non-scientific community, i.e. other health workers and patients.

De Swaan (2001: 78) discusses an important advantage of English as the global language of medicine claiming that nearly the whole of the world's scientific knowledge is stored in English, thus, "a universal corpus and standard of comparison is provided". But science cannot be regarded independent from the language in which it is expressed, and the historical and cultural implications should always be considered (cf. Siguan 2001). The English dominated medical communication and English as a sole language of European collaboration in the health sciences contradict the multilingual principle of the European Union. It can be considered as a violation of the linguistic human rights in the European Union. Phillipson (1993: 33) claims that in practice "some languages are more equal than others" in the Union, thus strengthening linguistic imperialism.

Some linguists point out that there is always a certain amount of linguistic purism (cf. 'the crumbling castle syndrome' in Aitchenson 1997) or 'moral panic' (cf. Cohen 1972) in non-English speaking countries. Speakers in countries of the 'expanding circle' (Kachru 1986), among them Hungarians, may consider that globalization and English pose a threat not only to their native language but also to the nation. Therefore, there is a certain amount of anxiety about the loss of national identity and economic power due to Englishization and/or Europeanization. There is also some fear of cultural imperialism due to the dominance of the English/American language and culture. Phillipson (2003: 80) poses the following question:

> "whether the pre-eminence of English in the scientific world is occurring at the expense of other languages of scholarship … and whether a single privileged language, along with the paradigms associated with it, represents a threat to other ways of thinking and their expression."

Some Hungarian linguists and scientists ask the question whether the predominance of English in sciences represents a threat to the Hungarian language and the Hungarian way of thinking as well (cf. Grétsy 1993; Balázs 2005). First language purists fear that the use of the second language with the first will either keep the first one from growing or debase it, or cause confusion in the speaker's mind. Second language purists may think the same. It might just be the case that both interlanguage and borrowing are needed for many reasons, one of which may be in order not to debase, erase, or cause cognitive confusion to either language.

The terminology of some medical disciplines lack Hungarian words and expressions. Some of the terms are not translated into Hungarian, they have no Hungarian equivalent, and the English terms are frequently used. Some of the Hungarian patterns of text and discourse are replaced by Anglo-American patterns concerning formulation of research results and theories. Therefore, some scholars (e.g. Fábián 2001; Zimányi 2002; Minya 2003; Bősze 2009) think that Hungarian medical researchers might lose the ability to talk about their specialty in Hungarian.

Bősze (2009: 75) describes 5 main arguments for the importance of preserving[60] the Hungarian medical language:

Hungarian medicine can exist only in Hungarian: the nationalistic approach is very important in the field of sciences, as Bessenyi[61] highlighted "each nation has become a scholar in its own language, and never in someone else's language" (my translation).

Complete, unambiguous dialogue is needed between doctors, doctors and nurses, and health workers, which can be achieved only in 'uncorrupted' Hungarian. Misunderstanding with serious consequences can be avoided only this way.

Use of the Hungarian medical language is a societal requirement. It is needed in health promotion, prevention of diseases and health education. But there is a tendency in the society to become more interested in recent achievements in medicine and biology as well. Therefore, Hungarian medical terms are needed as the foreign ones are 'useless' for this purpose. Information and education can be spread only in 'correct' Hungarian.

It is an obligation of Hungarian physicians to provide information to the patients prior to any medical intervention, and consent of the patient is needed for each intervention. Therefore, doctors should be able to inform patients about what their disease is, what the establishment of their diagnosis is based on, what treatment options are available, and what the advantage and disadvantage of each option is. The information should be provided to patients in Hungarian. A discharge report should be given to the patient after each hospital treatment, which should also be written in 'clear' and 'correct' Hungarian.

The Hungarian medical language is an important factor of the performance and competitiveness of the Hungarian language in general; therefore, it should be looked at as the means of competitiveness of the whole Hungarian discourse community.

The Hungarian medical community is in a situation of diglossia, in which English is considered to be the high language by many speakers, i.e. the language used in research and advanced academic teaching, while Hungarian is the low language, used for teaching at lower levels and for popularization. However, the bilingualism of physicians in general is unbalanced, and they have

60 Preserving, in Bősze's view, means preserving it free from Englishisms.

61 György Bessenyei was a Hungarian poet who lived in the 18th century. He wrote this frequently quoted statement in one of his pamphlets, *Magyarság* 'The Hungarian nation', in 1778.

to express their thoughts concerning medical research in a language in which their mastery is not as far-reaching as in their mother tongue. Therefore, there might be a great risk that their process of thinking and the development of ideas will be disadvantaged, having a negative impact on the quality of their Hungarian research.

Speakers and writers adapt to the predominant international patterns without realizing that in doing so they adopt a position in the linguistic power structure in which Hungarian will become subordinated (cf. writings by Bertók, Bősze, Donáth, Fehér, Grétsy, and Molnos). Changes in the structure of genres and genre patterns may occur, and as we have seen some changes have already occurred.

There has been a change in attitude toward the diagnosis and treatment of diseases in medicine (Bősze 2009): diseases are not defined through histology any more but based on their molecular categorization, and their genetic effects are also discussed. Medical knowledge is increasing rapidly, and there is a tendency for international unification and standardization: research is carried out on an international basis and a unified terminology has become necessary. Terminology and guidelines of certain specialties are defined and described by international committees. Medical thinking, treatment, research, and graduate and postgraduate education is formed by internationalization in medicine, which has become not only an ambition but a professional requirement.

Internationally English is the language of medical literature and of medical professionals, as international communication is possible only through one common language. As medicine is considered international, each detail of unification, terminology, definition is described in English, and, for example, newly discovered, identified molecules are given an English name. Therefore, recent knowledge and international medical guidelines are written in English.

An excellent command of English is nowadays essential for a clinical doctor because it is the international scientific language. The outcome is clear, Mélitz[62] (1999) argues, those who wish to reach a world audience will write in English. A physician writing in a 'minor' language necessarily has a much smaller chance of translation and international recognition. Therefore, those who strive to make a mark in their discipline try to publish in English.

The drawback of international English, according to some scholars, may be that the spreading of the English language has resulted in a mixed form of the English language spoken by millions, thus, the world language is simplified and deteriorates (cf. Hartman 1996). The Greek letters and Roman numbers are left out, which is explained by the fact that a lot of speakers are not familiar with them, and they also disturb the search programs in the Internet. Another

62 Jacques Mélitz is a researcher at CEPR (Centre de Recherche en Economie et Statistique, Paris).

disadvantage is the overuse of abbreviations and acronyms to save time and space, but they may actually take more time to interpret (cf. Bősze 2004).

English words and terms rule over national ones, English terms are borrowed and built in national languages, and they override national terms. Thus, the Hungarian medical language is lacking various terms, and the Hungarian medical language is ruled by the English words beside the Greek and Latin origin ones. These English words have no Hungarian equivalents; therefore, the Hungarian language is not appropriate for describing the technical terms of, for example, molecular biology (cf. writings by Bertók, Bősze, Fábián, Fehér, and Zimányi).

Hungarian purists fear that the Hungarian language of medicine is wasting, that is diluted by the English words, that morphologically assimilated loanwords are spreading, and that there is a tendency of overusing acronyms and abbreviations (cf. Bertók, Molnos, Mitsányi's writings). Therefore, the Hungarian language of medicine is becoming 'muddled' (cf. Zimányi 2004), Hungarian scientific publications and lectures are unclear, and misunderstanding can develop even in the daily life of physicians when talking to colleagues, other health workers or patients (cf. Bősze 2010).

Hungarian language purists claim that the orthography of the Hungarian medical language is 'corrupted', as it is full of English patterns. Englishized syntax is used and fashionable, impersonalized structures (cf. Fábián 1997; É. Kiss 2004; Molnos 2007). These authors suggest that this can originate from the lack of knowledge of the writers, or their wish to 'show off' their English competence, but it can also be due to the fact that the orthography of the Hungarian medical language is not regulated (Bősze 2002).

The modernization and development of the Hungarian language of medicine can be achieved only through publishing in Hungarian. Terminology and nomenclature do not develop spontaneously, but they are developed and sustained by the professionals working in that specific field (cf. Kiss 2009). The linguistic formulation (phenomena coding) is the task of the professionals as well as the spreading of recent information, data and knowledge. Scientific textbooks, university notes should be published in Hungarian, and university instruction should be performed in Hungarian (É. Kiss 2004).

One of the plausible dangers of the increasing use of English in the field of sciences is that it widens the rift between specialists and laypersons (cf. Hagstrom 2004): in the worst case, specialists will not be able to talk about their subject in their native tongue. This might lead to a breakdown in the communication between scientists and the public at large. This situation might be more threatening in case of medical experts: they may not be able to make themselves understood to their patients.

Viewing and constructing the world from one cultural point of view, however, may appear to be more normative and refined and, therefore, more conventionally accepted. The same constructs can be viewed from two or more world views in a rich bilingual and/or multicultural environment. In this case, one language might help the other, and sometimes the two together may create a new idea, image, thought, behavior, outlook, organization, and adaptation, and, thus, move culture to new adaptive places in the dynamics of cross-cultural life.

The level of awareness of language must be raised among scientists (cf. Gunnarson 2001). This is a requirement if native speakers are going to guide developments in the desired direction and not remain 'passive victims' of a linguistic power structure. Completely preventing external influence is impossible, and probably undesirable, but language policies should instead aim at adapting changes to the Hungarian context, to incorporate them into the traditional Hungarian patterns and structures. It is important to concentrate not only on the adaptation of words to our linguistic system but also take note of the more fundamental and perhaps more subtle text and discourse patterns.

An interlingual means of communication certainly has its merits but also involves a number of problems, such as disadvantages for lack of language proficiency, the diversity of cultures and their history, and the different structures and meanings of the various languages (cf. Bakró-Nagy 2009). In addition, national languages form national identities, and a nation may fear being foreignized by means of the Anglophone culture represented by the English language (cf. Fischer 2008).

The conclusion suggested by the material examined here is that linguistic Englishization in special fields of discourse is a more complex and nuanced process than it may appear at first sight. Many phenomena that are perceived as Englishisms do not, in fact, have the consequence of bringing the Hungarian language closer to the English language. In this sense, it demonstrates the paradox that linguistic globalisation often results in linguistic fragmentation (cf. the development of an interlanguage by Hungarian cardiologists) at the same time, which has the somewhat unexpected consequence of leading to a more complex and varied linguistic landscape.

Nevertheless, deficits in communication and information transfer between hospital-based physicians and primary care physicians are not substantial or ubiquitous. The discharge summary is a vital tool for communication and information transfer between members of the medical society. Cardiologists and family physician share a great deal of special medical knowledge and use the same interlanguage to communicate this knowledge. Both parties share the idea that the English language has become the lingua franca of medicine, they accept it and most of them have positive or neutral attitudes toward this phenomenon. They have developed a common language which is used in the written discourse of hospital discharge reports, and even if they do not speak English, family physicians are able to decode the message written in this interlanguage which has several English language contact-induced features.

Patients, however, do not speak this interlanguage, although the code has to be translated for them. The interviewed patients still seemed to have a neutral or even positive attitude toward the English language as the lingua franca of medicine. As generally they cannot distinguish between the Latin/Greek and English elements present in the language of medicine, they have no negative attitudes toward the English language. If they do not understand their discharge report or what physicians speak about, they attribute it generally to the lack of their own medical knowledge. However, according to the findings of the interviews, patients are generally satisfied with the explanations received from their health care providers.

We can conclude, however, that the discharge report is not written for the patients as they do not have the same linguistic code that physicians from all the three levels of care share or the medical knowledge behind it. Discharge reports are rather about the patients, and the interlanguage with the medical content should be 'translated', mediated toward the patients by members of the medical society at various levels, by both tertiary/secondary care physicians and primary care physicians.

6. Implications and suggestions for further research

Contact-induced changes can occur due to borrowing where native speakers of a language adopt vocabulary and structural features from another language (Thomason 1997b: 4). Every contact-induced change has a social component (e.g. the length or intensity of contact between the groups) (Winford 2003: 2), however, in some cases even prestige is relevant (Gal 1979), thus, speakers' attitudes should also be considered (Baker 1988).

As there is no geographical contact between the speakers of the two languages (English and Hungarian), the role of prestige and speakers' attitudes are the most important factors that should be investigated (Baker 1988). Thomason and Kaufman (1988:37) define borrowing as

"the incorporation of foreign features into a group's native language by speakers of that language: the native language is maintained but is changed by the addition of the incorporated features".

Incorporating material from one of the languages into the other, in our case from English into the Hungarian language of medicine, requires powerful social motives, which are shared by the members of the discourse community. But cross-linguistic influence cannot be fully attributed to prestigious reasons, it also fills a need or gap in the technical language under discussion (cf. Fasold 2006): new processes, inventions and concepts also have to be named, and linguistic borrowing can be an option for it.

Contact-induced changes are often one-sided, i.e. they may affect only a particular segment of a discourse community, and thus, the change will appear only in a particular dialect, jargon or in a specific register (cf. Maclean and Maher 2001). In the present study, English language contact-induced features have been examined in the Hungarian language of cardiology, which can be looked at as an interlanguage composed of mainly Hungarian vocabulary and grammar, plus Latin and English terms and other borrowed English structural features.

Classifications of the outcomes of language contact are useful and necessary, but focusing on the results can obscure the nature of the mechanisms and psycholinguistic processes that lie behind them (cf. Winford 2003). There are various degrees of language dominance and bilingualism, which may have consequences for the kind of contact-induced changes that occur in this specific register. Therefore, it is important to investigate the human factors, for example, speakers' attitudes and motivations, behind linguistic changes.

This book has aimed at analyzing the English language contact-induced features in a certain text type, the cardiological discharge report, and attempted to find the motives behind the contact linguistic phenomena by preparing semi-structured interviews with members of the medical community, and by interpreting the data gained from these interviews, which are focused on the language attitude of the interviewees.

The results of the study highlight the dominance of the English language in the Hungarian language of medicine, and especially of cardiology. It is a well-known fact that English has become the lingua franca of medicine (cf. Crystal 1997; Truchot 2002; Ammon 1998, 2001), and that first languages (e.g. Finnish, German, Polish, Spanish or Swedish, etc.) for medical purposes exhibit various English language contact-induced features.

On the one hand, this study has identified and analyzed these features in the language of cardiology through the investigation of discharge reports. Discharge reports are rarely investigated, as their availability is restricted due to their confidential nature; thus, the present research may provide a unique insight into a relatively unfamiliar written text type by analyzing and evaluating data with a contact linguistic approach.

On the other hand, the investigation of the attitudes of physicians has revealed that, in contrast to my previous hypothesis, there is no linguistic gap between tertiary/secondary care physicians, who may be considered bilingual speakers of Hungarian and English, and primary care physicians, for whom English competence is only a "beneficial advance". The two discourse communities use a common code, a medical interlanguage, which promotes understanding between them.

Patients' attitudes towards the dominance of the English language in medicine are also described in this book. Patients cannot be expected to achieve a high(er) command of English, especially in English for medical purposes, to be able to understand their own discharge reports. Thus, a consensus should be reached: making the content of hospital documents fully comprehensible not only to the physicians who write them, but also to patients who these reports are written about.

The language differences between members of the Hungarian medical community may lead to miscommunication in the future, especially between physicians and other health workers, as well as patients. Therefore, the necessity of language planning, especially through the promotion of publishing medical achievements in Hungarian, also needs to be considered. Language planning may also be employed by the Department of Health, university faculty leadership, as well as ambitious physicians and linguists to unify orthography rules of both loanwords and calques. Medical terminology need to be investigated, collected and made available to physicians in order to promote unification and standardization.

Another practical outcome of the research reported on in this book may be the information gained about the present language of medicine in Hungary, which might be utilized by the teachers of translation studies in teaching English–Hungarian medical translation. Awareness of future translators needs to be raised about the English language contact-induced features used by Hungarian medical writers, and the translators' responsibility for the development of Hungarian scientific terms needs to be highlighted.

The examination of language contact-induced features, as well as the attitude survey may also be helpful in the teaching of English for medical purposes, and the results can also provide medical English curricula and test designers with a better understanding of the language needs of Hungarian medical students.

7. Bibliography

Abbott, Pamela (ed.) 1990. *The sociology of the caring professions*. London: Falmer Press.

Aitcheson, Jean. 1997. *The language web: The power and problem of words*. Cambridge: Cambridge University Press.

Alberti, Gábor. 1996. Passziválási művelet a magyarban. [Passivization in Hungarian] In: Büky, László and Maleczky, Márta (eds.) *A mai magyar nyelv leírásának újabb módszerei II.* [Recent methods of describing current Hungarian 2] Szeged: University of Szeged, 7–46.

Alcaraz, Ariza. M. Á. and Navarro, Fernando. 2006. Medicine: Use of English. In: Brown, Keith (ed.) *Encyclopedia of language and linguistics*. (2nd edition). Volume 7. Amsterdam: Elsevier, 752–759.

Aldrich, Clarence Knight. 1999. *The medical interview: Gateway to the doctor–patient relationship*. (2nd edition). New York: The Parthenon Publishing Group.

Ammon, Ulrich. 1994. The present dominance of English in Europe: With an outlook on possible solutions to the European language problems. *Sociolinguistica,* 8: 1–14.

Ammon, Ulrich. 1998. *Ist Deutsch noch internationale Wissenschaftssprache? Englisch auch für die Lehre an deutschsprachigen Hochschulen*. Berlin: De Gruyter.

Ammon, Ulrich. 2001. English as a future language of teaching at German universities? A question of difficult consequences posed by the decline of German as a language of science. In: Ammon, Ulrich (ed.) *The Dominance of English as a language of science: Effects on other languages and language communities*. Berlin–New York: Mouton de Gruyter, 343–362.

Ammon, Ulrich and Hellinger, Marlis (eds.) 1992. *Status change of languages*. Berlin: Walter de Gruyter.

Anderson, Janet Byron. 1996. The language of eponyms. *Journal of the Royal College of Physicians London,* 30: 174–177.

Appel, René and Muysken, Pieter 1987. *Language contact and bilingualism.* New York: Edward Arnold.

Ardila, Alfredo. 2005. Spanglish, an anglicized Spanish dialect. *Hispanic Journal of Behavioral Sciences,* 1: 60–81.

Atkinson, Dwight. 1992. The evolution of medical research writing from 1735 to 1985: The case of the Edinburgh Medical Journal. *Applied Linguistics,* 13: 337–74.

Atkinson, Dwight. 1996. The philosophical transactions of the Royal Society of London, 1675–1975: A sociohistorical discourse analysis. *Language in Society,* 25: 333–71.

Atkinson, Paul. 1999. Medical discourse, evidentiality and the construction of professional responsibility. In: Sarangi, Srikant and Roberts, Celia (eds.) *Talk, work and institutional order: Discourse in medical, mediation and management settings.* Berlin: Mouton de Gruyter, 75–108.

Auer, Peter. 1984. *Bilingual conversation.* Amsterdam: John Benjamins.

Auer, Peter. 1985. The pragmatics of code-switching: A sequential approach. In: Milroy, Lesley and Muysken, Pieter (eds.) *One speaker, two languages: Cross disciplinary perspectives on code-switching.* Cambridge: Cambridge University Press, 115–135.

Auer, Peter (ed.) 1998. *Code-switching in conversation: Language, interaction and identity.* London: Routledge.

Backus, A. M. 1996. *Two in one: Bilingual speech of Turkish immigrants in the Netherlands.* Tilburg: Tilburg University Press.

Baker, Colin. 1988. *Key issues in bilingualism and bilingual education.* Clevedon: Multilingual Matters.

Baker, Colin. 1992. *Attitudes and language.* Clevedon/Philadelphia: Multilingual Matters.

Baker, Colin. 1993. *Foundations of bilingual education and bilingualism*. Clevedon: Multilingual Matters.

Bakewell, David. 1992. Publish in English, or perish? *Nature,* 356: 648.

Bakró-Nagy, Marianne. 2009. *A jövő a múltból múltból tekintve. A magyar nyelv a határon innen és túl.* [Looking back to the future: The Hungarian language in and outside Hungary.] A jövőkutatás helye a 21. században. A jövőkutatás fejlődése és tudományterületi kapcsolatai. VII. Magyar (Jubileumi) Jövőkutatási Konferencia. [Future research in the 21st century. 7th (Jubilee) Conference on Future Research] Győr: Palatia Kiadó és Nyomda, 39–47.

Balázs, Géza. 1998. *Magyar nyelvkultúra az ezredfordulón.* [Hungarian language culture at the turn of the millennium]. Budapest: A–Z Kiadó.

Balázs, Géza. 2005. *"A magyar nyelv elémozdításáért..." – Vitairat a nyelvművelésért.* ["For the development of the Hungarian language..." – A polemical essay on language cultivation]. Budapest: Akadémiai Kiadó.

Baldauf, Richard and Jernudd, Björn H. 1987. Academic communication in a foreign language: The example of Scandinavian psychology. *Review of Applied Linguistics*. 41: 220–224.

Balint, Michael. 1957. *The doctor, his patient, and the illness*. New York: International Universities Press.

Bamgbose, Ayo. 2001. World Englishes and globalization. *World Englishes,* 20: 357–363.

Bartha, Csilla. 1993. *Egy amerikai magyar közösség nyelvhasználatának szociolingvisztikai megközelítései*. [Sociolinguistic approaches to the study of language use of an American–Hungarian community] Budapest. PhD dissertation.

Bartha, Csilla. 1998. *A szociolingvisztika alapjai* [The basics of sociolinguistics]. Budapest: Department of Contemporary Hungarian, Faculty of Arts, Eötvös Loránd University.

Bartha, Csilla. 1999. *A kétnyelvűség alapkérdései*. [The basic questions of bilingualism] Budapest: Nemzeti Tankönyvkiadó.

Bartha, Csilla. 2007. Nyelvi attitűdök és a nyelvcsere. [Language attitudes and languge shift] In: Benő, Attila, Fazakas, Emese and Szilágyi, N. Sándor (eds.) *Nyelvek és nyelvváltozatok. Köszöntő kötet Péntek János tiszteletére.* [Languages and language variaties: Festschrift for János Péntek] Kolozsvár: Anyanyelvápolók Erdélyi Szövetsége, 84–101.

Barton, Ellen. 2000. The interactional practices of referrals and accounts in medical discourse: compliance and expertise. *Discourse Studies,* 2: 259–281.

Barton, Ellen. 2006. Medical specialty encounters. In: Brown, Keith (ed.) *Encyclopedia of language and linguistics.* (2nd edition). Volume 7. Amsterdam: Elsevier, 732–742.

Bartos, Huba. 2009. The syntax of Hungarian -vA adverbial participles. In: É. Kiss, Katalin (ed.): *Adverbs and adverbial adjuncts at the interfaces.* Berlin/New York: Mouton de Gruyter, 75–102.

Bates, Stephen R. and Jenkins, Laura. 2007. Teaching and learning of ontology and epistemology in political science. *Politics,* 1: 55–63.

Bazerman, Charles. 1988. *Shaping written knowledge: The genre and activity of the experimental article in science.* Madison: University of Wisconsin Press.

Bazerman, Charles. 1998. Emerging perspectives on the many dimensions of scientific discourse. In: Martin, James R. and Veel, Robert. (eds.) *Reading science: Critical and functional perspectives on discourses of science.* London: Routledge, 15–28.

Bazerman, Charles and Paradis, James (eds.) 1991. *Textual dynamics of the professions: Historical and contemporary studies of writing in professional communities.* Madison: University of Wisconsin Press.

Beck, Ulrich. 1997. *Was ist Globalisierung?* Frankfurt/M: Suhrkamp.

Beisecker, Analee and Beisecker, Thomas. 1990. Patient information-seeking behaviors when communicating with doctors. *Medical Care,* 28: 19–28.

Belazi, Heidi, Rubin, Edward and Toribio, Almeida J. 1994. Code switching and x-bar theory: The functional head constraint. *Linguistic Inquiry,* 2: 221–237.

Bellmann, Gunter. 1971. *Slavoteutonica.* Berlin/New York: de Gruyter.

Benfield, John R. 2007. Cardiothoracic surgeons divided by a common language. *Annals of Thoracic Surgery,* 84: 363–364.

Benfield, John R. 2006. How authors can cope with the burden of English as an international language. *Chest,* 129: 1728–1730.

Benfield, John R. and Howard, K.M. 2000. The language of science. *European Journal of Cardiothoracic Surgery,*18: 642–648.

Benő, Attila. 2000. A magyar–román nyelvi érintkezés jelentéstani kérdései. [Semantic interferences in Hungarian-Romanian language contact] Kolozsvár: Babes Bolyai University MS.

Benő, Attila and Szilágyi, N. Sándor. 2005. Hungarian in Romania. In: Fenyvesi, Anna (ed.) *Hungarian language contact outside Hungary: Studies on Hungarian as a minority language.* IMPACT. Volume 20. Amsterdam–Philadelphia: John Benjamins Publishing Company, 133–162.

Bernsten, Jan. 1990. The integration of English loans in Shona: Social correlates and linguistic consequences. East Lansing: Michigan State University. PhD dissertation.

Betz, Werner. 1939. Lehnwörter und Lehnprägungen im Vor- und Frühdeutschen. [Loanwords and In: Friedrich, Mauer and Friedrich, Stroh (eds.) *Deutsche Wortgeschichte.* Berlin: Schmidt, 127–147.

Betz, Werner. 1974. Lehnwörter und Lehnprägungen im Vor- und Frühdeutschen. Volume I. Berlin/ New York: de Gruyter, 135–163.

Bhatia, Viyah K. 1993. *Analysing genre: Language use in professional settings.* London: Longman.

Biber, Douglas. 1995. *Dimensions of register variation: A cross-linguistic comparison.* New York: Cambridge University Press.

Bickerton, Derek. 1977. Pidginization and creolization: Language acquisition and language universals. In: Valdman, Albert (ed.) *Pidgin and creole languages.* Bloomington: Indiana University Press, 44–69.

Bickerton, Derek. 1981. *Roots of language.* Ann Arbor: Karoma.

Bilan de l'année. 1996. *Fédération Canadienne des Sciences Humaine*. http://www.fedcan.ca/ftpFiles/documents/annualreport2007.pdf . Access: 23 June, 2008

Bloomfield, Leonard. 1933. *Language*. (Revised from the 1914 edition) New York: Holt.

Blum-Kulka, Shoshana, House, Juliane and Kasper, Gabriele. 1989. The CCSARP coding manual. In: Blum-Kulka, Shoshana, House, Juliane and Kasper, Gabriele (eds.) *Cross-cultural pragmatics: Requests and apologies*. Norwood, NJ: Ablex, 273–294.

Bolton, Kingsley. 2004. World Englishes. In: Davies, Alan and Elder, Catherine (eds.) *The handbook of applied linguistics*. Malden, Ma.: Blackwell Publishing, 367–396.

Bondebjerg, Ib. 2003. Culture, media and globalisation. In: *Humanities – essential research for Europe*. Copenhagen: Danish Research Council for the Humanities, 71–88.

Bonnano, Michael. 1982. Women's language in the medical interview. In: Pietro, Robert D. (ed.) *Linguistics and the profession*. Norwood: Ablex, 27–38.

Bonnano, Michael. 1995. *Hedges in the medical intake interview: Discourse task, gender and role*. Washington, D.C.: Georgetown University. PhD dissertation.

Bősze, Péter. 2002. Gondolatok az orvosi nyelv magyarításáról. [Some thoughts on Hungarianizing the medical language] *Magyar Orvosi Nyelv,* 1: 2–5.

Bősze, Péter 2004. Gondolatok az orvosi nyelv magyarításáról. [Some thoughts on Hungarianizing the medical language] In: Balázs, Géza (ed.) *A magyar nyelvi kultúra jelene és jövője*. [The presence and future of Hungarian language culture] Budapest: Magyar Tudományos Akadémia.

Bősze, Péter. 2009. A magyar orvosi nyelv fejlesztése: Lehetőségek, kötelességek. [Developing the Hungarian medical language: Possibilities and obligations]. *Magyar Tudomány*, 1: 75–85

Bősze, Péter (ed.) 2010. *A magyar orvosi nyelv tankönyve*. [The Hungarian language of medicine – A coursebook]. Budapest: Medicina Könyvkiadó.

Bősze, Péter and Palkovits, Miklós. 2006. *Tudományos közlemények írása, szerkesztése és értékelése (Útmutató orvosi közlemények írói, olvasói és bírálói számára).* [Writing, editing and evaluating scientific articles: Instructions to authors, readers and reviewers of medical papers] Budapest: NOK.

Bourhis, R., Roth, S. and MacQueen, G. 1989. Communication in the hospital setting: A survey of medical and everyday language use amongst patients, nurses and doctors. *Social Science and Medicine,* 28: 339–346.

Britten, Nicky. 1995. Qualitative research: Qualitative interviews in medical research. *British Medical Journal,* 311: 251–253.

Brock, Dan W. and Wartman, Steven A. 1990. When competent patients make irrational choices. *New England Journal of Medicine,* 322: 1595–1599.

Brown, Penelope and Levinson, Stephen C. 1987. *Politeness: Some universals in language usage*. Cambridge: Cambridge University Press.

Buda, Béla. 2002. Gondolatok a magyar orvosi szaknyelv kérdéséhez. [Some thoughts concerning the Hungarian language of medicine] *Magyar Orvosi Nyelv,* 2: 6–71.

Burchfield, Robert. 1985. *The English language.* Oxford: Oxford University Press.

Bussmann, Hadumod. 1996. *Routledge dictionary of language and linguistics*. London: Routledge.

Buvári, Márta. 2001. Mondjuk magyarul! [Let's say it in Hungarian] *Édes Anyanyelvünk,* 3: 13.

Byrne, Patrick S. and Long, B. E. L. 1976. *Doctors talking to patients*. London: Her Majesty's Stationery Office.

Campbell, Lyle. 1998. *Historical linguistics: An introduction.* Edinburgh: Edinburgh University Press.

Cannon, Sue. 1989. Social research in stressful settings: Difficulties for the sociologist studying the treatment of breast cancer. *Sociology of Health and Illness,* 11: 62–77.

Cargile, Aaron C. and Bradac, J. J. 2001. Attitudes toward language: A review of speaker-evaluation research and a general process model. In: Gudykunst, William B. (ed.) *Communication Yearbook,* 25: 347–82.

Carmi, Amnon. 2002. Human rights in medicine and law. In: Carmi, Amnon and Wax, Harry (eds.) *Patients' rights*. Tel Aviv: Yozmot Publication Ltd.

Carmichael, Cathie. 2000. Conclusions: Language and national identity in Europe. In: Barbour, Stephen and Carmichael, Cathie (eds.) *Language and nationalism in Europe*. Oxford: Oxford University Press, 280-289.

Carstensen, Busse. 1993. *Anglizismen-Wörterbuch: Der Einfluß des Englischen auf den deutschen Wortschatz nach 1945*. Band 1 A-E. Berlin: de Gruyter.

Chaitchik, Samario, Kreitler, Shulamith, Shared, Shlomo, Schwartz, Idit, and Rosin, Roni. 1992. Doctor–patient communication in a cancer ward. *Journal of Cancer Education,* 7: 41.

Chandler-Burns, Robert M. 1997. *Non-native writing instruction for medical purposes*. Paper presented at the 1997 meeting of International Teachers of English to Speakers of Other Languages. Orlando, FL.

Christy, Nicholas P. 1979. Medspeak. *New England Journal of Medicine,* 301: 508.

Cicourel, Aaron. 1974. *Theory and method in a study of Argentine fertility*. New York: Wiley.

Cicourel, Aaron. 1981. Language and medicine. In: Ferguson, Charles and Heath, Shirley (eds.) *Language in the USA*. New York: Cambridge University Press, 407–429.

Cicourel, Aaron. 1983. Hearing is not believing: Language and the structure of belief in medical communication. In: Fisher, Sue and Todd, Dundas Alexandra (eds.) *The social organization of doctor–patient communication*. Washington, DC: Center for Applied Linguistics, 221–239.

Clyne, Michael. 1982. *Multilingual Australia*. Melbourne: River Seine.

Clyne, Michael. 1991. *Community languages*. Cambridge: Cambridge University Press.

Clyne, Michael. 1992. (ed.) *Pluricentric languages. Differing norms in different nations*. Berlin/New York: Mouton de Gruyter.

Clyne, Michael. 2003. *Dynamics of language contact: English and immigrant languages*. Cambridge: Cambridge University Press.

Cohen, Stanley. 1972. *Folk devils and moral panics*. London: MacGibbon and Kee.

Connor, Ulla and Kaplan, Robert B. (eds.) 1987. *Writing across languages: Analysis of L2 text*. England and Reading, Wokingham, MA: Addison–Wesley.

Cook, Vivian. 1991. *Second language learning and language teaching*. Edward Arnold/ Hodder Headline Group: Melbourne.

Cooper, Lisa A., Roter, Debrah L. Johnson, RachelL. Ford, Daniel E. Steinwachs, Donald M. and Powe, Neil R. 2003. Patient-centered communication, ratings of care, and concordance of patient and physician race. *Annals of Internal Medicine,* 139: 907–915.

Cooper, Robert. L. and Fishman, Joshua. 1974. The study of language attitudes. *Linguistics,* 136: 5–19.

Cordella, Marisa. 2004. *The dynamic consultation: A discourse analytical study of doctor–patient communication in Chilean Spanish*. Amsterdam: Benjamins.

Corder, S. Pit. 1975. *The study of interlanguage*. Paper presented at AILA Congress. Stuttgart.

Corder, S. Pit. 1981. *Error analysis and interlanguage*. London: Oxford University Press.

Coulmas, Florian. 1991. European integration and the idea of the national language. Ideological roots and economic consequences. In: Coulmas, Florian (ed.) *A language policy for the European Community. Prospects and quandaries*. Berlin: Mouton de Gruyter, 1–43.

Council of Europe. 2001. *Linguistic diversity for democratic citizenship in Europe.* Strasbourg: Éditions du Conseil de l'Europe.

Coupland, Nikolas. 2007. *Style: Language variation and identity*. Cambridge: Cambridge University Press.

Crane, John A. 1997. Patient comprehension of doctor-patient communication on discharge from the emergency department. *Journal of Emergency Medicine,* 1: 1–7.

Creswell, John W. 2005. Educational research: Planning, conducting, and evaluating quantitative and qualitative research. Upper Saddle River, NJ: Pearson.

Crichton, Michael. 1975. Medical obfuscation: Structure and function. *New England Journal of Medicine,* 293: 1257–1259.

Crossgrove, William, Schleissner, Margaret and Voigts, Linda E. (eds.) 1998. Early science and medicine. *Journal for the Study of Science, Technology and Medicine in the Pre-Modern Period.* Special Issue: The vernacularization of science, medicine, and technology in late medieval Europe, 3: 81–87.

Crystal, David. 1987. *The Cambridge encyclopedia of language*. Cambridge: Cambridge University Press.

Crystal, David. 1995. *The Cambridge encyclopedia of the English language.* Cambridge: Cambridge University Press.

Crystal, David. 1997. *English as a global language*. Cambridge: Cambridge University Press.

Csapó, József. 1971. English sporting terminology in Hungarian. *Angol Filológiai Tanulmányok,* 5: 5–50.

Csedő, Károly. 2005. Tények és javaslatok. [Facts and recommendations.] In: Kontra, Miklós (ed.) *Sültgalamb: Magyar egyetemi tannyelvpolitika.* [Waiting for a dead man's shoes? Hungarian language policy concerning language of instruction at the university level] Somorja/Dunaszerdahely: Lilium Aurum Könyvkiadó, 125–129.

Cselovszkyné Tarr, Klára. 1999. Tabu és eufemizmus az egészségügy nyelvében. Ph.D. értekezés. [Taboo and euphemism in the language of health care] *Medicina et Linguistica*. Különszám. Budapest: Semmelweis Orvostudományi Egyetem. PhD dissertation.

Csernicskó, István. 1998. *A magyar nyelv Ukrajnában (Kárpátalján).* [The Hungarian language in Ukraine (Subcarpathia)]. Budapest: Osiris Kiadó és MTA Kisebbségkutató Műhely.

Csernicskó, István and Fenyvesi, Anna. 2000. The sociolinguistic stratification of Hungarian in Subcarpathia. *Multilingua,* 19: 95–122.

Davies, Alan. 1989. Is international English an interlanguage? *TESOL Quarterly,* 3: 447–467.

Davis, Lennard. 1995. *Enforcing normalcy: Disability, deafness, and the body.* London: Verso.

Davis, Lennard (ed.) 2006. *The disability studies reader*. New York: Routledge.

De Groot, Anette M. B. and Kroll, Judith F. (eds.) 1997. *Tutorials in bilingualism: Psycholinguistic perspectives.* Mahwah, NJ: Erlbaum.

de Swan, Abraham. 2001. English in the social sciences. In: Ammon, Ulrich (ed.) *The Dominance of English as a Language of Science: Effects on other languages and language communities.* Berlin–New York: Mouton de Gruyter, 71–84.

De Vries, John. 1999. Language acquisition, language shift and immigrant integration. The experience of foreign-born adults in Canada. In: Halli, Shivalingappa and Driedger, Leo (eds.) *Immigrant Canada.* Toronto: University of Toronto Press, 261–281.

DeBakey, Lois. 1966. Language and the physician. *Archives of Surgery,* 92: 964–972.

DeLancey, Scott. 1981. An interpretation of split ergativity and related patterns. *Language,* 57: 626–657.

Del Valle, Sandra. 2003. *Language rights and the law in the United States.* Clevedon: Multilingual Matters.

Deme, László. 1956. *Magyarázat helyesírási szabályzatunk új (10.) kiadásához.* [Explanation to the new (10th) edition of our orthography] Budapest: Akadémiai Kiadó.

Demeter, Éva. 2005. A szakmai diskurzus a személyiség tükrében. [Professional discourse and the individual]. *Porta Lingua.* Debrecen: Debreceni Egyetem, 31–48.

Denzin, Norman and Lincoln, Yvonna. 2005. *Handbook of qualitative research.* (3rd edition). Thousand Oaks, California: Sage.

di Cicco-Bloom, Barbara and Crabtree, Benjamin. 2006. The qualitative research interview. *Medical Education,* 40: 314–321.

DiPietro, Robert J. 1977. Codeswitching as a verbal strategy among bilinguals. In: Eckman, Fred Robert (ed.) *Current themes in linguistics: Bilingualism, experimental linguistics and language typologies.* Washington, DC: Hemisphere.

Di Sciullo, Anne-Marie, Muysken, Pieter. and Singh, Rajendra. 1986. Government and code-mixing. *Journal of Linguistics,* 22: 1–24.

Dirckx, John H. 1983. *The language of medicine. Its evolution, structure, and dynamics.* New York: Praeger.

Dirckx, John H. 2001.The synthetic genitive in medical eponyms: Is it doomed to extinction? *Panacea,* 5: 15–24.

Dirckx, John H. 2006. Anatomical nomenclature: History. In Brown, Keith (ed.) *Encyclopedia of language and linguistics.* (2nd edition). Volume 1. Amsterdam: Elsevier, 244–252.

Dorian, Nancy (ed.) 1989. *Investigating obsolescence: Studies in language contraction and death.* Cambridge: Cambridge University Press.

Dörnyei, Zoltán. 2001. *Teaching and researching motivation.* Harlow: Longman.

Dörnyei, Zoltán. 2006. Individual differences in second language acquisition. *AILA Review,* 19: 42–68.

Dörnyei, Zoltán, Csizér, Kata and Németh, Nóra. 2006. *Motivation, language attitudes and globalization: A Hungarian perspective*. Clevedon-Buffalo-Toronto: Multilingual Matters Ltd.

Douglas, Jack. 1985. *Creative interviewing*. Beverly Hills, Ca: Sage.

Dubois, Betti Lou. 1981. The construction of noun phrases in biomedical journal articles. In: Hoedt, Jorgen, Lundquist, Lita, Picht, Heribert and Qvistgaard, Jacques (eds.) *Pragmatics and LSP*. Copenhagen: Copenhagen School of Economics, 49–67.

Duckworth, David. 1977. Zur terminologischen und systematischen Grundlage der Forschung auf dem Gebiet der englisch-deutschen Interferenz. Kritische Übersicht und neuer Vorschlag. In: Kolb, Herbert and Lauffer, Hartmut (eds.) *Sprachliche Interferenz. Festschrift für Werner Betz zum 65. Geburtstag.* Tübingen: Niemeyer, 36–56.

Duran, Richard P. (ed.) 1981. *Latino language and communicative behavior.* Norwood: Ablex Press.

Dürmüller, Urs. 1989. Attitudes towards English as a possible lingua franca in Switzerland. *York Papers in Linguistics,* 14: 3–17.

Dürmüller, Urs. 1992. The changing status of English in *Switzerland*. In: Ammon, Ulrich. and Hellinger, Marlis (eds.) *Status change of languages*. Berlin/New York: Mouton de Gruyter, 335–370.

Duszak, Anna (ed.) 1997. *Trends in linguistics: Culture and styles of academic discourse*. Berlin: Mouton de Gruyter.

É. Kiss Katalin. 2002. Negative quantifiers and specificity. In: Kenesei, István and Siptár, Péter (eds.) *Approaches to Hungarian 8*. Budapest: Akadémiai Kiadó, 39–60.

É. Kiss, Katalin. 2004. *Anyanyelvünk állapotáról*. Budapest: Osiris.

É. Kiss, Katalin, Kiefer, Ferenc and Siptár, Péter. 2003. *Új magyar nyelvtan.* [New Hungarian grammar] Budapest: Osiris Kiadó.

Edwards, John. 1982. Language attitudes and their implications among English speakers. In: Ryan, Ellen Bouchard and Giles, Howard (eds.) *Attitudes towards language variation: Social and applied contexts*. London: Edward Arnold, 20–33.

Edwards, John. 1994. *Multilingualism*. London/New York: Routledge.

Egger, Matthias, Zellweger-Zähner, T., Schneider, M., Junker, C., Lengeler, C. and Antes, G. 1997. Language bias in randomised controlled trials published in English and German. *The Lancet,* 350: 326–329.

Eggins, Suzanne and Martin, J.R. 1997. Genre and registers of discourse. In: van Dijk, Teun A. (ed.) *Discourse as Structure and Process*. London: Sage, 230–256.

Ellis, Rod. 1985. *Understanding second language acquisition*. Oxford: Oxford University Press.

Engel, George L. 1977. The need for a new medical model, a challenge for new medicine. *Science,* 196: 129–136.

Erling, Elizabeth J. 2004. *Globalization, English and the German university classroom: A sociolinguistic profile of students of English*. PhD Thesis. University of Edinburgh.

ESC 2008 Final Congress Programme. Access: February 15, 2008 http://www.eurostroke.org/ni_general_information.htm.

Europeans and their languages. 2006. http://www.scibd.com/doc/322326/ebs-243-en Access: December 17, 2007.

Fábián, Pál. 1993. Szaknyelvi helyesírási szabályzataink mérlege. [Considerations of our regulations on spelling of technical vocabulary] *Magyar Nyelvőr,* 117: 595–599.

Fábián, Tamás. 2006. *Betegjogi képviseleti rendszer Magyarországon*. (Szószóló Alapítvány). [The represention system of patients'rights in Hungary]. Access: December 30, 2006. http://www.szoszolo.hu/06tanulmanyaink/frindex.htm

Fairclough, Norman. 1989. *Language and power*. London: Longman.

Fairclough, Norman. 1995. *Critical discourse analysis*. Boston: Addison Wesley.

Fairclough, Norman. 2006. *Language and globalization*. London: Routledge.

Farkas, Judit and Kniezsa, Veronika. 2002. Hungarian. In: Görlach, Manfred (ed.) *English in Europe*. Oxford: Oxford University Press, 277–290.

Fasold, Ralph. 1984. *The sociolinguistics of society*. Oxford: Basil Blackwell.

Fasold, Ralph. 2006. *An introduction to language and linguistics*. Cambridge: Cambridge University Press.

Fehér, János. 1997. Az orvosi szakirodalmi nyelv rövid története. [A short history of the language of medical literature]. *Orvosi Hetilap,* 138: 2685.

Fenyvesi, Anna. 1995a. Hungarian diglossia in Slovakia: A new linguistic approach. *Budapest Review of Books,* 2: 37–39.

Fenyvesi, Anna. 1995b. Language contact and language death in an immigrant language: The case of Hungarian. *University of Pittsburgh Working Papers in Linguistics,* 3: 1–117.

Fenyvesi, Anna. 1998. Patterns of borrowing and language attrition: American Hungarian in McKeesport, Pennsylvania. In: De Groot, Casper and Kenesei, István (eds.) *Papers from the Amsterdam conference: Approaches to Hungarian* 6. Szeged: JATE Press, 229–249.

Fenyvesi, Anna. 2005. Hungarian in the United States. In: Fenyvesi, Anna (ed.) *Hungarian language contact outside Hungary: Studies on Hungarian as a minority language*. IMPACT. Volume 20. Amster-dam–Philadelphia: John Benjamins Publishing Company, 265–318.

Fenyvesi, Anna. 2006. Contact effects in Toledo Hungarian: Quantitative findings. In: Watson, Greg and Hirvonen, Pekka (eds.) *Finno-Ugric language contacts*. Frankfurt am Main: Peter Lang, 157–177.

Ferguson, Charles A. 1959. Diglossia. *Word,* 15: 325–340.

Fergusson, Gibson. 2006. *Language planning and education.* Edinburgh: Edinburgh University Press.

Ferguson, Gibson. 2009. Issues in researching English as a lingua franca: A conceptual enquiry. *International Journal of Applied Linguistics,* 2: 117–135.

Field, Fredric W. 2002. *Linguistic borrowing in bilingual context.* Amsterdam: John Benjamins Publisher.

Fielding, G. and Evered, C. 1980. The influence of patients' speech upon doctors. In: St. Clair, Robert N. and Giles, Howard (eds.) *The social and psychological contexts of language.* Hillsdale, NJ: Erlbaum, 51–72.

Fielding, Robert. 1995. *Clinical communication skills.* Hong Kong: Hong Kong University Press.

Filipović, Rudolf (ed.) 1990. *The English element in European languages.* Volume 3. Zagreb: Institute of Linguistics.

Filipović, Rudolf. 1996. English as a word donor to other languages of Europe. In: Hartmann, R. (ed.) *The English language in Europe.* Exeter: Intellect, 37–46.

Fink, Hermann. 1968. *Amerikanismen im Wortschatz der deutschen Tagespresse.* Dissertation. Johannes Gutenburg Universität.

Fischer, Roswitha. 2008. Introduction: Studying Anglicisms. In: Fischer, Roswitha and Pulaczewska, Hanna (eds.) *Anglicisms in Europe: Linguistic diversity in a global context.* New Castle upon Tyne: Cambridge Scholars Publishing, 1–15.

Fisher, Sue and Todd, Alexandra D. 1983. *The social organization of doctor–patient communication.* Washington, D.C.: Center for Applied Linguistics.

Fishman, Joshua. 1964. Language maintenance and language shift as fields of inquiry. *Linguistics,* 9: 32–70.

Fishman, Joshua (ed.) 1966. *Language loyalty in the United States: The maintenance and perpetuation of non-English mother tongues by American ethnic and religious groups.* The Hague: Mouton.

Fishman, Joshua. 1971. The sociology of language: An interdisciplinary social science approach to language in society. In: Fishman, Joshua (ed.) *Advances in the sociology of language*. Volume 1. Mouton: The Hague, 217–258.

Fishman, Joshua (ed.) 1985. *The rise and fall of the ethnic revival.* Berlin: Mouton de Gruyter.

Fishman, Joshua. 1989. Language and ethnicity in minority sociolinguistic perspective. Philadelphia: Multilingual Matters.

Fishman, Joshua. 1991. Reversing language shift: Theory and practice of assistance to threatened languages. Clevedon: Multilingual Matters.

Fishman, Joshua. 1996. Summary and interpretation: Post-imperial English 1940–1990. In: Fishman, Joshua A., Conrad, Andrew W. and Rubal-Lopez, Alma (eds.) Post-imperial English. Berlin/ New York: Mouton de Gruyter, 623–641.

Fishman, Joshua. 1997. The multilingual apple: Languages in New York (with Ofelia Garcia). Berlin: Mouton de Gruyter.

Fishman, Joshua. 1998. The new linguistic order. Foreign Policy, 113: 26–40.

Fishman, Joshua. 2000. Bilingualism with and without diglossia; diglossia with and without bilingualism. In: Wei, Li (ed.) The bilingualism reader. London: Routledge, 81–88. (Source: Fishman, Joshua. 1967. Bilingualism with and without diglossia; diglossia with and without bilingualism. Journal of Social Issues, 2: 29–38.)

Flick, Uwe. 2002. An introduction to qualitative research. London: Sage.

Foddy, William. 1993. Constructing questions for interviews and questionnaires. Cambridge: Cambridge University Press.

Foley, William. 1997. Anthropological linguistics: An introduction. Oxford: Blackwell Publishing.

Fowler, Roger. Linguistic criticism. Oxford: Oxford University Press.

Freidson, Eliot. 1961. Patients' views of medical practice. New York: Russell Sage Foundation.

Freidson, Elit. 1970. Profession of medicine: A study of the sociology of applied knowledge. New York: Dood Mead Inc.

Freidson, Elit. 1975. Doctoring together: A study of professional social control. New York: Elsevier.

Freidson, Eliot. 1986. Professional powers: A study of the institutionalization of formal knowledge. Chicago: University of Chicago Press.

French, Roger. 2003. Medicine before science: The business of medicine from the Middle Ages to the Enlightenment. Cambridge: Cambridge University Press.

Gal, Susan. 1979. Language shift: Social determinants of linguistic change in bilingual Austria. New York: Academic Press.

Galtung, Johan. 1980. The true worlds: A transnational perspective. New York: The Free Press.

Gardner, Howard. 2004. Changing minds - The art and science of changing our own and other people's minds. Massachusetts: Harvard Business School Press.

Gardner, Robert C. 1985. Social psychology and second language learning: The role of attitudes and motivation. London: Edward Arnold.

Gardner, Robert C. and Lambert, Wallace E. 1959. Motivational variables in second language acquisition. Canadian Journal of Psychology, 13: 266–272.

Gardener-Chloros, Penelope. 1995. Code-switching in community, regional and national repertoires: The myths of discreteness of linguistic systems. In: Milroy, Leslie and Muysken, Pieter (ed.) One speaker two languages. Cross disciplinary perspectives on code-switching. Cam-bridge: Cambridge University Press, 68–89.

Gardner, Robert C. and MacIntyre, P. D. 1991. An instrumental motivation in language study: Who says it isn't effective. *Studies in Second Language Acquisition,* 13: 57–72.

Garfinkel, Harold. 1967. Studies in ethnomethodology. Englewood Cliffs, NJ: Prentice–Hall.

Geeraerts, Dirk. 1997. Diachronic prototype semantics. A contribution to historical lexicology. Oxford: Clarendon.

Giles, Howard. 1977. Language, ethnicity and intergroup relations. London: Academic Press.

Giles, Howard and Billings, A. C. 2004. Assessing language attitudes: Speaker evaluation studies. In: Davies, Alan and Elder, Catherine (eds.) The handbook of applied linguistics. Malden: Blackwell Publishing, 187–210.

Giles, Howard and Pierson, H. D. 1988. Social inferences from language proficiency in Hong Kong: A reinterpretation of Hui and Yam. British Journal of Social Psychology, 27: 279–81.

Goebl, Hans, Nelde, Peter H., Starý, Zdenek and Wölck, Wolfgang (eds.) 1996. Kontaktlinguistik/Contact Linguistics/Linguistique de Contact: Ein internationales Handbuch zeitgenössischer Forschung/ An International Handbook of Contemporary research/ Manuel inter-national des recherches contemporaines. 1. Berlin–New York: Walter de Gruyter.

Göncz, Lajos. 1999. A magyar nyelv Jugoszláviában (Vajdaságban). [The Hungarian language in Yugoslavia (Vojvodina)]. Budapest/Újvidék: Osiris – Forum Kiadó.

Göncz, Lajos. 2001. Az egyes és a többes szám használata Kárpát-medencei magyar beszélőközösségeknél [The use of the singular and plural inHungarian speech communities in the Carpathian Basin]. Pszichológia, 4: 371–391.

Gönye, Anikó. 1999. *Az orvos rendelőintézeti nyelvhasználatának elemzése szociolingvisztikai szempontok alkalmaz*ásával. [An analysis of the language use of the physician at the outpatient clinic] Budapest: ELTE. PhD dissertation.

Görlach, Manfred (ed.) 2001. A dictionary of European Anglicisms: A usage dictionary of Anglicisms in sixteen European languages. Oxford: Oxford University Press.

Görlach, Manfred (ed.) 2002a. English in Europe. Oxford: Oxford University Press.

Görlach, Manfred (ed.) 2002b. Annotated bibliography of European Anglicisms. Oxford: Oxford University Press.

Gottlieb, Henrik. 1997. Subtitles, translation and idioms. Copenhagen: University of Copenhagen.

Graddol, David. 1997. The future of English? London: British Council.

Graddol, David. 2006. English next. Why global English may mean the end of 'English as a Foreign Language'. London: The British Council.

Grétsy, László. 1993. Nemzetközpontú nyelvművelés. [Nation centered language cultivation]. Magyar Nyelvőr, 117: 402–404.

Grétsy, László. 1996. Az orvosi szaknyelvről – az orvosi szaknyelvért. [On medical English – for medical English] Magyar Tudomány, 9: 1140–1141.

Grétsy, László. 2001. Globalizáció és anyanyelv. [Globalization and mother tongue] Magyar Orvosi Nyelv, 1: 20–3.

Grétsy, László. 2002a. Nemzetösszetartónk: az anyanyelv. [Native tongue as the cohesion of the nation] In: V. Raisz, Józsa and Zimányi, Árpád (eds.) Feladatok és módszerek az anyanyelvi nevelésben a XXI. század elején. [Tasks and methods in Hungarian language teaching at the beginning of the 21st century] Magyar Nyelvtudományi Társaság, Budapest, 15–21.

Grétsy, László. 2002b. A szaknyelvek nyelvújításáért. [For the language reform of technical language]. Magyar Nyelvőr, 126: 275–283.

Grétsy, László and Kemény, Gábor (eds.) 1996. Nyelvművelő kéziszótár. [Dictionary of language cultivation]. Budapest: Auktor Könyvkiadó.

Grétsy, László and Kovalovszky, Miklós (eds.). 1983 and 1985. Nyelvművelő kézikönyv I. és II. [Language cultivation handbook, Vols 1 and 2]. Budapest: Akadémiai Kiadó.

Grétsy, Zsombor. 2004. Az orvosi nyelv magyarítása: Stratégiai kérdések a magyar orvosi szaknyelvben. [Translating medical language into Hungarian: Strategic issues in the Hungarian language of medicine] In: Balázs, Géza (ed.) *A magyar nyelvi kultúra jelene és jövője* I. [The present state and future of Hungarian language culture]. Budapest: MTA Társadalomkutató Központ, 311–325.

Grosjean, Francois. 1982. Life with two languages: An introduction to bilingualism. Cambridge, MA: Harvard University Press.

Grosjean, Francois and Soares, C. 1986. Processing mixed language: Some preliminary findings. In: Vaid, Jyotsna (ed.) Language processing in bilinguals: Psycholinguistic and neuropsychological perspectives. Hillsdale, New Jersey: Lawrence Erlbaum.

Grzega, Joachim. 2002. Some aspects of modern diachronic onomasiology. Linguistics, 40: 1021–1045.

Gumperz, John. 1962. Types of linguistic communities. Anthropological Linguistics, 1: 28–40.

Gumperz, John. 1964. Hindi-Punjabi code-switching in Delhi. In: Lunt, H. (ed.) Proceedings of the Ninth International Congress of Linguists. The Hague: Mouton, 1115–1124.

Gumperz, John. 1982. Discourse strategies. Cambridge: Cambridge University Press.

Gunnarsson, Britt-Louise. 2001. Swedish tomorrow – A product of the linguistic dominance of English? In: Boyd, Sally and Huss, Leena (eds.) Managing multilingualism in a European nation-state. Challenges for Swedish. Current Issues in Language and Society. 7/1. Clevedon: Multilingual Matters Ltd, 51–69.

Gunnarsson, Britt-Louise. 2006. Medical discourse: Sociohistorical construction. In: Brown, Keith (ed.) Encyclopedia of language and linguistics. (2nd edition). Volume 7. Amsterdam: Elsevier, 709–717.

Gunnarsson, Britt-Louise and Bäcklund, Ingegerds (eds.) 1995. Writing in academic contexts. TEFA 11. Forskningsgruppen för text-och facksprakstudier. Uppsala: Uppsala University, 30–53.

Gunnarsson, Britt-Louise, Linell, Per and Nordberg, Bengt. 1997. The construction of professional discourse. London: Longman.

Gyarmathi, Sámuel. 1799. Affinitas lingvae hvngaricae cvm lingvis fennicae originis grammatice demonstrata. Nec non vocabvlaria dialectorvm tataricarvm et slavicarvm cvm hvngarica comparata. Göttingae.

Haarmann, Harald and Holman, Eugene. 2001. The impact of English as a language of science in Finland. In: Ammon, Ulrich (ed.) The dominance of English as a language of science: Effects on other languages and language communities. Berlin–New York: Mouton de Gruyter, 229–260.

Hadlow, Jan and Pitts, Marian. 1991. The understanding of common health terms by doctors, nurses and patients. Social Science and Medicine, 32: 193–196.

Hagstrom, Cynthia. 2004. The language of doctors and patients. In: Edward, Finegen and Rickford, John R. (eds.) Language in the USA: Themes for the twenty-first century. Cambridge: Cambridge University Press, 445–462.

Halliday, Michael Alexander K. 1988. On the language of physical science. In: Ghadessy, Mohsen (ed.) Registers of written English: Situational factors and linguistic features. London/New York: Pinter Publishers, 162–178.

Halliday, Michael Alexander K. and Martin, J.R. 1993. Writing science. Literacy and discursive power. London: The Falmer Press.

Hamers, Josiane F. and Blanc, Michel H. A. 1990. Bilinguality and bilingualism. Cambridge: Cambridge University Press.

Hammersley, Martyn. 1990. Reading ethnographic research: A critical guide. London: Longsman.

Hammersley, Martyn. 1992. What's wrong with ethnography? Methodological explorations. London: Longmans.

Hänsch, Holger and Fleck, Eckart. 2006. New possibilities for communication between hospital cardiologists and general practitioners. Disease Management and Health Outcomes. 14. Supplement, 1: 19–22.

Hansen, Klaus, Uwe, Carls and Lucko, Peter. 1996. Die Differenzierung des Englischen in nationale Varianten. Berlin.

Harris, Alice and Campbell, Lyle. 1995. Historical syntax in cross-linguistic perspective. Cambridge: Cambridge University Press.

Hartig, Matthias. 1980. Soziolinguistik für Anfänger. Hamburg: Hoffmann und Campe.

Hartmann, Reinhardt. 1996. Introduction. In: Hartmann, Reinhardt (ed.) The English language in Europe. Oxford: Intellect,1–2.

Haugen, Einar. 1950. The analysis of linguistic borrowing. Language, 26: 210–231.

Haugen, Einar. 1953. The Norwegian language in America: A study in bilingual behavior. Bloomington: Indiana University Press. (Reprinted in 1969).

Haugen, Einar. 1958. Languages in contact. In: Siversten, E. (ed.) Proceedings of the Eighth International Congress of Linguists. Oslo: Oslo University Press, 771–785.

Haugen, Einar. 1972. The ecology of language. Stanford, California: Stanford University Press.

Hawkins, John A. 1986. A comparative typology of English and German: Unifying the contrasts. London/Sydney: Croom Helm.

Heath, Jeffrey. 1989. From code-switching to borrowing: A case study of Moroccan Arabic. London/New York: Kegan Paul International.

Heine, Bernd and Kuteva, Tania. 2008. Constraints on contact induced linguistic change. Journal of Language Contact. Thema, 2: 57–90.

Heine, Bernd, Kuteva, Tania and Mufwene, Salikoko S. 2005. Language contact and grammatical change. Cambridge: Cambridge University Press.

Heller, Klaus. 1970. Der Wortschatz unter dem Aspekt des Fachwortes – Versuch einer Systematik. In: Wissenschaftliche Zeitschrift der Karl-Marx-Universität Leipzig. GS Reihe 19, 531–544. Reprinted in: von Hahn, W. 1981. Fachsprachen. Darmstadt: Wissenschaftliche Buchgesellschaft, 218–238.

Heller, Monica (ed.) 1988. Code switching: Anthropological and sociolinguistic perspectives. Berlin: Mouton de Gruyter.

Heller, Monica. 1999. Linguistic minorities and modernity: A sociolinguistic ethnography. London: Longman.

Herzog, George. 1941. Culture change and language shifts in the Pima vocabulary. In: Spier, Leslie, Hallowell, A.Irving and Newmann, S. Stanley (eds.) Language, culture and personality: Essays in Memory of Edward Sapir. Menasha, Wisconsin: Sapir Memorial Publication Fund, 66–74.

Hock, Hans. 1991. Principles of historical linguistics. Berlin: Mouton de Gruyter.

Hockett, Charles. 1958. A course in modern linguistics. New York: Macmillan.

Hoffmann, Charlotte. 1991. An introduction to bilingualism. New York: Longman.

Hope, Terry E. 1971. Lexical borrowing in the romance languages. Oxford: Basil Blackwell.

Hopper, Robert and Williams, Fredrick. 1973. Speech characteristics and employability. Speech Monographs, 46: 296–302.

Horváth, Julia and Siloni, Tal. 2005. Active lexicon: Adjectival passives. Paper presented at GLOW 28: Semitic Syntax Workshop. University of Geneva.

Horváth, Katalin and Lizanec, Péter. 1993. A kárpátaljai magyar nyelvjárások főbb sajátosságairól [On the most important characteristics of regional dialects of Hungarian in Subcarpathia]. In Lizanec, Péter and Horváth, Katalin (eds.). Az Ungvári Hungarológiai Intézet tudományos gyűjteménye [A scholarly collection of the Užhorod Hungarian Studies Institute]. Budapest/Ungvár: Intermix, 57–74.

House, Juliane. 2005. Englisch als 'Lingua Franca'. Eine Bedrohung für die deutsche Sprache? In: Motz, Markus (ed.) Englisch oder Deutsch in internationalen Studiengängen. Frankfurt: Lang, 53–55.

Huddleston, Rodney and Pullum, Geoffrey K. 2002. The Cambridge grammar of the English language. Cambridge: Cambridge University Press.

Hui, Harry C. and Yam, Yat-Ming. 1987. Effects of language proficiency and physical attractiveness on person perception. British Journal of Social Psychology, 26: 257–61.

Hyland, Ken. 1998. Persuasion and context: The pragmatics of academic metadiscourse. Journal of Pragmatics, 30: 437–455.

Hyland, Ken. 2000. Disciplinary discourses: Writer stance in research articles. In: Candlin, Christopher N. and Hyland, Ken (eds.) Writing: Texts, processes and practices. Harlow: Addison Wesley Longman, 99–121.

Hymes, Dell. 1964. Introduction: Toward ethnographies of communication. *American Anthropologist,* 6: 1–34.

Hymes, Dell. 1971. Pidginization and creolization of languages. Cambridge: Cambridge University Press.

Hymes, Dell. 1974. Foundations in sociolinguistics: An ethnographic approach. London: Longman.

Iedema, Rick. 2006. Medicine and health: Inter- and intraprofessional communication. In: Brown, Keith (ed.) Encyclopedia of language and linguistics. (2nd Edition). Volume 7. Amsterdam: Elsevier, 745–752.

Jacobson, Roman (ed.) 1989. Codeswitching as a worldwide phenomenon. New York: Peter Lang.

Jernudd, Björn. 1989. The texture of language purism: An introduction. Berlin: Mouton de Gruyter.

Jespersen, Otto. 1955. Growth and structure of the English language. (9th edition) Indiana: Doubleday.

Jespersen, Otto. 1964. Language. Its nature, development and origin. New York: W.W. Norton and Company.

Johanson, Lars. 1992. Strukturelle Faktoren in türkischen Sprachkontakten. (Sitzungsberichte der Wissenschaftlichen Gesellschaft an der Johann Wolfgang Goethe-Universität Frankfurt am Main. 5) Stuttgart: Franz Steiner, 169–299.

Johanson, Lars. 2002. Structural factors in Turkic language contacts. Translated by Karam, V. Richmond: Curzon.

Johnson, Diane and Murray, John. 1985. Do doctors really mean what they say? In: Enright, D. J. (ed.) Fair of speech: The uses of euphemisms. Oxford: Oxford University Press, 151–158.

Joint Commission on the Accreditation of Healthcare Organizations. Joint Commission on the Accreditation of Healthcare Organizations' Comprehensive Accreditation Manual for Hospitals 2004 [Management of Information; IM 6.10 element 7]. Oakbrook Terrace, Il.

Joseph, John E. 2001. Globalization and the spread of English: The long perspective. Journal of Southeast Asian Education, 2: 212–240.

Joshi, Aravind. 1985. Processing of sentences with intrasentential codeswitching. In: Dowty, David, Karttunen, Lauri and Zwicky, Arnold (eds.) Natural language parsing. Cambridge: Cambridge University Press, 190–205.

Juaristi, Patxi, Reagan, Timothy and Tonkin, Humphrey. 2008. Language diversity in the European Union. An overview. In: Arzoz, Xabier (ed.) Respecting linguistic diversity in the European Union. Amsterdam: John Benjamins, 47–72.

Kabakchi, V. Victor. 1998. Osnovy angloyazychnoi mezhkul'turnoi kommunikatsii. St. Petersburg: Russian State Pedagogical University Press.

Kabakchi, V. Victor. 2000. Unexplored type of translating activity: Inner translation. Studia Linguistica. Cognitive-pragmatic and expressive language functions. St. Petersburg: Trigon.

Kachru, Braj. 1979. The Englishization of Hindi: Language rivalry and language change. In: Rauch, Irmengard and Carr, Gerald (eds.) Linguistic method: Essays in honor of Herbert Penzl. The Hague: Mouton.

Kachru, Braj. 1985. Standards, codification and sociolinguistic realism: The English language in the outer circle. In: Quirk, Randolph and Widdowson, H. (eds.) English in the world: Teaching and learning the language and literatures. Cambridge: Cambridge University Press, 11–36.

Kachru, Braj. 1986. The alchemy of English: The spread, function and models of non-native Englishes. Oxford: Pergamon.

Kachru, Braj. 1992. World Englishes: Approaches, issues and resources. Language Teaching, 25: 1–14.

Kachru, Braj and Nelson, C. 1996. World Englishes. In: McKay, Sandra and Hornberger, Nancy (eds.) Sociolinguistics and language teaching. Cambridge: Cambridge University Press, 71–101.

Kaplan, Robert. 2001. English the accidental language of science? In: Ammon, Ulrich. (ed.) The Dominance of English as a language of science: Effects on other languages and language communities. Berlin–New York: Mouton de Gruyter, 3–26.

Kasper, Gabriele and Blum-Kulka, Shoshana. 1993. Interlanguage pragmatics. Oxford: Oxford University Press.

Katz, Daniel. 1960. The functional study of attitudes. Public Opinion Quarterly, 24: 163–204.

Kenesei, István, Vago, Robert. M. and Fenyvesi, Anna. 1998. Hungarian (Descriptive grammars series). London: Routledge.

Kenesei, István. 2000. Szavak, szófajok, toldalékok [Word, parts of speech and suffixes]. In: Kiefer, Ferenc (ed.) Strukturális magyar nyelvtan, [A stuctural Hungarian grammar] 3: 75–136. Budapest: Akadémiai Kiadó.

Keresztes, Csilla. 2003. Az angol nyelv hatása a magyar szakmai nyelvre. [The influence of the English language on the Hungarian professional languages]. In: Tóth, Szergej (ed.) Nyelvek és kultúrák találkozása. [The meeting of languages and cultures]. Szeged: Officina Press Kft, 168–172.

Keresztes, Csilla. 2006a. A többségi nyelv hatása a kisebbségi szaknyelvekre. Az erdélyi magyar orvosi nyelv. [The influence of the majority language on minority technical languages: The Hungarian medical language in Transylvania]. In: Benő, Attila and Szilágyi N., Sándor (eds.) Nyelvi közösségek – nyelvi jogok. [Language communities – language rights]. Kolozsvár: Anyanyelvápolók Erdélyi Szövetsége, 177–185.

Keresztes, Csilla. 2006b. Lektorálás a szakfordító képzésben: Kontaktushatásra létrejött nyelvi változatok azonosítása javító olvasáskor. [Proof reading in the translator course. Identifying language contact-induced features]. In: Demeter, Éva and Solymosi, Mária (eds.) *Szegedi Nyelvi Mozaik*. [Language mosaic in Szeged]. Szeged: Szegedi Tudományegyetem Idegennyelvi Központ, 101–112.

Keresztes, Csilla. 2007a. Nyelvi kontaktushatások vizsgálata szakszövegek fordításakor. [Examining language contact-induced features when translating special purpose texts]. In: Porta Lingua. Silye, Magdolna (ed.) *Szaknyelvoktatásunk – határokon átívelő híd*. [Special purpose language teaching – bridging borders]. Debrecen: Debreceni Egyetem, 295–301.

Keresztes, Csilla. 2007b. Slip of the doctor's eye: Recognizing English contact-induced features in Hungarian medical texts. In: Lengyel, Zsolt and Navracsics, Judit (eds.) *Second language lexical processes*. Clevedon/Buffalo/Toronto: Multilingual Matters, 83–97.

Keresztes, Kálmán. 1975. *Hungarian postpositions vs. English prepositions: A contrastive study. The Hungarian–English contrastive linguistics project*. Working Papers No. 7. East European Projects. Arlington, Virginia: Center for Applied Linguistics.

Keszler, Borbála. 1993. *Fejezetek az európai írásjelhasználat történetéből*. Budapest: ELTE BTK Mai Magyar Nyelvi Tanszéke.

Keszler, Borbála. 2004. A XVII. századi nyelvújítás és a magyar orvosi nyelv. [Language reform in the 17th century and the Hungarian language of medicine]. *Magyar Nyelvőr*, 128: 494–501.

Kevin MD.com http://www.kevinmd.com/blog/2007/04/defensive-medicine.html

King, M. H. and Barber, S.G. 1991. Towards better discharge summaries: brevity and structure. *West of England Medical Journal*, 2: 40–41.

King, Ruth. 2000. *The lexical basis of grammatical borrowing: A Prince Edward Island case study*. Amsterdam: John Benjamins.

Kirk, Jerome and Miller, Marc. 1986. *Reliability and validity in qualitative research*. London: Sage.

Kirkness, Alan. 1984. Aliens, denziens, hybrids and natives: foreign influence on the etymological structure of German vocabulary. In: Russ, Charles V. J. (ed.) *Foreign influences on German*. Dundee: Lochee.

Kirkness, Alan. 1997. Eurolatin and English today. *English Today,* 1: 3–8.

Kiss, Jenő. 2009. A tudományos nyelvek, az anyanyelv és az értelmiségi elit. [Languages of science languages, native tongue and the intellectual elite] *Magyar Tudomány,* 1: 67–73.

Klaudy, Kinga. 1997. *Fordítás I. Bevezetés a fordítás elméletébe* [Translation I. Introduction to the theory of translation]. Budapest: Scholastica.

Kloss, Heinz. 1929. *Nebensprachen: Eine sprachpolitische Studie über die Beziehungen eng verwandter Sprachgemeinschaften (Niederländisch, Deutsch, Jiddisch, Afrikaans, Friesisch, Pennsylvaniadeutsch).* Wien: Braumüller.

Komlósy, András. 1994. Complements and adjuncts. In: Kiefer, Ferenc and É. Kiss, Katalin (eds.) *Syntax and Semantics 27. The syntactical structure of Hungarian*. Budapest, 91–178.

Kontra, Miklós. 1981. *A nyelvek közötti kölcsönzés néhány kérdéséről, különös tekintettel 'elangolosodó' orvosi nyelvünkre*. [On the question of borrowing from different languages, with special respect to our 'Anglicized' medical jargon]. Nyelvtudományi Értekezések, 109. Budapest: Akdémiai Kiadó.

Kontra, Miklós. 1982. Medical languages in contact: English and Hungarian. *Angol Filológia Tanulmányok* [Hungarian Studies in English] XV. Debrecen: Kossuth Lajos Tudományegyetem, 75–89.

Kontra, Miklós. 1990. *Fejezetek a South Bend-i magyar nyelvhasználatból.* [The Hungarian language as spoken is South Bend, Indiana]. Budapest: MTA Nyelvtudományi Intézete.

Kontra, Miklós. 1992. Hungarians turned gateniks in 1990. *American Speech,* 67: 216–222.

Kontra, Miklós. 1997a. Angol nyelvi és kulturális imperializmus és magyar tanárképzés. [English language imperialism and culture, and Hungarian teacher training]. *Modern Nyelvoktatás,* 3: 3–14.

Kontra, Miklós. 1997b. On the right to use the language of one's choice in Slovakia. *Canadian Centre for Linguistic Rights Bulletin,* 4: 5–8.

Kontra, Miklós. 2001. Exchange: Disinformation on English in Hungary. *World Englishes,* 20: 113–114.

Kontra, Miklós (ed.). 2003. *Nyelv és társadalom a rendszerváltáskori Magyarországon.* Budapest: Osiris Kiadó.

Kontra, Miklós. 2006. Sustainable linguicism. In: Hinskens, Frans (ed.) *Language variation – European perspectives.* Amsterdam: John Benjamins, 97–126.

Kontra, Miklós. 2008. *Linguistic prejudice in Budapest and its correlates.* Paper presented at Sociolinguistics Symposium 17, Amsterdam, 5 April 2008.

Kontra, Miklós. 2009. Nyelvi genocídium az oktatásban a Kárpát-medencében. [Linguistic genocide in education in the Carpathian Basin] *Fórum Társadalomtudományi Szemle,* 4: 67–76.

Kontra, Miklós, Nekvapil, Jirí and Kielkiewicz-Janowiak, Agnieszka. 2010. Sociolinguistics in Hungary, the Czech Republic and Poland. In: Ball, Martin J. (ed.) *The Routledge handbook of sociolinguistics around the world.* Abingdon, Oxon: Routledge, 359–371.

Kontra, Miklós, Phillipson, Robert, Skutnabb-Kangas, Tove and Várady, Tibor (eds.) 1999. *Language: A right and a resource. Approaching linguistic human rights.* Budapest: Central European University Press.

Korchmáros, Valéria. M. 2006. *Hungarian step by step. Hungarian grammar - not only for Hungarians*. Szeged: Hungarian and Central European International Studies Center University of Szeged.

Kozma, László and Fóris, Ágota. 2002. Kultúra és nyelv a globalizációs folyamatban. [Culture and language in the process of globalization]. *Tudásmenedzsment,* 2: 3–14.

Kress, Gunther. 1986. Language in the media: The construction of the domains of public and private. *Media, Culture and Society,* 8.

Kripalani, Sunil, LeFevre, Frank and Phillips, Christopher O. 2007. Deficits in communication and information transfer between hospital-based and primary care physicians: Implications for patient safety and continuity of care. *Journal of American Medical Association,* 297: 831–841.

Kurtán, Zsuzsa. 2003. *Szakmai nyelvhasználat*. [Specific purpose language use]. Budapest: Nemzeti Tankönyvkiadó.

Kuteva, Tania and Heine, Bernd. 2003. On contact-induced grammaticalization. *Studies in language,* 3: 529–572.

Labov, William. 1966. *The social stratification of English in New York City*. Washington, DC: Centre for Applied Linguistics.

Labov, William. 1971. The notion of 'system' in creole languages. In: Hymes, Dell (ed.) *Pidginization and creolization of languages*. Cambridge: Cambridge University Press, 447–472.

Labov, William. 1972. *Sociolinguistic patterns*. Philadelphia: The University of Pennsylvania Press.

Laczkó, Tibor. 1995. *The syntax of Hungarian noun phrases. A lexical–functional approach*. MetaLinguistica 2. Frankfurt am Main: Peter Lang.

Laczkó, Tibor. 1999. A comprehensive analysis of three Hungarian participles. In: Bird, S., Carnie, A., Haugen, J. and Norquest, P. (eds.) *WCCFL 18 Proceedings*. Somerville: MA: Cascadilla Press, 272–284.

Laczkó, Krisztina and Mártonfi, Attila. 2005. *Helyesírás* [Orthography]. Budapest: Osiris Kiadó.

Ladegaard, Hans. 2000. Language attitudes and sociolinguistic behavior: Exploring attitude –behavior relations in language. *Journal of Sociolinguistics,* 4: 214–233.

Lakoff, Robin. 1972. Language in context. *Language,* 48: 907–927.

Lambert, Wallace E. 1967. A social psychology of bilingualism. *Journal of Social Issues,* 23: 91–109.

Lambert, Wallace E., Hodgson, R., Gardner, R. C. and Fillenbaum, S. 1960. Evaluational reactions to spoken languages. *Journal of Abnormal and Social Psychology,* 60: 44–51.

Lance, Donald M. 1975. Spanish–English code-switching. In: Cohen, Eduardo Hernandez-Chavez and Beltramo, Anthony (ed.) *El lenguaje de los chicanos.* Arlington, Virginia: Center for Applied Linguistics, 138–153.

Langslow, David. 1989. Latin technical language: Synonyms and Greek words in Latin medical terminology. *Transactions of the Philological Society,* 1: 33–53.

Langslow, David. 2000. *Medical Latin in the Roman Empire.* Oxford and New York: Oxford University Press.

Langslow, David. 2004. Etymology and history: For a study of medical language in Indo-European. In: Penney, J.H.W and Davies, Alan M. (eds.) *Indo-European Perspectives.* Oxford: Oxford University Press, 30–47.

Lanstyák, István. 1998. *A magyar nyelv szlovákiai változatainak sajátosságai.* [Characteristics of Hungarian language varieties in Slovakia]. Dunaszerdahely: Lilium Aurum.

Lanstyák, István. 2000. *A magyar nyelv Szlovákiában.* [The Hungarian language in Slovakia]. Budapest, Pozsony: Osiris Kiadó, Kalligram Könyvkiadó, MTA Kisebbségkutató Műhely.

Lanstyák, István. 2006. *Nyelvből nyelvbe: Tanulmányok a szókölcsönzésről, kódváltásról és fordításról.* [From one language into the other: Studies on borrowing, code-switching and translation]. Pozsony: Kalligram Könyvkiadó.

Lanstyák, István and Szabómihály, Gizella 1996. Contact varieties of Hungarian in Slovakia: A contribution to their description. *International Journal of the Sociology of Language*, 120: 111–130.

Lanstyák, István and Szabómihály, Gizella. 1997. *Magyar nyelvhasználat – iskola – kétnyelvűség (Nyelvi változók a szlovákiai és magyarországi középiskolások néhány csoportjának magyar nyelvhasználatában).* [Hungarian language use, schools and bilingualism: Language variants in the Hungarian language use of secondary school students in Slovakia and Hungary]. Pozsony: Kalligram Kiadó.

Le Page, Robert B. and Tabouret-Keller, A. 1985. *Acts of identity: Creole-based approaches to language and ethnicity*. Cambridge: Cambridge University Press.

Lee, Ching Ying, Yan, C. Yen, and Tsai, Chiu-Fan. 2006. Application of code-switching in medical communication: Institutional context of nursing practitioners. In: *Proceedings of the 2nd Annual English Conference of the Applied English Department.* Taipei County: Tung Nan Institute of Technology, 13–28.

Leenen, Henk, Gevers, Sjef and Pinet, Genevieve (eds.) 1993. *The rights of patients in Europe: A comparative study*. Deventer/Boston: Kluwer Law and Taxation Publishers.

Lefebvre, Claire. 1985. Grammaires en contact: Définition et perspectives de recherche. *Revue québécoise de Linguistique,* 14: 11–47.

Lengyel, Csaba and Fazekas, Tamás. 2009. A szerzett hosszú-QT-szindróma és a torsades de pointes kamrai tachycardia [Acquired long-QT-syndrome and torsadesde pointes ventricular tachycardia]. In: Fazekas, Tamás, Merkely, Béla, Papp, Gyula and Tenczer, József (eds.) Klinikai szív-elektrofiziológia és aritmológia [Clinical cardiac electrophysiology and arrhythmology]. Budapest: Akadémiai Kiadó, 673–724.

Lesznyák, Ágnes. 2004. *Communication in English as an international lingua franca: an exploratory case study.* Norderstedt: Books on Demand, GmbH.

Levitt, Theodore. 1983. The globalization of markets. *Harvard Business Review,* 61: 92–102.

Lewis, P. D. 1975. *Adjectives in descriptive anatomy*. Department of Linguistics and Phonetics. University of Leeds. MA/ELT Thesis.

Ligeti, Lajos. 1976. A magyar nyelv török kapcsolatai és ami körülöttük van. [The Turkic connections of Hungarian and what surrounds them] *Magyar Nyelv*, 72: 11–27 and 129–136.

Lippi-Green, Rosina. 1997. *English with an accent: Language, ideology, and discrimination in the United States*. New York: Routledge.

Loveday, Leo J. 1996. *Language contact in Japan: A socio-linguistic history*. Oxford: Clarendon Press.

Lowe, R., Schwartzman, J., Freeman, J., Quinn, L. and Zuckerman, S. 1998. Doctor talk and diabetes: Towards an analysis of the clinical construction of chronic illness. *Social Science and Medicine,* 47: 1267–1276.

Lozsádi, Károly and Czuriga, István. 2009. A kardiológia áttekintő története [Historical overview on Cardiology]. Budapest: Medicina.

Lyons, John. 1968. *Introduction to theoretical linguistics*. London: Cambridge University Press.

Maclean, Joan and Maher, John. 2001. Medical language. In: Mesthrie, Rajend (ed.) *Concise encyclopaedia of sociolinguistics*. Amsterdam: Elsevier, 256–259.

MacSwan, Jeff. 2005. Codeswitching and generative grammar: A critique of the MLF model and some remarks on "modified minimalism." *Bilingualism: Language and Cognition,* 1: 1–22.

Magay, Tamás. 1977. A chapter in the history of English lexicography in Hungary. The "concise dictionary of the English and Hungarian languages". *Angol Filológiai Tanulmányok,* 11: 19–27.

Mageean, R. J. 1986. Study of "discharge communications" from hospital. *British Medical Journal Clinical Research Edition,* 293: 1283–1284.

Maher, John. 1986. State of the art: English for medical purposes. *Language Teaching,* 2: 112–145.

Mahootian, Shahrzad. 1993. *A null theory of code-switching*. PhD dissertation. Northwestern University.

Manner, Paul A. 2007. Practicing defensive medicine: Not good for patients or physicians. at *http://www.aaos.org/news/bulletin/janfeb07/clinical2.asp.*

Martin, Emily. 1992. AES Distinguished lecture: The end of the body? *American Ethnology*, 19: 121–140.

Martinez, Glenn. 2008. Language-in-healthcare policy, interaction patterns, and unequal care on the U.S.-Mexico border. *Language Policy,* 7: 345–363.

Master, Peter. 1991. Active verbs with inanimate subjects in scientific prose. *ESP Journal,* 10: 15–33.

Mattingly, Cheryl. 1998. In search of the good: Narrative reasoning in clinical practice. *Medical Anthropology Quarterly,* 12: 273–297.

McArthur, Tom. 1998. A mutually defining circle of words: Some reflections on the making of the Longman Lexicon of Contemporary English. In: McArthur, Tom (ed.) *Living words: language, lexicography, and the knowledge revolution*. Exeter: University of Exeter Press.

McGroarty, Mary. 1996. Language attitudes, motivation and standards. In: McKay, Sandra and Hornberger, Nancy (eds.) *Sociolinguistics and language teaching*. Cambridge: Cambridge University Press, 3–46.

McLuhan, Marshall. 1969. *Understanding media: The extension of man*. New York: New American Library.

Medgyes, Péter. 1993. The national L2 curriculum in Hungary. *Annual Review of Applied Linguistics,* 13: 24–36.

Medgyes, Péter and Kaplan, Robert. 1992. Discourse in a foreign language: The example of Hungarian scholars. *International Journal of the Sociology of Language,* 98: 67–100.

Medgyes, Péter and László, Mónika. 2001. The foreign English competence of Hungarian scholars: Ten years later. In: Ammon, Ulrich (ed.) *The dominance of English as a language of science: Effects on other languages and language communities*. Berlin/New York: Mouton de Gruyter, 261–286.

Meier, Diane E., Back, Anthony L. and Morrison, R. Sean. 2001. The inner life of physicians and care of the seriously ill. *Journal of the American Medical Association,* 286: 3007–3014.

Mesthrie, Rajend. 1995. Review of J.K. Chambers, sociolinguistic theory. *English World-Wide,* 16: 2.

Mészáros, Ágnes. 2009. A magyar egészségbiztosítási szakszókincs kialakulásának és módosulásának vizsgálata. [Investigating the development and changes in the vocabulary of Hungarian health insurance] *Alkalmazott Nyelvtudomány,* 1–2: 17–34.

Miethaner, Ulrich. 2000. Orthographic transcriptions of non-standard varieties: The case of earlier African-American English. *Journal of Sociolinguistics,* 4: 534–560.

Milroy, John. 1992. A social model for the interpretation of language change. In: Rissanen, Matti (ed.) *History of Englishes: New methods and interpretations in historical linguistics*. Berlin: Mouton de Gruyter, 72–91.

Mintz, David. 1992. What's in a word: The distancing function of language in medicine. *Journal of Medical Humanities,* 4: 223–233.

Minya, Károly. 2003. *Mai magyar nyelvújítás. Szókészletünk módosulása a neologizmusok tükrében a rendszerváltozástól az ezredfordulóig*. [Recent language reform in Hungary. Changes in our lexicon considering neologisms from 1989 to 2000]. Segédkönyvek a nyelvészet tanulmányozásához. [Handbooks in linguistics]. XVI. Budapest: Tinta Könyvkiadó.

Modiano, Marko. 1999. Standard English(es) and educational practices for the world's lingua franca. *English Today,* 15: 3–13.

Molnos, Angéla. 2007. Gyógyítsunk magyarul! [We should treat patients in Hungarian] Debrecen: A Lélektani Szaknyelv Megújításáért Alapítvány.

Montalt, Vicent and Davies, Maria Gonzalez. 2007. *Medical translation step by step*. Manchester: St. Jerome Publishing.

Moore, Kate and Varantola, Krista. 2005. Anglo–Finnish contacts: Collisions and collusions. In: Anderman, Gunilla and Rogers, Margaret (eds.) *In and out of English: For better, for worse?* Clevedon: Multilingual Matters Ltd, 133–52.

Moravcsik, Edith. A. 1978. Language contact. In: Greenberg, Joseph Harold (ed.) *Universals of human language*. 1. Stanford: Stanford University Press, 94–122.

Mühlhauser, Peter. 1986. *Pidgin and creole linguistics*. Oxford: Basil Blackwell.

Murray, Heather and Dingwall, Silvia. 2001. The dominance of English at European universities. In: Ammon, Ulrich (ed.) *The dominance of English as a language of science: Effects on other languages and language communities*. Berlin–New York: Mouton de Gruyter, 85–112.

Muysken, Pieter. 1985. Linguistic dimensions of language contact: The state of the art in interlinguistics. *Rev. québécoise de Linguistique,* 14: 49–76.

Muysken, Pieter. 1999. Three processes of borrowing: borrowability revisited. In: Extra, Guus and Verhoeven, Ludo (eds.) *Bilingualism and migration*. Berlin/New York: Mouton de Gruyter, 229–246.

Muysken, Pieter. 2000. *Bilingual speech: A typology of code-mixing*. Cambridge: Cambridge University Press.

Myers, Greg. 1989. The pragmatics of politeness in scientific articles. *Applied Linguistics,* 1: 1–35.

Myers, Greg. 1990. *Writing biology: Texts in the social construction of scientific knowledge*. Madison: University of Wisconsin Press.

Myers-Scotton, Carol. 1993. *Dueling languages: Grammatical structure in code-switching*. Oxford: Clarendon Press.

Myers-Scotton, Carol. 1997. Code-switching. In: Coulmas, Florian (ed.) *The handbook of sociolinguistics*. Oxford: Blackwell Publishing, 217–237.

Myers-Scotton, Carol. 2002. *Contact linguistics: Bilingual encounters and grammatical outcomes*. Oxford: Oxford University Press.

Myers-Scotton, Carol and Jake, Janice L. 2000. Matching lemmas in a bilingual language competence and production model: Evidence from intrasentential code-switching. In: Wei, Li (ed.) *The bilingualism reader*. London/New York: Routledge, 281–318.

Nádasdy, Ádám. 1989. Consonant length in recent borrowings into Hungarian. *Acta Linguistica Hungarica,* 1–4: 195–213.

Nádasdy, Ádám. 2002. Mi az angol? [What is the English language?] *Magyar Narancs,* 11/14.

Náray-Szabó, Gábor and Sztáray, Bálint. 2001. Tizedesvessző vagy tizedespont? Viták-vélemények. [Decimal comma or point? Dis-cussions and opinions]. *Magyar Tudomány,* 5: 595.

Navarro, F. A. 1996. Englisch oder Deutsch? Die Sprache der Medizin aufgrund der in der Deutschen Medizinischen Wochenschrift erschienen Literaturangaben (1920 bis 1995). *Deutsche Medizinische Wochenschrift,* 121: 1561–1566.

Nelde, Peter Hans. 1997. Language conflict. In: Coulmas, Florian (ed). *The handbook of sociolinguistics*. Oxford: Blackwell, 285–300.

Nelde, Peter Hans. 2002. Language contact. In: Kaplan, Robert B. (ed.) *The Oxford Handbook of Applied Linguistics*. Oxford/New York: Oxford University Press, 325–334.

Nelde, Peter Hans, Strubell, M. and Williams, G. 1996. *Euromosaic: Production and reproduction of minority language groups in the EU.* European Commission, Luxembourg.

New Jersey Administrative Code Title 8 chapter 43G. Hospital Licensing Standards. 101-102 quoting N.J.S.A. 26:2H-1 et seq. Access: January 27, 2005.
http://www.nj.gov/health/healthfacilities/documents/ac/njac43g_hoslicstd.pdf.

Ngũgĩ, Thiong. 1998. *Penpoints, gunpoints, and dreams: Towards a critical theory of the arts and the state in Africa*. Oxford: Oxford University Press.

Nicol, Janet (ed.) 2001. *One mind, two languages: Bilingual language processing.* Oxford: Blackwell Press.

Nylenna, Magne, Riis, Povl and Karlsson, Yngve. 1994. Multiple blinded reviews of the same two manuscripts: Effects of referee characteristics and publication language. *Journal of the American Medical Association,* 272: 149–151.

Odlin, Terence. 1989. *Language transfer: Cross-linguistic influence in language learning*. Cambridge: Cambridge University Press.

Ogden, David J. 2007. Time to drop eponyms: Curbing medicalese is the issue. *British Medical Journal,* 335: 528.

Ong, L.M.L., de Haes, J.C., Itoos, A.M. and Lammes, F.B. 1995. Doctor–patient communication: A review of the literature. *Social Science and Medicine,* 40: 903–918.

Onysko, Alexander. 2005. English code-switching in the German news-magazine *Der Spiegel. TRANS. Internet-Zeitschrift für Kulturwissenschaften*. 16.

Onysko, Alexander. 2007. *Anglicisms in German. Borrowing, lexical productivity, and written codeswitching*. Berlin: de Gruyter.

Országh, László. 1968. The life and death of English words in the Hungarian language. *The New Hungarian Quarterly,* 31: 180–188.

Országh, László. 1977. Angol eredetű elemek a magyar szókészletben. [English elements in the Hungarian lexicon]. *Nyelvtudományi Érte-kezések.* [Linguistic Studies]. 93. Budapest: Akadémiai Kiadó.

Oxford, Rebecca L. and Shearin, Jill. 1994. Language learning motivation: Expanding the theoretical framework. *Modern Language Journal,* 78: 12–28.

Oxford, Rebecca L. 1996. Employing a questionnaire to assess the use of language learning strategies. *Applied Language Learning,* 1–2: 25–45.

Pap, Leo. 1949. *Portuguese–American speech*. New York: King's Crown.

Parsons, Talcott. 1951. *The social system*. Glencoe, Il: Free Press.

Parsons, Talcott. 1958. Definitions of health and illness in the light of American values and social structure. In: Jaco, E. Gartley (ed.) *Patients, physicians and illness*. New York: Free Press.

Parsons, Talcott. 1978. *Action theory and the human condition*. New York: Free Press.

Patton, Michael Q. 1987. *How to use qualitative methods in evaluation*. London: Sage.

Paul, Hermann. 1880. *Prinzipien der Sprachgeschichte*. Halle: Max Niemeyer. (Translated into English by Strong, H. A. in 1970. *Prin-ciples of the history of language*. College Park: McGroth Publishing Company).

Pauwels, Anne. 1986. *Immigrant dialects and language maintenance in Australia*. Dordrecht: Foris.

Peckham, Donald, Kalocsai, Karolina, Kovács, Emőke and Sherman, Tamás. 2008. *English and multilingualism, or English only in a multilingual Europe?* Szeged: University of Szeged, MS.

Pendleton, David and Hasler, John (eds.) 1983. *Doctor – patient communication*. New York: Academic Press.

Pennycook, Alaister. 1995. *The cultural politics of English as an interna-tional language*. London/New York: Longman.

Pennycook, Alastair. 2003. Global Englishes, rip slyme, and performativity. *Journal of Sociolinguistics,* 4: 513–533.

Péntek, János. 1997. Kontaktusjelenségek és folyamatok a magyar nyelv kisebbségi változataiban. [Contact induced features and processes in the Hungarian minority languages] *Nyelv- és Irodalomtudományi Közlemények,* 1: 37–50.

Péntek, János (ed.) 2004. *Magyarul megszólaló tudomány*. [Science in Hungarian]. Budapest: Lucidus Kiadó.

Péntek, János and Benő, Attila. 2003. Nyelvi jogok Romániában. [Language rights in Romania]. In: Nádor, Orsolya and Szarka, László (eds.) *Nyelvi jogok, kisebbségek, nyelvpolitika Kelet–Közép–Európában.* [Language rights, minorities and language policy in East Central Europe]. Budapest: Akadémiai Kiadó, 123–147.

Petzold, Ruth and Berns, Margie. 2000. Catching up with Europe: Speakers and functions of English in Hungary. *World Englishes,* 19: 113–124.

Pfaff, Carol. 1979. Constraints on language mixing: Intrasentential code-switching and borrowing in Spanish/English. *Language,* 2: 291–318.

Phillipson, Robert. 1992. *Linguistic imperialism.* Oxford: Oxford University Press.

Phillipson, Robert. 2001. *English yes, but equal language rights first.* Access: July 17, 2007.
http://www.guardian.co.uk/theguardian/2001/apr/19/guardianweekly.guardianweekly1

Phillipson, Robert. 2003. *English-only Europe? Challenging language policy.* London/New York: Routledge.

Phillipson, Robert. 2006. English, a cuckoo in the European higher education nest of languages? *European Journal of English Studies,* 1: 13–32.

Phillipson, Robert. 2008. The linguistic imperialism of neoliberal empire. *Critical Inquiry in Language Studies,* 1: 1–43.

Phillipson, Robert. 2009. *Some partner languages are more equal than others.* Presented at the Bamako International Forum on Multilingualism, organized by the African Academy of languages (www.acalan.org), Bamako, Mali, 19–21 January 2009.

Phillipson, Robert and Skutnabb-Kangas, Tove. 1996. English-only world-wide, or language ecology? *TESOL Quarterly.* In: Ricento, Thomas and Hornberger, Nancy (eds.) Special–Topic Issue: Language Planning and Policy, 429–452.

Pigg, Stacy Leigh. 1996. The credible and the credulous: the question of villager's belief in Nepal. *Cultural Anthropology,* 11: 160–201.

Pique-Angordans, Jordi and Posteguillo, Santiago. 2006. Medical discourse and academic genres. In: Brown, Keith (ed.) *Encyclopedia of language and linguistics.* (2nd edition). Volume 6. Amsterdam: Elsevier, 649–657.

Pogarell, Reiner and Schröder, Markus. 1999. *Wörterbuch überflüssiger Anglizismen*, IFB Verlag: Paderborn.

Polenz, Peter. 1967. Fremdwort und Lehnwort sprachwissenschaftlich betrachtet. *Muttersprache,* 77: 65–80.

Poplack, Shana. 1980. Sometimes I'll start a sentence in English y termino en espanol. *Linguistics,* 18: 581–616.

Poplack, Shana (ed.) 2000. *The English history of African American English.* Oxford: Blackwell.

Poplack, Shana and Meecham, Marjory. 1998. Introduction: How languages fit together in code-mixing. *International Journal of Bilingualism,* 2: 127–139.

Poplack, Shana and Sankoff, David. 1984. Borrowing: The synchrony of integration. *Linguistics,* 22: 99–135.

Preston, Dennis. 2004. Language with an attitude. In: Chambers, J.K., Trudgill, Peter and Schilling-Estes, Natalie (eds.) *The handbook of language variation and change.* Malden: Blackwell Publishing, 40–67.

Prince, Ellen. 1988. On pragmatic change: The borrowing of discourse functions. *Journal of Pragmatics,* 12: 505–518.

Proshina, Z. G. 2001. *Angliiskii yazyk i kul'tura Vostochnoi Azii.* Vladivostok: Far Eastern University Publ.

Putnam, Hilary. 1975. The meaning of "meaning". In: Gunderson, Keith (ed.) *Language, mind and knowledge.* Minneapolis: University of Minnesota Press, 215–271.

Rajadurai, Joanne. 2007. Intelligibility studies: a consideration of empirical and ideological issues. *World Englishes,* 1: 87–98.

Raley, Rita. 1998. *What is global English?* Access: December 20, 2007. http://www.english.ucsb.edu/faculty/rraley/index2.html.

Ramanathan, Vaidehi. 2009. Introduction to thematic issue: Language policies and health. *Language Policy,* 1: 1–7.

Rando, Gaetano. 1973. A quantitaive analysis of the use of Anglicisms in written standard Italian during the1960s. *Italica*, 1: 73–82.

Rannut, Mart. 2004. *Language planning in Estonia: Past and present*. Working Paper 16. Ciemen/Mercator.

Rao, Pratibha, Andrei, Anca, Fried, Alvin, Gonzalez, David and Shine, Daniel. 2005. Assessing quality and efficiency of discharge summaries. *American Journal of Medical Quality,* 6: 337–343.

Rébék-Nagy, Gábor. 1997. *Modulation of authors' claims in the introduction and discussion sections of medical research articles*. Birmingham: Aston University. MSc dissertation.

Reed, Carroll E. 1948. The adaption of English to Pennsylvania German morphology. *American Speech,* 23: 239–44.

Richards, Ivor Armstrong. 1943. *Basic English and its uses*. London: Kegan Paul, Trench, Trubner and Co.

Riska, Elianne. 2001. Health professions and occupations. In: Cockerham, William C. (ed.) *The Blackwell companion to medical sociology*. Malden: Blackwell Publisher, 144–159.

Roberts, Celia. 2006. Doctors and patients in multilingual settings. In: Brown, Keith (ed.) *Encyclopedia of language and linguistics*. (2nd edition). Volume 7. Amsterdam: Elsevier, 741–748.

Roberts, G.V. 1994. Nurse/patient communication within a bilingual health care setting. *British Journal of Nursing,* 2: 60–67.

Robertson, Roland. 1992. *Globalization: Social theory and global culture*. London: Sage.

Rogers, Carl R. 1957. The necessary and sufficient conditions of therapeutic personality change. *Journal of Consulting Psychology,* 21: 95–103.

Romaine, Suzanne. 1989. *Pidgin and creole languages*. London: Longman.

Romaine, Suzanne. 2003. Multilingualism. In: Aronoff, Mark and Rees-Miller, Janie (eds.) *The handbook of linguistics*. Oxford: Blackwell Publishing, 512–533.

Ross, Malcolm D. 1988. *Proto Oceanic and the Austronesian languages of western Melanesia. Pacific Linguistics. C–98*. Canberra: The Australian National University.

Ross, Malcolm D. 2003. Metatypy. In: Brown, Keith (ed.) *Encyclopedia of language and linguistics*. Volume 7. Oxford: Elsevier, 429–432.

Rothkopf, David. 1997. In praise of cultural imperialism. *Foreign policy,* 38–53.

Rounds, Carol. 2009. *Hungarian: An essential grammar*. Oxon: Routledge.

Rounds, Patricia. 1982. *Hedging in written academic discourse: Precision and flexibility.* Mimeo: The University of Michigan.

Sackley, Catherine M. and Pound, Kate. 2002. Stroke patients entering nursing home care: a content analysis of discharge letters. *Clinical Rehabilitation,* 16: 736–740.

Sager, Juan C., Dungworth, David and McDonald, Peter F. 1980. *English special languages: principles and practice in science and technology*. Wiesbaden: Oscar Brandstetter Verlag.

Sajnovics, János. 1770 *Demonstratio. Idioma Ungarorum et Lapponum idem esse*. Tyrnavia.

Salager-Meyer, Francoise. 1994. Hedges and textual communicative function in medical English written discourse. *English for Specific Purposes,* 2: 149–170.

Salager-Meyer, Francoise, Ariza, Alcaraz and Zambrano, Nahirana. 2003. The scimitar, the dagger and the glove: Intercultural differences in the rhetoric of criticism in Spanish, French and English medical discourse (1930–1995). *English for Specific Purposes,* 22: 223–247.

Samarin, William J. 1968. Lingua francas of the world. In: Fishman, Joshua (ed.) *Readings in the Sociology of Language*. The Hague: Mouton, 660–672.

Sándor, Klára. 2000. National feeling or responsibility: The case of the Csángó language revitalization. *Multilingua,* 19: 141–168.

Sándor, Klára. 2001. Nyelvművelés és ideológia. [Language cultivation and ideology]. In: Sándor, Klára (ed.) Nyelv, nyelvi jogok, oktatás. [Language, language rights and education]. Szeged: JGyF Kiadó. 153–216.

Sankoff, Gilian. 1980. Multilingualism in Papua New Guinea. In: Sankoff, Gilian (ed.) *The social life of language*. Philadelphia: University of Pennsylvania Press.

Sankoff, David. 1998. A formal production-based explanation of the facts of code-switching. *Bilingualism, language and cognition,* 1: 39–50.

Sankoff, Gilian. 2004. Linguistic outcomes of language contact. In: Chambers, J.K., Trudgill, Peter and Schilling-Estes, Nancy (eds.) *The handbook of language variation and change*. Malden: Blackwell Publishing, 638–669.

Sankoff, David and Poplack, Shana. 1981. A formal grammar for code-switching. *Papers in Linguistics: International Journal of Human Communication,* 1: 3–45.

Sapir, Edward. 1921. *Language*. New York: Harcourt Brace and Company.

Scheele, Brigitte and Groeben, Norbert. 1988. *Dialog–Konsens–Methoden zur Rekonstruktion Subjektiver Theorien.* Tübingen: Francke.

Scheler, Manfred. 1977. *Der englische Wortschatz.* Berlin: Schmidt.

Schmidt, Johannes. 1872. *Die Verwandtschaftsverhältnisse der indogermanen Sprachen*. Weimar.

Schneider, Edgar W. 2004. Investigating variation and change in written documents. In: Chambers, J.K., Trudgill, Peter and Schilling-Estes, Nancy (eds.). *The handbook of language variation and change.* Malden: Blackwell Publishing, 67–97.

Schuchardt, Hugo. 1928. *Schuchardt Brevier: Ein Vadmecum der allgemeinen prachwissenschaft.* Halle: Niemeyer.

Schuchardt, Hugo. 1884. *Slawo–Deutsches und Slawo–Italienisches. Dem Herrn Franz von Miklosich zum 20. November 1883*. Graz: Leuschner/Lubensky.

Schumann, John H. 1975. Affective factors and the problem of age in second language acquisition. *Language Learning,* 205–235.

Scotton, Carol. Myers and Ury, William. 1977. Bilingual strategies: The social functions of code-switching. *International Journal of the Sociology of Language,* 13: 5–20.

Seliger, Herbert W. and Shohamy, E. 1989. *Second language research methods.* Oxford: Oxford University Press.

Selinker, Larry. 1972. Interlanguage. *IRAL (International Review of Applied Linguistics in Language Teaching),* 10: 209–231.

Semenets, O. E. 1985. *Sotsial'nyi kontekst i yazykovoe razvitie: Territorial'naya i sotsial'naya differentsiatsiya angliiskogo yazyka v razvivayuschikhsia stranakh.* Kiev: Vyscha Shkola.

Sensing, Jozien and Dronkers, Johan. 1991. Instrumental and affective aspects of physician behavior. *Medical Care,* 30: 283–297.

Shapiro, Michael C. and Schiffman, Harold F. 1981. *Language and society in South Asia.* Delhi: Motilal Banarsidass.

Shome, Raka and Hegde, Radha S. 2002. Postcolonial approaches to communication: Charting the terrain, engaging the intersections. *Communication Theory,* 12: 249–270.

Siguan, Miguel. 2001. English and the language of science: On the unity of language and the plurality of languages. In: Ammon, Ulrich (ed.) *The dominance of English as a language of science: Effects on other languages and language communities.* Berlin/New York: Mouton de Gruyter, 59–70.

Silva-Corvalan, Carmen. 1994. *Language contact and change: Spanish in Los Angeles*. Oxford: Oxford University Press.

Silverman, David. 1987. *Communication and medical practice*. Thousand Oaks: Sage.

Silverman, David. 2000. *Interpreting qualitative data: Methods for analysing talk, text and interaction*. London: Sage.

Sinclair, John. 1990. *English grammar*. London: Harper-Collins Publishers.

Skeleton, J. 1997. How to tell the truth in the British Medical Journal: Patterns of judgement in the 19th and 20th centuries. In: Markkanen, Raija and Scroder, Hartmut (eds.) *Hedging and discourse. Approaches to the analysis of a pragmatic phenomenon in academic texts*. Berlin: Walter de Gruyter, 42–63.

Skutnabb-Kangas, Tove. 1984. *Bilingualissn or not: The education of minorities.* Clevedon: Multilingual Matters.

Skutnabb-Kangas, Tove. 1996. Educational language choice – multilingual diversity or monolingual reductionism? In: Hellinger, Marlis and Ammon, Ulrich (eds.) *Contrastive sociolinguistics*. Berlin/New York: Mouton de Gruyter, 175–204.

Skutnabb-Kangas, Tove. 2000. *Linguistic genocide in education, or world-wide diversity and human rights?* Mahwah: Lawrence Erlbaum Associates, Inc. Publishers.

Skutnabb-Kangas, Tove. 2001. The globalisation of (educational) language rights. *International Review of Education,* 3–4: 201–219.

Solomon, J.K., Maxwell, R.B. and Hopkins, A.P. 1995. Content of a discharge summary from a medical ward: Views of general practitioners and hospital doctors. *Royal College of Physicians London,* 29: 307–310.

Sorensen, Arthur. 1967. Multilingualism in the North West Amazon. *American Anthropologist,* 69: 670–84.

Spatz, H., Engel, J., Holzel, D. and Jauch, K.W. 2001. The surgical discharge summary: A lack of substantial clinical information may affect the postop treatment of rectal cancer patients. *Langenbecks Archives of Surgery,* 386: 350–356.

Spitzmüller, Jürgen. 2005. *Metasprachdiskurse. Einstellungen zu Anglizismen und ihre wissenschaftliche Rezeption*. Berlin: de Gruyter.

Sridhar, S. N. and Sridhar, Kamal. 1980. The syntax and psycholinguistics of bilingual code mixing. *Canadian Journal of Psychology,* 4: 409–418.

Stanforth, Anthony William. 1984. Against the tide – the influence of German on English. In: Russ, Charles V. J. (ed.) *Foreign influences on German,* 109–125.

Steffen, Therese. 2002. Between transnationalism and globalization: Kara Walker's cultural hybridities. In: Ilmberger, Frances and Robinson, Alan (eds.) *Globalization*. Tübingen: Gunter Narr Verlag, 89–111.

Strevens, Patar. 1980. *Teaching English as an international language: From practice to principle.* Oxford: Pergamon Press.

Studdert, David M., Mello, Michelle M., Sage, William M., DesRoches, Catherine M., Peugh, Jordon, Zapert, Kinga and Brennan, Troyen A. 2005. Defensive medicine among high-risk specialist physicians in a volatile malpractice environment. *Journal of the American Medical Association.* 293:2609-2617.

Swales, John. 1981. *Aspects of article introductions*. Aston Monographs. No.1. The University of Aston, Language Studies Unit.

Swales, John. 1985. *Episodes in English*. Oxford: Pergamon Press.

Swales, John. 1990. *Genre analysis: English in academic and research settings.* Cambridge: Cambridge University Press.

Swales, John. 1997. English as Tyrannosaurus rex. *World Englishes,* 16: 373–382.

Szepesy, Gyula. 1986. *Nyelvi babonák*. [Language myths] Budapest: Gondolat.

Taavitsainen, Irma. 1994a. On the evolution of scientific writings from 1375 to 1675: Repertoire of emotive features. In: Fernández, Francisco, Fuster, Miguel and Calvo, Juan Jose (eds.) *English historical linguistics*. Amsterdam: John Benjamins, 329–342.

Taavitsainen, Irma. 1994b. Subjectivity as a text–type marker in historical stylistics. *Language and Literature,* 3: 197–212.

Taavitsainen, Irma. 2001. Language History and the Scientific Register. In: Diller, Hans Jürgen and Görlach, Manfred (eds.) *Towards a history of English as a history of genres*. Heidelberg: C. Winter, 185–202.

Taavitsainen, Irma. 2006. Medical communication, lingua franca. In: Brown, Keith (ed.) *Encyclopedia of language and linguistics*. (2nd edition). Volume 7. Amsterdam: Elsevier, 643–644.

Taavitsainen, Irma and Pahta, Paivi. 2000. Conventions of professional writing: The medical case report in a historical perspective. *Journal of English Linguistics,* 28: 60–76.

Taavitsainen, Irma and Pahta, Paivi. 2003. English in Finland, globalization, language awareness and questions of identity. *English Today,* 4: 3–15.

Tardy, Christine. 2004. The role of English in scientific communication: lingua franca or Tyrannosaurus rex? *Journal of English for Academic Purposes,* 3: 247–269.

Task Force on Aboriginal Languages and Cultures. 2005. *Towards a New Beginning. A foundational report for a strategy to revitalize First Nation, Inuit and Métis languages and cultures*. Report to the Minister of Canadian Heritage, June 2005. Ottawa: Aboriginal Languages Directorate. www.aboriginallanguagestaskforce.ca. Access: 15th August, 2008

ten Have, Paul. 1989. The Consultation as a genre. In: Torode, Brian (ed.) *Text and talk as social practice.* Dordrecht/Providence R.I.: Foris, 115–135.

ten Have, Paul. 2001. *Sequential structures in doctor–patient interaction: Ethnomethodology and history.* Paper presented at the conference 'Structure and emergence of professionalized "Praxis"'. J. W. Goethe Universität, Frankfurt, Germany, September 26 – 28. http://www2.fmg.uva.nl/emca/seqstruct.htm. Access: July 12, 2007.

Thomason, Sarah Grey. 1997a. On mechanisms of interference. In: Eliasson, Stig and Jahr, Ernst H. (eds.) *Language and its ecology: Essays in memory of Einar Haugen*. Berlin: de Gruyter, 181–207.

Thomason, Sarah Grey. 1997b. On the unpredictability of contact effects. Access: March 31, 2008. http://www-personal.umich.edu/~thomason/papers/unpred.pdf.

Thomason, Sarah Grey. 2001. *Language contact: An introduction.* Edinburgh and Washington, DC: Edinburgh University Press and Georgetown University Press.

Thomason, Sarah Grey. 2003. Contact as a source of language change. In: Janda, Richard D. and Joseph, Brian D. (eds.) *A handbook of historical linguistics*. Oxford: Blackwell, 687–712.

Thomason, Sarah Grey. 2005. Typological and theoretical aspects of Hungarian in contact with other languages. In: Fenyvesi, Anna (ed.) *Hungarian language contact outside Hungary: Studies on Hungarian as a minority language*. IMPACT. Volume 20. Amsterdam–Philadelphia: John Benjamins Publishing Company, 11–28.

Thomason, Sarah Grey. 2009. Why universals versus contact-induced change? In: Markku, Filppula (ed.) *Vernacular universals and language contacts: evidence from varieties of English and beyond*. London: Taylor and Francis, 349–362.

Thomason, Sarah Grey and Kaufman, Thomas. 1988. *Language contact, creolization and genetic linguistics*. Berkeley, CA: University of California Press.

Todd, Loreto. 1987. *An introduction to linguistics*. Beirut: York Press.

Tompa, József (ed.). 1969–1970. *A mai magyar nyelv rendszere I., II* [The structure of present day Hungarian, Vols 1 and 2]. Budapest: Akadémiai Kiadó.

Tóth, Mária. 1987. *Az orvosi szakszókincs fejlődésének története az orvosi helyesírás tükrében.* [History of the development of medical vocabulary reflected in medical orthography] Budapest. MA thesis.

Tóthfalusi, István. 1998. Hogy mi ne legyünk angol nyelvi gyarmat. [That we should not be an English–language colony]. *Magyar Nyelvőr,* 122: 403–417.

Trask, Robert Lawrence. 1993. *A dictionary of grammatical terms in linguistics*. New York: Routledge.

Treanor, Paul. 1999. *Making Europe multilingual*. Access: May 30, 2006. http://www.heise.de/tp/english/inhalt/te/1155/1.html.

Truchot, Claude. 2001. The languages of science in France: Public debate and language policies. In: Ammon, Ulrich (ed.) *The dominance of English as a language of science: Effects on other languages and language communities.* Berlin/New York: Mouton de Gruyter, 167–176.

Truchot, Claude. 2002. *Language policy division directorate of school, out-of-school and higher education.* Strasbourg: DGIV Council of Europe.

Trudgill, Peter. 1992. *Introducing language and society*. London: Penguin.

Tsuda, Yukio. 1994. The diffusion of English: Its impact on culture and communication. *Keio Communication Review,* 16: 49–61.

Unseld, Dieter Werner. 2006. Angol–magyar: Magyar–angol orvosi szótár [English–Hungarian: Hungarian–English medical dictionary]. Budapest: Medicina Könyvkiadó Zrt.

Untermann, Jürgen. 1978. *Etymologie und Terminus technicus*. Unpublished manuscript.

Valdes-Fallis, Guadalupe. 1976. Code-switching in bilingual Chicano poetry. *Hispania*, 59: 877-886.

Van Coetsem, Frans. 1988. *Loan phonology and the two transfer types in language contact.* Dordrecht: Foris.

van Leeuwen, Thed N., Moed, Henk F., Tussen, Robert J.W., Visser, Martin S. and van Raan, Anthony F.J. 2001. Language biases in the coverage of the Science Citation Index and its consequences for international comparisons of national research performance. *Scientometrics,* 51: 335–346.

van Naerssen, M. Margaret. 1985. Medical records: One variation of physicians' language. *International Journal of the Sociology of Language,* 5: 43–73.

Vandenbroucke, Jan P. 1989. On not being born a native speaker of English. *British Medical Journal,* 298: 1461–1462.

Véghelyi, Péter and Csink, Tamás (eds.). 1971. Angol–magyar orvosi szótár [English–Hungarian medical dictionary]. Budapest: Terra.

Véghelyi, Péter and Csink, Tamás (eds.). 1971. Magyar–angol orvosi szótár [Hungarian–English medical dictionary]. Budapest: Terra.

Vegni, Elena, Mauri, Emanuela and Moja, Egido. 2004. Stories of doctors with patients in pain. A qualitative research on physicians' perspective. *Supportive Care in Cancer,* 13: 18–25.

Vegni, Elena, Visioli, Sonia and Moja, Egido. 2005. When talking to the patient is difficult: The physician's perspective. *Communication and medicine,* 2: 69–76.

Vegni, Elena, Zannini, L., Visioli, Sonia and Moja, Egido. 2001. Giving bad news: A GPs' narrative perspective. *Supportive Care in Cancer,* 9: 390–396.

Venuti, Lawrence. 1995. *The translator's invisibility*. London and New York: Routledge.

Viereck, Wolfgang. 1986. The influence of English on German in the past and in the Federal Republic of Germany. In: Vierick, Wolgang and Bald, W. Dietrich (eds.) *English in contact with other languages: Studies in honour of Broder Carstensen on the occasion of his 60th birthday*. Budapest: Akadémiai Kiadó, 107–128.

Viereck, Wolfgang. 1996. English in Europe: Its nativisation and use as a lingua franca, with special reference to German speaking countries. In: Hartmann, Reinhard (ed.) *The English language in Europe*. Exeter: Intellect, 16–24.

Vildomec, Veroboj. 1963. *Multilingualism*. Leyden: A.V. Sythoff.

Vogt, H. Friedrich. 1954. Language contacts. *Word,* 2–3: 365–374.

Wang, Yan. and Bai, Y. 2007. A corpus-based syntactic study of medical research article titles. *Science Direct,* 35: 388–399.

Warta, Vilmos. 2006. Szerzői hang. Angol nyelvű orvosi esetismertetések műfajelemzése korpusznyelvészeti módszerekkel. [Author's voice: Analysing English medical case reports by corpus linguistic methods] Pécs: Pécsi Tudományegyetem. PhD dissertation.

Wear, Andrew, French, R.K. and Lonie, Iain.M. 2009. *The medical renaissance.* Cambridge: Cambridge University Press.

Weinreich, Uriel. 1953. *Languages in contact.* New York: Linguistic Circle of New York.

Weinreich, Uriel. 1988. *Wege der Sprachkultur.* Stuttgart: Deutscher Taschenbuch Verlag.

Weinreich, Uriel, Labov, William and Herzog, Marvin. 1968. Empirical foundations for a theory of language change. In: Lehmann, Winfred and Malkiel, Yakov (eds.) *Directions for historical linguistics.* Austin: University of Texas Press, 97–195.

Weiss, Andreas von. 1959. *Hauptprobleme der Zweisprachigkeit.* Heidelberg.

Wells, David. 1986. *The Penguin dictionary of curious and interesting numbers.* Middlesex, England: Penguin Books.

West, Candace. 1984. *Routine complications: Troubles with talk between doctors and patients.* Bloomington: Indiana University Press.

West, Candace. 1990. Not just "doctors' orders": Directive–response sequences in patients' visits to women and men physicians. *Discourse and Society,* 1: 85–113.

Wexler, Paul. 1974. *Purism and language. A case study in modern Ukrainian and Belorussian nationalism (1840-1967).* Bloomington: Indiana University Press.

Whitney, William Dwight. 1881. On mixture in language. *Transactions of the American Philological Association*, 12: 5–26.

Wierzbicka, Anna. 1991. *Cross-cultural pragmatics: The semantics of human interaction.* Berlin: Mouton de Gruyter.

Wilce, James. M. 2009. Medical discourse. *Annual reviews of anthropology,* 38: 199–215.

Winford, Donald. 2003. *An introduction to contact linguistics.* Malden, MA: Blackwell.

WHO (World Health Organization). 2009. Media centre. Access: 22 December 2009. http://www.who.int/mediacentre/factsheets/fs317/en/index.html

Wodak, Ruth. 1997. Discourse–sociolinguistics and the study of doctor–patient interaction. In: Gunnarson, Britt-Louise, Linnel, Per and Nordberg, Bengt (eds.) *The construction of professional discourse*. London: Longman 173–200.

Woolford, Ellen. 1983. Bilingual code-switching and syntactic theory. *Linguistic Inquiry,* 14: 520–536.

Wright, Sue. 2003. *Language policy and language planning: From nationalism to globalization.* Houndmills, Basingstoke and New York: Palgrave Macmillan.

Yang, Wenliang. 1990. *Anglizismen im Deutschen: am Beispiel des Nachrichtenmagazins 'Der Spiegel'.* Tübingen: Niemeyer.

Yanoff, Karin Lindblad. 1988. *The rhetoric of medical discourse: An analysis of the major genres*. University of Pennsylvania. PhD thesis.

Zámbori, Anett. 2004. *The roles of English in scientific communication in Europe; English in academic activities of Hungarian engineers*. Szeged: University of Szeged. MA thesis.

Zethsen, Karen Korning and Askehave, Inger. 2006. Medical communication Professional–lay. In: Brown, Keith (ed.) *Encyclopedia of language and linguistics*. (2nd edition) Volume 3. Amsterdam: Elsevier, 644–649.

Zhang, Yawei (ed.) 2008. *Encyclopedia of global health.* London: Sage Publications.

Zimányi, Árpád. 2003. A szaknyelvi helyesírás-tervezés újabb feladataiból. *Magyar Nyelvőr,* 1: 12–23.

Zimányi, Árpád. 2004. Some aspects of the influence of English on the Hungarian language. In: Kurtán, Zsuzsa and Zimányi, Árpád (eds.) *A nyelvek vonzásában. Köszöntő kötet Budai László 70. születésnapjára* [Attracted by languages: Festschrift to László Budai on his 70th birthday]. Eger–Veszprém: Veszprémi Egyetemi Kiadó, 180–186.

Zimányi, Árpád. 2006. *Nyelvhasználat, nyelvváltozás.* [Language use and language change] Pandora Könyvek. 4. Eger: Líceum Kiadó.

Zsilinszky, Éva. 2003. Az angol vonatkozású elemek újabb etimológiai szótárainkban. [English related elements in recent Hungarian etymological dictionaries]. *Nyelvtudományi Értekezések.* 153. Budapest: Akadémiai Kiadó.

Zuluaga, Ospina Alberto. 1980. *Introducción al estudio de las expresiones fijas.* Studia Romanica et Linguistica. 10. Frankfurt-am-Main, Berne, Cirencester: Peter Lang.

8. Appendices

Appendix 1: Components of the English hospital discharge report/summary

The Discharge Summary is a concise summary of hospitalization to the PCP[63] who will follow the patient in clinic after his/her hospital stay or the admitting doctor at next hospitalization.[64]
The major parts of the discharge summary are the following:

- Patient's name, medical record number, date of birth or age of the patient
- Admission and discharge dates
- Principal diagnoses on admission
- Discharge diagnoses
- Consultants
- Procedures
- Complications
- History and hospital course
- Discharge plan
- Medications at discharge
- Issues to be addressed at follow-up
- CC (physician(s) who will see patient in follow-up)

63 PCP means the primary care physician.

64 Definition and data taken from OU-Tulsa Department of Internal Medicine Discharge Summary Format http://tulsa.ou.edu/im/Discharge%20Summary%20Guide.pdf and http://www.uth.tmc.edu/uth_orgs/hcpc/procedures/volume2/chapter4/discharge-04.htm. Access: 15 August, 2007.

Appendix 2: The Hungarian hospital discharge report/summary

The hospital/clinical discharge report is the summary of the patient's data containing the reason for admission, major medical findings, procedures, treatment, patient's condition on discharge, special advice given to the patient or the relatives (follow-up, medication). The hospital discharge report is the history and hospital course of the patient.
The major parts of the discharge summary[65] are the following:

- Personal data of the patient
- Admission date
- Past history
- Present history
- Condition on admission
- Investigations (laboratory and imaging studies)
- Management
- Diagnoses
- Clinical course
- Medications
- Signatures

65 Based on guidelines given in MEES (*Magyar egészségügyi ellátási standardok* [Hungarian health care standards]) cf. website http://www.eum.hu.

Appendix 3: Informed consent

I, ..., hereby grant permission to dr. Csilla Keresztes, member of the English–Hungarian Medical Translator Group, Faculty of Medicine at the University of Szeged to tape-record the interview in which I talk to her, and I also grant her permission to use the information generated from this interview in her applied linguistics PhD research. I give my consent to her to publish these data in a written form and/or to present these data at a conference. However, my personal demographic data, or a combination of them on the basis of which my personality could be positively identified (e.g. name, sex, age and occupation) will be accessible only for Csilla Keresztes, and no third party are they available to in any form.

----

signature of the participant

Szeged

Date: 2009

Appendix 4: Beleegyező nyilatkozat

Alulírott .... hozzájárulok, hogy Keresztes Csilla az SZTE ÁOK Angol-magyar Orvosi Szakfordítóképző Csoportjának munkatársa saját alkalmazott nyelvészeti PhD kutatásához hangfelvételen rögzítse és utána kutatásai céljára felhasználja a beszélgetés során elhangzó információt. Azaz hozzájárulok, hogy a nyert adatokból származó összefüggéseket írott formában megjelentesse, illetve azok konferenciaelőadás formájában elhangozzanak. Azonban a rám vonatkozó konkrét személyi adataim, illetve azok olyan kombinációja, melyek alapján kilétem egyértelműen beazonosítható lenne, (név, nem, kor, foglalkozás), csak dr. Keresztes Csilla számára elérhetőek, harmadik személy semmilyen formában nem juthat hozzá

____

Közreműködő

Szeged, 2009. ....

Appendix 5: Interview questions for tertiary care cardiologists

Background information on the research:

This survey is part of an applied linguistic PhD research the aim of which is to describe the Hungarian language of medicine, especially the language of cardiological discharge reports. The direct aim of the research is to reveal the various linguistic features in this text type and to analyze them, and the indirect aim is to prepare students who take part in the medical translator course more extensively by having a thorough knowledge of the real language use of the physicians' discourse community.

Personal data of the participant:

- Sex:
- Age:
- Occupation (post):
- Language knowledge:

Questions of the semi-structured interview:

1. When, how and in how many hours per week did you start learning English?
2. Have you studied English for medical purposes? If yes, when and how?
3. Have you been to an English speaking country? When? How much time did you spend there? Did you work or research there as a physician?
4. How important is the English language in your profession?
5. How/ For what do you use the English language? (speaking to colleagues, in scientific research, talking to patients)
6. What do you think of the fact that English has become the international lingua franca of medicine?

7. Do you like that English has become the lingua franca of medicine? Can you benefit from it? What are the advantages of it for you?
8. Are there any disadvantages?
9. Do you think that a doctor who cannot speak English is at a disadvantage?
10. As English is not your first language, have you ever felt the disadvantage of it during professional work? Could you give me an example of it?
11. Which language do you prefer reading, publishing or presenting/listening to a presentation in?
12. Can you mention an example for using English words/abbreviations when you speak/write in Hungarian? Do you use English structures, do you "think in English"?
13. Please, think of a situation when you explain a hospital discharge report to your patient. What do you tell thc patient in a different way?
14. What do patients remark on? What don't they understand when reading their medical report?
15. Have your colleagues in secondary or primary care ever asked you to explain them the discharge report written by you? What did you have to write differently?

Proof reading task:

1. Instruction before handing over the text:
   Please, read this Hungarian hospital discharge report and underline everything in the text that you would write differently.
2. After underlining all the items that would be changed, comments should be made:

2.1. How would you write the underlined part? Why have you decided to change it? What didn't you like in it?

2.2. If the interviewer thinks that the interviewee skipped an Anglicism, she asks a direct question: Is this part all right? Do you like it? Why haven't you changed it?

Appendix 6: Interview questions for primary care physicians

Background information on the research:

This survey is part of an applied linguistic PhD research the aim of which is to describe the Hungarian language of medicine, especially the language of cardiological discharge reports. The direct aim of the research is to reveal the various linguistic features in this text type and to analyze them, and the indirect aim is to prepare students who take part in the medical translator course more extensively by having a thorough knowledge of the real language use of the physicians' discourse community.

Personal data of the participant:

- Sex:
- Age:
- Occupation (post):
- Language knowledge:

Questions of the semi-structured interview:

1. Have you learned English?
2. When, how and in how many hours per week did you learn English?
3. Have you studied English for medical purposes? If yes, when and how?
4. Have you been to an English speaking country? When? How much time did you spend there? Did you work there as a physician?
5. How important is the English language in your profession?
6. How/ For what do you use the English language? (speaking to colleagues , in scientific research, talking to patients)

7. What do you think of the fact that English has become the international lingua franca of medicine? Do you like it? Can you benefit from it? What are the advantages of it for you?
8. Are there any disadvantages?
9. Do you think that a doctor who cannot speak English is at a disadvantage?
10. As English is not your first language, have you ever felt the disadvantage of it during professional work? Could you give me an example of it?
11. Which language do you prefer reading/listening to a medical presentation in?
12. Can you mention an example for using English words/abbreviations when you speak/write in Hungarian? Do you use English structures, do you "think in English"?
13. Please, think of a situation when you explain a hospital discharge report to your patient. What do you tell the patient in a different way?
14. What do patients remark on? What don't they understand when reading their medical report?
15. Do your colleagues working in tertiary care use expressions or abbreviations the meaning of which you don't know or you are uncertain about? Can you give me an example?

Proof reading task:

1. Instruction before handing over the text:
   Please, read this Hungarian hospital discharge report and underline everything in the text that you would write differently.
2. After underlining all the items that would be changed, comments should be made:

2.1. How would you write the underlined part? Why have you decided to change it? What didn't you like in it?

2.2.If the interviewer thinks that the interviewee skipped an Anglicism, she asks a direct question: Is this part all right? Do you like it? Why haven't you changed it?

Appendix 7: Interview questions for patients

Background information on the research:

This survey is part of an applied linguistic PhD research the aim of which is to describe the Hungarian language of medicine, especially the language of cardiological discharge reports. The direct aim of the research is to reveal the various linguistic features in this text type and to analyze them, and the indirect aim is to prepare students who take part in the medical translator course more extensively by having a thorough knowledge of the real language use of the physicians' discourse community.

Personal data of the participant:

- Sex:
- Age:
- Occupation (post):
- Language knowledge:

Questions of the semi-structured interview:

1. Have you studied English?
2. When, how and in how many hours per week did you learn English?
3. Have you been to an English speaking country? When? How much time did you spend there?
4. What do you think of the fact that English has become the international lingua franca of medicine?
5. Do you like that English has become the lingua franca of medicine? Can you benefit from it? What are the advantages of it for you?
6. What are the disadvantages of it for you?
7. Do you think that a doctor who cannot speak English is at a disadvantage?

8. Please, think of a situation when you talked to your doctor about your hospital discharge report. Was there anything that you could not understand from the doctor's explanation?
9. Do doctors use any expressions or abbreviations in the discharge report that you don't understand or you are uncertain about? Could you give me an example for it?

Reading task:

1. Instruction before handing over the text:

Please, read this Hungarian hospital discharge report and underline everything in the text that you don't understand or you are uncertain about.

2. After reading and underlining the selected items, comments should be made:

2.1. If the interviewer thinks that the interviewee skipped an Anglicism, she asks a direct question: Is this part all right? Do you like it? Why haven't you changed it?

Appendix 8: Interjúkérdések klinikai kardiológusoknak

Háttérinformáció a kutatásról:

A vizsgálat egy alkalmazott nyelvészeti PhD kutatás részét képezi, melyben arra keressük a választ, hogy milyen a magyar orvosi szaknyelv, ezen belül, azt vizsgáljuk, hogy mi jellemzi a kardiológiai zárójelentések nyelvhasználatát. A kutatás közvetlen célja a különféle nyelvi jelenségek feltárása és értelmezése, közvetett célja pedig a szakfordító képzésben résztvevő orvostanhallgatók alaposabb nyelvi felkészítése a szakma tényleges nyelvhasználata ismeretében.

Az interjúalany adatai:

- Neme:
- Kora:
- Foglalkozása (beosztása):
- Nyelvtudás:

Irányított interjú kérdései:

1. Mikor, hogyan, hány órában kezdett el angolul tanulni?
2. Tanult-e angol szaknyelvet? Ha igen, mikor, hogyan?
3. Járt-e angol nyelvterületen? Mikor? Mennyi időt töltött ott? Orvosként is kutatott/dolgozott ott?
4. Munkája során mennyire fontos az angol nyelv ismerete?
5. Hogyan/mire használja az angol nyelvet? (kollégákkal a napi gyakorlatban, a tudományos életben, betegekkel)
6. Ön hogyan ítéli meg azt, hogy az angol nyelv vált az orvostudomány nemzetközi nyelvévé?

7. Jó ez így vagy nem? Ön érzi-e ennek a jó oldalát? Ön szerint milyen pozitív következménye(i) van(nak) ennek?
8. Van-e valami negatív következménye is?
9. Mit gondol, hátrányt szenved az az orvos, aki nem beszél/tud angolul?
10. Ön tanulta az angol nyelvet, nem az anyanyelve az angol. Került-e munkája során valaha hátrányba emiatt? Fejtse ki/mondjon rá példát.
11. Ön legszívesebben melyik nyelven olvas szakirodalmat, publikál, tart/hallgat előadást?
12. Tud példát mondani arra, amikor magyarul beszél/ír és angol szavakat, rövidítéseket használ közben, angolos szerkezeteket alkalmaz, angolul/angolosan gondolkodik?
13. Kérem, gondoljon egy olyan helyzetre, amikor a betegével átbeszéli a zárójelentést, diagnózist. Mit mond a betegnek másként?
14. Mi tűnik fel a betegeknek, mit tapasztalt, mi az, amit nem értenek az orvosi jelentésekből?
15. Kapott-e olyan visszajelzést a járóbetegellátásból vagy a háziorvostól, hogy a kolléga valamit nem értett az Ön által írt zárójelentésből? Mi az, amit másként kellett írnia?

Feladatmegoldás:

1. Instrukció a szöveg átadása előtt:

Olvassa át ezt a magyar nyelvű zárójelentést, és húzza alá, mi az, amit Ön másként írna.

2. A feladat megoldása után kommentálja a saját változtatásait:

2.1. Miként mondaná, írná másként ezt a részt? Miért döntött így? Mit nem szeretett benne?

2.2. Ha kimaradt olyan megfogalmazás, ami szerintem javítható/javítandó anglicizmus lenne, rákérdezek arra: Ez a rész itt rendben van? Tetszik? Ezt miért nem változtatta?

Appendix 9: Interjúkérdések háziorvosoknak

Háttérinformáció a kutatásról:

A vizsgálat egy alkalmazott nyelvészeti PhD kutatás részét képezi, melyben arra keressük a választ, hogy milyen a magyar orvosi szaknyelv, ezen belül, azt vizsgáljuk, hogy mi jellemzi a kardiológiai zárójelentések nyelvhasználatát. A kutatás közvetlen célja a különféle nyelvi jelenségek feltárása és értelmezése, közvetett célja pedig a szakfordító képzésben résztvevő orvostanhallgatók alaposabb nyelvi felkészítése a szakma tényleges nyelvhasználata ismeretében.

Az interjúalany adatai:

- Neme:
- Kora:
- Foglalkozása:
- Nyelvtudása:

Irányított interjú kérdései:

1. Tanult-e angol nyelvet?
2. Mikor, hogyan, hány órában kezdett el angolul tanulni?
3. Tanult-e angol szaknyelvet? Ha igen, mikor, hogyan?
4. Járt-e angol nyelvterületen? Mikor? Mennyi időt töltött ott? Orvosként is dolgozott ott?
5. Munkája során mennyire fontos az angol nyelv ismerete?
6. Hogyan/mire használja az angol nyelvet? (kollégákkal a napi gyakorlatban, a tudományos életben, betegekkel)

7. Ön hogyan ítéli meg azt, hogy az angol nyelv vált az orvostudomány nemzetközi nyelvévé? Jó ez így vagy nem? Ön érzi-e ennek a jó oldalát? Ön szerint milyen pozitív következménye(i) van(nak) ennek?
8. Van-e valami negatív következménye is?
9. Mit gondol, hátrányt szenved az az orvos, aki nem beszél/tud angolul?
10. Ön tanulta az angol nyelvet, nem az anyanyelve az angol. Került-e munkája során valaha hátrányba emiatt? Fejtse ki/mondjon rá példát.
11. Ön legszívesebben melyik nyelven olvas szakirodalmat, hallgat esetleg tart előadást?
12. Tud példát mondani arra, amikor magyarul beszél/ír és angol szavakat, rövidítéseket használ közben, angolos szerkezeteket alkalmaz, angolul/angolosan gondolkodik?
13. Kérem, gondoljon egy olyan helyzetre, amikor a betegével átbeszéli annak kórházi zárójelentését, diagnózisát. Mit mond a betegnek másként?
14. Mi tűnik fel a betegeknek, mit tapasztalt, mi az, amit nem értenek az orvosi jelentésekből?
15. Használnak-e a klinikai kardiológusok olyan kifejezéseket, rövidítéseket, amit Ön nem ért vagy amelynek a jelentésében bizonytalan? Tudna példát mondani?

<u>Feladatmegoldás:</u>

1. Instrukció a szöveg átadása előtt:

Olvassa át ezt a magyar nyelvű zárójelentést, és húzza alá, mi az, amit Ön másként írna.

2. A feladat megoldása után kommentálja a saját változtatásait:

2.1. Miként mondaná, írná másként ezt a részt? Miért döntött így? Mit nem szeretett benne?

2.2. Ha kimaradt olyan megfogalmazás, ami szerintem javítható/javítandó anglicizmus lenne, rákérdezek arra: Ez a rész itt rendben van? Tetszik? Ezt miért nem változtatta meg?

Appendix 10: Interjúkérdések betegeknek

Háttérinformáció a kutatásról:

A vizsgálat egy alkalmazott nyelvészeti PhD kutatás részét képezi, melyben arra keressük a választ, hogy milyen a magyar orvosi szaknyelv, ezen belül, azt vizsgáljuk, hogy mi jellemzi a kardiológiai zárójelentések nyelvhasználatát. A kutatás közvetlen célja a különféle nyelvi jelenségek feltárása és értelmezése, közvetett célja pedig a szakfordító képzésben résztvevő orvostanhallgatók alaposabb nyelvi felkészítése a szakma tényleges nyelvhasználata ismeretében.

Az interjúalany adatai:

- Neme:
- Kora:
- Foglalkozása:
- Nyelvtudása:

Irányított interjú kérdései:

1. Tanult-e angol nyelvet?
2. Mikor, hogyan, hány órában kezdett el angolul tanulni?
3. Járt-e angol nyelvterületen? Mikor? Mennyi időt töltött ott?
4. Ön hogyan ítéli meg azt, hogy az angol nyelv vált az orvostudomány nemzetközi nyelvévé?
5. Jó ez így vagy nem? Ön érzi-e ennek a jó oldalát? Ön szerint milyen pozitív következménye(i) van(nak) ennek?
6. Van-e valami negatív következménye is?
7. Mit gondol, hátrányt szenved az az orvos, aki nem beszél/tud angolul?

8. Kérem, gondoljon egy olyan helyzetre, amikor az orvosával átbeszélték az Ön zárójelentését, diagnózisát. Volt-e valami, amit nem értett a magyarázatból?
9. Használnak-e a klinikai zárójelentésekben olyan kifejezéseket, rövidítéseket, amit Ön nem ért vagy amelynek a jelentésében bizonytalan? Tudna példát mondani?

Feladatmegoldás:

1. Instrukció a szöveg átadása előtt:

Olvassa át ezt a magyar nyelvű zárójelentést, és húzza alá, mi az, amit Ön nem ért/melynek jelentésében nem biztos.

2. A feladat megoldása után kommentálja a saját változtatásokat:

2.1. Ha kimaradt olyan megfogalmazás, ami szerintem javítható/javítandó anglicizmus lenne, rákérdezek arra: Ez a rész itt rendben van? Tetszik? Ezt miért nem változtatta meg?

Appendix 11: Rights and Obligations of Patients (According to Act CLIV of 1997 on Health)

The Right to Information

Section 13

(1) The patient shall have a right to complete information provided in an individualized form.

(2) The patient shall have a right to receive detailed information on:

- his state of health, including its medical evaluation,
- the recommended examinations and interventions,
- the possible benefits and risks of performing or not performing the recommended examinations and interventions,
- the planned dates for performing the examinations and interventions,
- his right to decide in respect of the recommended examination or intervention,
- the possible alternative procedures and methods,
- the course of care and the expected outcome,
- additional services, and
- the recommended lifestyle.

(3) The patient has a right to pose additional questions during information and subsequently.

(4) The patient shall have a right to be informed of the results or eventual failure, or unexpected outcomes and their reasons, after an examination or intervention has been performed in the course of his care.

(5) The legally incapable patient or a patient with reduced disposing capacity shall also have a right to information corresponding to his age and mental state.

(6) The patient shall have a right to know the identity, qualifications and professional status of those directly providing services.

(7) The conditions necessary for the assertion of the rights to information shall

be provided by the agency running the healthcare facility.
(8) The patient shall have a right to be informed in a way which is comprehensible for him, with regard to his or her age, education, knowledge, state of mind and his wish expressed on the matter. If necessary and if possible, the services of an interpreter or a sign language interpreter shall be supplied for the provision of information.

Section 14

(1) A patient with full disposing capacity may waive the right of being informed, except in cases when he must be aware of the nature of his illness in order not to endanger the health of others. If an intervention takes place at the patient's initiative and not for therapeutic purposes, such waiver of the right of being informed shall only be valid in writing.
(2) The patient with full disposing capacity shall have a right to designate a person in writing or in any other credible manner who is to be informed in his stead.
(3) The patient shall have a right to be informed even in cases where his consent is not otherwise a condition for initiating medical care.

The Right to Become Acquainted With the Medical Record

Section 24

(1) A patient shall have the right to become acquainted with the data contained in the medical record prepared on him or her, and shall have the right to request information on his or her health care data, with regard to the contents of Section 135.
(2) The health care provider shall dispose of the medical record, while the patient shall dispose of the data contained therein.

(3) The patient shall have the right to
a) be informed of the management of the data related to the medical treatment,

b) become acquainted with the health care data relating to him,
c) gain access to the medical record and to receive copies thereof at his own expense,
d) be given a discharge summary upon discharge from the healthcare institution (Section 137),
e) receive a written summary or abridged opinion of his health data for justified purposes, at his own expense.

(4) A patient shall have the right to initiate completion or correction of the medical record relating to him, that he deems to be inaccurate or incomplete, which shall be entered in the medical record by the attending physician, or by another person handling such data, together with his professional opinion. The erroneous health care data may not be deleted following the entry thereof, and shall be corrected in such a way that the data entered originally can be established.
(5) If the medical record prepared of a patient also contains information concerning another person's right to confidentiality, the right of inspection and other right set forth in subsection (3) may only be exercised in respect of the part thereof relating to the patient.
(6) The right to inspect the medical record of a person with no disposing capacity shall be exercised by a person as defined in Subsections (1) and (2) of Section 16.
(7) In the course of health care delivered for his current condition, a patient shall have the right to give written authorization to a person designated by him to inspect the medical record relating to him and to have copies made thereof.
(8) Following the conclusion of the patient's medical treatment, only the person being authorized by the patient in a fully conclusive private deed shall have the right to inspect the medical record and to have a copy made thereof.
(9) During a patient's lifetime, or following his death, the spouse, a lineal kin, a sibling or common law spouse shall have the right to become acquainted with

the health care data, upon written request, if

27. such health data is required in order to

27. identify a reason that might influence the life or health of the spouse, a lineal kin, a sibling or common law spouse, or

28. provide healthcare to the persons set forth in Subparagraph aa); and

b) there are no other ways to become acquainted with such health data or to establish them by inference.

(10) In the case set forth in Subsection (9), only those health data may be learnt that are directly related to the reason defined in Paragraph a) of Subsection (9). Information on the health data shall be provided by the patient's attending physician, or the director of medical services of the healthcare provider, in keeping with the requirements on the provision of medical information, if necessary, based on consultation with the attending physician of the claimant.

(11) In the case of a patient's death, his legal representative, close relative, or heir shall have the right, upon written request, to become acquainted with health data that is, or may be, related to the cause of death, and data that is related to the medical treatment preceding death, furthermore to inspect the medical record and to be provided by copies thereof, at his own cost.

(12) The detailed rules of handling and protecting healthcare and related personal data shall be established by a separate law.

Appendix 12: World Health Organization, WHO Regional Office for Europe, Declaration on the Promotion of Patients' Rights in Europe, reprinted in 45 International Digest of Health Legislation 411 (1995).

2. INFORMATION

2.1 Information about health services and how best to use them is to be made available to the public in order to benefit all those concerned.

2.2 Patients have the right to be fully informed about their health status, including the medical facts about their condition; about the proposed medical procedures, together with the potential risks and benefits of each procedure; about alternatives to the proposed procedures, including the effect of non-treatment; and about the diagnosis, prognosis and progress of treatment.

2.3 Information may only be withheld from patients exceptionally when there is good reason to believe that this information would without any expectation of obvious positive effects cause them serious harm.

2.4 Information must be communicated to the patient in a way appropriate to the latter's capacity for understanding, minimizing the use of unfamiliar technical terminology. If the patient does not speak the common language, some form of interpreting should be available.

Appendix 13: Statistics on borrowed lexical features

Descriptive statistics 1

	N	Minimum	Maximum	Sum	Mean	Standard deviation
Prevalence in the given discharge report	400	.00	49.00	4066.00	10.1650	6.43127
Valid N (listwise)	400					

Descriptive Statistics 2

Shortened version of researched items

	N	Minimum	Maximum	Sum	Mean	Standard deviation
ALP	400	0	5	197	.49	.776
attack	400	0	1	2	.01	.071
block	400	0	6	178	.45	1.158
blockoló	400	0	1	7	.02	.131
blokk	400	0	3	50	.13	.424
blokkoló	400	0	2	5	.01	.132
bypass	400	0	2	9	.02	.179
cholesterinszegény	400	0	2	22	.06	.239
cirkulátor	400	0	1	18	.05	.208
csúcsgradiens	400	0	3	8	.02	.199
defibrillátor	400	0	1	6	.02	.122
detektálható	400	0	2	8	.02	.157
diffuse	400	0	2	17	.04	.225
diffúz	400	0	2	43	.11	.362
diszkomfort	400	0	1	2	.01	.071
diszkonnektál	400	0	1	7	.02	.131
dyscomfort	400	0	1	4	.01	.100
elektív	400	0	3	56	.14	.413
elongált	400	0	1	3	.01	.086
entrainment	400	0	1	5	.01	.111
falmozgászavar	400	0	5	90	.23	.534
flatternt	400	0	1	1	.00	.050
flow	400	0	3	36	.09	.377
flowt	400	0	1	2	.01	.071
flow-val	400	0	1	2	.01	.071
flutter	400	0	5	96	.24	.784
fluttern	400	0	3	31	.08	.370
Giga/L	400	0	35	542	1.36	3.666
gócjel	400	0	1	14	.04	.184

góctünet	400	0	1	49	.12	.328
GOT	400	0	5	217	.54	.700
göbmentes	400	0	1	42	.11	.307
GPT	400	0	5	203	.51	.641
grafttal	400	0	1	1	.00	.050
guided	400	0	1	1	.00	.050
guiding	400	0	3	8	.02	.186
HDL	400	0	2	98	.25	.436
hemiblock	400	0	3	10	.03	.199
hormon	400	0	1	2	.01	.071
hospitalizáció	400	0	1	3	.01	.086
INR	400	0	6	260	.65	.930
in-stent	400	0	4	6	.02	.212
invazív	400	0	3	18	.05	.261
kaliberekvivalens	400	0	1	8	.02	.140
kaliberingadozó	400	0	1	2	.01	.071
kalóriaszegény	400	0	0	0	.00	.000
kinking	400	0	1	3	.01	.086
koleszterinszegény	400	0	1	31	.08	.268
kontúregyenetlenség	400	0	1	5	.01	.111
kőmentes	400	0	1	4	.01	.100
kőreflexió	400	0	2	8	.02	.157
LAD	400	0	10	355	.89	1.365
LBBB	400	0	2	21	.05	.245
LDL	400	0	2	96	.24	.450
left main	400	0	1	5	.01	.111
LMWH	400	0	2	9	.02	.165
lobmentes	400	0	1	50	.13	.331
magasvérnyomás-betegség	400	0	1	72	.18	.385
mapping	400	0	1	2	.01	.071
MCH	400	0	10	248	.62	1.449
MCHC	400	0	5	124	.31	.725
mid-LAD	400	0	6	21	.05	.430
mmol/L	400	0	29	704	1.76	4.176
monitorizálás	400	0	2	13	.03	.216
MPV	400	0	5	124	.31	.714
nem-inzulin dependens cukorbetegség	400	0	1	1	.00	.050
NIDDM	400	0	1	14	.04	.184
non-sustained	400	0	1	2	.01	.071
NYHA	400	0	1	7	.02	.131
pace	400	0	13	194	.49	1.493
pacemaker	400	0	11	177	.44	1.390
Pacemaker Ambulancia	400	0	2	2	.01	.100
pacemaker tasak	400	0	1	7	.02	.131
pacemakerek	400	0	1	25	.06	.242
panaszmentes	400	0	4	74	.19	.449
panaszmentesen	400	0	1	25	.06	.242

PCR	400	0	2	3	.01	.112
PM	400	0	6	138	.35	.915
potassium	400	0	1	5	.01	.111
pozicionáltunk	400	0	1	1	.00	.050
provokálható	400	0	2	4	.01	.122
puff	400	0	4	12	.03	.243
PW	400	0	4	74	.19	.460
RDA	400	0	6	147	.37	.880
re-entry	400	0	1	5	.01	.111
regisztrál	400	0	2	23	.06	.244
rezidens	400	0	2	93	.23	.457
Ritmuszavar Ambulancia	400	0	1	1	.00	.050
scan	400	0	2	5	.01	.132
scanek	400	0	1	2	.01	.071
SEC	400	0	11	375	.94	1.681
SGOT	400	0	1	29	.07	.260
SGPT	400	0	2	29	.07	.269
shock	400	0	3	16	.04	.262
shockkal	400	0	1	4	.01	.100
shunt	400	0	2	4	.01	.122
sick	400	0	3	7	.02	.193
sodium	400	0	1	9	.02	.148
sokk	400	0	1	9	.02	.148
SPECT	400	0	2	12	.03	.198
spike	400	0	1	4	.01	.100
spike-ok	400	0	1	2	.01	.071
spray	400	0	2	15	.04	.203
sprayre	400	0	1	3	.01	.086
standard	400	0	1	6	.02	.122
STD	400	0	2	13	.03	.191
STEMI	400	0	3	12	.03	.233
stent	400	0	14	243	.61	1.649
stentben	400	0	2	13	.03	.216
stentelést	400	0	1	2	.01	.071
stentet	400	0	2	19	.05	.256
stenttől	400	0	2	5	.01	.132
steroid	400	0	1	5	.01	.111
strainjelek	400	0	1	2	.01	.071
stressz	400	0	1	3	.01	.086
stroke	400	0	2	24	.06	.294
study	400	0	2	4	.01	.122
szoros vérnyomáskontroll	400	0	1	3	.01	.086
szövődménymentesen	400	0	1	22	.06	.228
teszt	400	0	1	14	.04	.184
tilt	400	0	1	3	.01	.086
TIMI	400	0	2	22	.06	.259
upgrade	400	0	1	4	.01	.100
vitamin	400	0	2	10	.03	.172

zsírszegény	400	0	1	2	.01	.071
Valid N (listwise)	400					

FSC
www.fsc.org
MIX
Papier | Fördert
gute Waldnutzung
FSC® C083411

Kolibri 360 GmbH
Ferdinand-Jühlke-Straße 7
99095 Erfurt, Deutschland
produktsicherheit@kolibri360.de